Chronic Pancreatitis

Zhao-Shen Li • Zhuan Liao
Jian-Min Chen • Claude Férec
Editors

Chronic Pancreatitis

From Basic Research to Clinical Treatment

SSTP

Springer

Editors
Zhao-Shen Li
Department of Gastroenterology
Changhai Hospital
Shanghai, China

Zhuan Liao
Changhai Hospital
Department of Gastroenterology
Shanghai, China

Jian-Min Chen
INSERM
Brest, France

Claude Férec
INSERM UMR 1078
Brest, France

ISBN 978-981-10-4513-4   ISBN 978-981-10-4515-8 (eBook)
DOI 10.1007/978-981-10-4515-8

The print edition is not for sale in China Mainland. Customers from China Mainland please order the print book from: Shanghai Scientific and Technical Publishers.

Library of Congress Control Number: 2017951646

Printed on acid-free paper

This Springer imprint is published by Springer Nature
The registered company is Springer Nature Singapore Pte Ltd.
The registered company address is: 152 Beach Road, #21-01/04 Gateway East, Singapore 189721, Singapore

Preface

Chronic pancreatitis is an irreversible complex disorder of the pancreas characterized by chronic progressive pancreatic inflammation and fibrosis, resulting in the failure of exocrine and endocrine function. Since 1788, when Thomas Cawley first reported a patient with alcoholic chronic pancreatitis whose pancreas was widely calcified, a huge number of studies have been carried out on pancreatitis providing us with a much deeper understanding of the pathogenesis of this debilitating condition.

Chronic Pancreatitis is a concise guide to the clinical diagnosis and management of chronic pancreatitis. It will focus on various key aspects of the condition, such as the etiology, pathogenesis, epidemiology, molecular genetics, diagnosis, endoscopic and surgical treatment, and prognosis. It will also include a series of typical case presentations that together provide a fairly comprehensive synopsis of the disease. This book has been written by more than 30 world-renowned experts, mainly from China, France, Denmark, Germany, India, Italy, Japan, Singapore, the United Kingdom, and the United States. We believe that it will be an ideal reference work not only for researchers but also for the physicians and surgeons who care for patients with acute or chronic pancreatitis.

The magnificent support of the research teams from Changhai Hospital in Shanghai and Institut National de la Santé et de la Recherche Médicale (INSERM) in Brest is gratefully acknowledged. We thank Dr. Wen-Bin Zou for the executive editor's work, and Mr. Bin Hu of Springer for his skillful editing and production work. Finally, we thank our families for their encouragement and understanding while we put this volume together.

Abbreviations

ACP	Alcoholic chronic pancreatitis
ADHs	Alcohol dehydrogenases
AIP	Autoimmune pancreatitis
ALDHs	Aldehyde dehydrogenases
ANA	Anti-nuclear antibody
ANG2	Angiopoietin-2
AP	Acute pancreatitis
ARP	Acute recurrent pancreatitis
BiP	Immunoglobulin-binding protein
BMI	Body mass index

BT-PABA	*N*-benzoyl-L-tyrosyl-*p*-aminobenzoic acid
CA19-9	Carbohydrate antigen 19-9
CAD	Computer-aided diagnosis
CASR	Calcium-sensing receptor
CCK	Cholecystokinin
CE-EUS	Contrast enhancement EUS
CEL	Carboxy ester lipase
CEL-HYB	CEL-Hybrid
CFA	Coefficient of fat absorption
CFTR	Cystic fibrosis transmembrane conductance regulator
CLDN2	Claudin-2
COX	Pain management
CP	Chronic pancreatitis
CPA1	Carboxypeptidase A1
CT	Computed tomography
CTLA-4	Cytotoxic T-lymphocyte-associated protein 4
CTRC	Trypsin-degrading enzyme chymotrypsin C
CTSB	Cathepsin B
DBTC	Dibutyltin dichloride
DCP	DC-plasma emission
DP	Distal pancreatectomy
DPP-4	Dipeptidyl peptidase-4
DPPHR	Duodenum-preserving pancreatic head resection
EDXRF	Energy dispersive x-ray fluorescence
ERCP	Endoscopic retrograde cholangiopancreatography
ERS	Endoplasmic reticulum stress
EST	Endoscopic sphincterotomy
ESWL	Endoscopy and shock-wave lithotripsy
EUS	Endoscopic ultrasonography
EUS-FNA	Endoscopic ultrasound-guided fine needle aspiration
EUS-FNA/B	EUS-guided fine need aspiration/biopsy
EUS-TCB	EUS-guided Tru-cut biopsy
FAEEs	Fatty acids to fatty ethyl esters
FCPD	Fibrocalculous pancreatic diabetes
FE1	Fecal elastase-1
FNA	Fine needle aspiration
FOV	Field of view
FSE	Fast sequence echo
GEL	Granulocytic epithelial lesion
GIP	Glucose-dependent insulinotropic polypeptide
GLP-1	Glucagon-like peptide 1
GP-2	Glycoprotein-2
GPI	Glycophophatidyl inositol
GWAS	Genome-wide association study
HbA1c	Glycosylated hemoglobin A1c
HP	Hereditary pancreatitis
HU	Hounsfield units
ICDC	International Consensus Diagnostic Criteria

IDCP	Idiopathic duct-centric chronic pancreatitis
Ig	Immunoglobulin
IgG4	Immunoglobulins G4
IL-1β	Interleukin-1β
IL-6	Interleukin-6
INSPPIRE	INternational Study Group of Pediatric Pancreatitis: In Search for a CuRE
IPMN	Intraductal papillary mucinous neoplasm
LAVA	Liver acquisition with volume acceleration
LF	Lactoferrin
lpr	Lymphoproliferation
LPS	Lipopolysaccharides
LPSP	Lymphoplasmacytic sclerosing pancreatitis
LTF	Lactotransferrin
MAC	Membrane attack complex
MCP-1	Monocyte chemoattractant protein 1
MCT	Medium chain triglycerides
MFP	Mass forming pancreatitis
miRNA	microRNA
mMCP-1	mutant MCP-1
MODY	Maturity-onset diabetes of the young
MPD	Main pancreatic duct
MRCP	Magnetic resonance cholangiopancreatography
MRI	Magnetic resonance imaging
NACP	Nonalcoholic chronic pancreatitis
NAHR	Nonallelic homologous recombination
NBT-PABA test	*N*-benzoyl-L-tyrosyl-*p*-aminobenzoic acid test
NF-kB	Nuclear factor kappa B
NMD	Nonsense-mediated mRNA decay
NMDA	*N*-methyl-D-aspartic acid
NO	Nitrogen oxide
NOS	Not otherwise specified
OGTT	Oral glucose tolerance test
OOI	Other organ involvement
PanIN	Pancreatic intraepithelial neoplasia
PCKD	Polycystic kidney disease
PD	Pancreatoduodenectomy
PDAC	Pancreatic ductal adenocarcinoma
Pdwk1 and 2	Pancreatitis and diabetes mellitus in WBN/Kob locus 1 and 2
PEI	Pancreatic exocrine insufficiency
PERK	Protein kinase R-line endoplasmic reticulum kinase
PERT	Pancreatic enzyme replacement therapy
PST	Pancreatic stimulation test
PGs	Prostaglandins
PLT	Pancreolauryl test
poly I:C	Polyinosinic:polycytidylic acid
PP	Polypeptide

PPARg	Peroxisome proliferator-activated receptor-g
PPPD	Pancreatoduodenectomy
PRSS1	Anionic trypsinogen1
PRSS2	Anionic trypsinogen2
PSCs	Pancreatic stellate cells
PSL	Prednisolone
PSP	Pancreatic stone protein
PSTI	Pancreatic secretory trypsin inhibitor
PTP	Pancreatic thread protein
RAP	Recurrent acute pancreatitis
reg gene	Regenerating gene
SEM	Scanning electron microscopy
SGLT2	Sodium/glucose cotransporter 2
SIR	Standardized incidence ratio
S-MRCP	Secretin-enhanced magnetic resonance cholangiopancreatography
SNPs	Single nucleotide polymorphisms
SNRIs	Serotonin–noradrenaline reuptake inhibitors
SPINK1	Kajal type 1 serine protease inhibitor
SS-FSE	Single shot fast sequence echo
T1DM	Type 1 diabetes mellitus
T_1WI	T_1-weighted imaging
T2DM	Type 2 diabetes mellitus
T_2WI	T_2-weighted imaging
T3cDM	Type 3c diabetes mellitus
TAMs	Tumor-associated macrophages
TCAs	Tricyclic antidepressants
TCF7L2	Transcription factor 7-like 2
TCP	Tropical calcific pancreatitis
TE	Echo time
TGF β1	Transforming growth factor β1
TNBS	Trinitrobenzene sulfonic acid
TPIAT	Total pancreatectomy with islet auto-transplantation
TR	Single shot fast sequence echo
TUS	Transabdominal ultrasound
US	Ultrasonography
VNTR	Variable number tandem repeat
WBN/Kob	Wistar-Bonn/Kobori
XBP1s	X-box binding protein-1

Shanghai, China Zhao-Shen Li
Shanghai, China Zhuan Liao
Brest, France Jian-Min Chen
Brest, France Claude Férec

Contents

1 **A Short History of Research into Chronic Pancreatitis** 1
Wen-Bin Zou, David N. Cooper, Zhuan Liao, Jian-Min Chen, and Zhao-Shen Li

2 **Definition and Classification of Chronic Pancreatitis** 7
Xin-Ying Tang, Zhuan Liao, and Zhao-Shen Li

3 **The Epidemiology of Chronic Pancreatitis** 13
Qian-Qian Zhu, Quan-Cai Cai, Luo-Wei Wang, Zhuan Liao, and Zhao-Shen Li

4 **Etiology of Chronic Pancreatitis** 21
Raffaele Pezzilli

5 **The Pathogenesis of Chronic Pancreatitis** 29
Jakob Lykke Poulsen, Søren Schou Olesen, Asbjørn Mohr Drewes, Bo Ye, Wei-Qin Li, Ali A. Aghdassi, Matthias Sendler, Julia Mayerle, and Markus M. Lerch

6 **Pathogenetics of Chronic Pancreatitis** 63
Zhuan Liao, Zhao-Shen Li, David N. Cooper, Claude Férec, and Jian-Min Chen

7 **Diagnosis of Chronic Pancreatitis** 79
Xin-Ying Tang, An-Jing Zhao, Jin Yu, Jin-Huan Lin, Wen-Bin Zou, Zhuan Liao, Zhao-Shen Li, Song Su, Mao-Jin Xu, Jutta Keller, Peter Layer, Yun Bian, Jian-Ping Lu, Li Wang, Liang-Hao Hu, Lei Xin, Jian-Wei Zhu, Fei Jiang, and Zhen-Dong Jin

8 **Conservative Management of Chronic Pancreatitis** 119
Yang-Yang Qian, Zhuan Liao, and Zhao-Shen Li

9 **Endoscopic Management of Chronic Pancreatitis** 125
Boon Eu Andrew Kwek, Tiing Leong Ang, and Amit Maydeo

10 **Surgical Treatment of Chronic Pancreatitis** 137
Sui-Zhi Gao and Gang Jin

11 Special Types of Chronic Pancreatitis 141
Atsushi Masamune, Atsushi Kanno, Tooru Shimosegawa, Prachand Issarapu, Sumit Paliwal, Seema Bhaskar, Giriraj Ratan Chandak, Maisam Abu-El-Haija, and Aliye Uc

12 Chronic Pancreatitis and Pancreatic Cancer 179
Xiang-Yu Kong and Ke-Ping Xie

13 Typical Cases of Chronic Pancreatitis 191
Jin-Huan Lin, Liang-Hao Hu, Jia-Yun Chen, Wen-Bin Zou, Zhuan Liao, and Zhao-Shen Li

Index 205

Contributors

Maisam Abu-El-Haija Division of Gastroenterology, Hepatology and Nutrition, Cincinnati Children's Hospital Medical Center, Cincinnati, OH, USA

Ali A. Aghdassi Department of Medicine A, University Medicine Greifswald, Greifswald, Germany

Tiing Leong Ang Department of Gastroenterology and Hepatology, Changi General Hospital, Singapore, Singapore

Seema Bhaskar Genomic Research on Complex Diseases (GRC Group), CSIR-Centre for Cellular and Molecular Biology, Hyderabad, Telangana, India

Yun Bian Department of Radiology, Changhai Hospital, The Second Military Medical University, Shanghai, China

Department of Radiology, The 411st Hospital of Chinese PLA, Shanghai, China

Quan-Cai Cai Center for Clinical Epidemiology and Evidence-Based Medicine, Changhai Hospital of Second Military Medical University, Shanghai, China

Giriraj Ratan Chandak Genome Research on Complex Diseases (GRC Group), CSIR-Centre for Cellular and Molecular Biology, Hyderabad, Telangana, India

Jia-Yun Chen Department of Gastroenterology, Changhai Hospital, The Second Military Medical University, Shanghai, China

Jian-Min Chen Institut National de la Santé et de la Recherche Médicale (INSERM), Brest, France

Etablissement Français du Sang (EFS)—Bretagne, Brest, France

Faculté de Médecine et des Sciences de la Santé, Université de Bretagne Occidentale (UBO), Brest, France

David N. Cooper Institute of Medical Genetics, School of Medicine, Cardiff University, Cardiff, UK

Asbjørn Mohr Drewes Department of Gastroenterology and Hepatology, Centre for Pancreatic Diseases, Mech-Sense, Clinical Institute, Aalborg University Hospital, Aalborg, Denmark

Claude Férec Institut National de la Santé et de la Recherche Médicale (INSERM), Brest, France

Etablissement Français du Sang (EFS)—Bretagne, Brest, France

Laboratoire de Génétique Moléculaire et d'Histocompatibilité, Centre Hospitalier Universitaire (CHU) Brest, Hôpital Morvan, Brest, France

Faculté de Médecine et des Sciences de la Santé, Université de Bretagne Occidentale (UBO), Brest, France

Sui-Zhi Gao Department of Pancreatic Surgery, Changhai Hospital, The Second Military Medical University, Shanghai, China

Chinese Institute of Pancreatic Diseases, Shanghai, China

Liang-Hao Hu Department of Gastroenterology, Changhai Hospital, The Second Military Medical University, Shanghai, China

Shanghai Institute of Pancreatic Diseases, Shanghai, China

Prachand Issarapu Genome Research on Complex Diseases (GRC Group), CSIR-Centre for Cellular and Molecular Biology, Hyderabad, Telangana, India

Fei Jiang Department of Gastroenterology, Changhai Hospital, The Second Military Medical University, Shanghai, China

Gang Jin Department of Pancreatic Surgery, Changhai Hospital, The Second Military Medical University, Shanghai, China

Chinese Institute of Pancreatic Diseases, Shanghai, China

Zhen-Dong Jin Department of Gastroenterology, Changhai Hospital, The Second Military Medical University, Shanghai, China

Atsushi Kanno Division of Gastroenterology, Tohoku University Graduate School of Medicine, Sendai, Japan

Jutta Keller Department of Internal Medicine, Israelitic Hospital, Hamburg, Germany

Xiang-Yu Kong Department of Gastroenterology, Shanghai Changhai Hospital, Shanghai, China

Boon Eu Andrew Kwek Department of Gastroenterology and Hepatology, Changi General Hospital, Singapore, Singapore

Peter Layer Department of Internal Medicine, Israelitic Hospital, Hamburg, Germany

Markus M. Lerch Department of Medicine A, University Medicine Greifswald, Greifswald, Germany

Wei-Qin Li Department of General Surgery, Jinling Hospital, Medical School of Nanjing University, Nanjing, China

Zhao-Shen Li Department of Gastroenterology, Changhai Hospital, The Second Military Medical University, Shanghai, China

Shanghai Institute of Pancreatic Diseases, Shanghai, China

Zhuan Liao Department of Gastroenterology, Changhai Hospital, The Second Military Medical University, Shanghai, China

Shanghai Institute of Pancreatic Diseases, Shanghai, China

Jin-Huan Lin Department of Gastroenterology, Changhai Hospital, The Second Military Medical University, Shanghai, China

Jian-Ping Lu Department of Radiology, Changhai Hospital, The Second Military Medical University, Shanghai, China

Atsushi Masamune Division of Gastroenterology, Tohoku University Graduate School of Medicine, Sendai, Japan

Amit Maydeo Baldota Institute of Digestive Sciences, Global Hospital, Mumbai, India

Julia Mayerle Department of Medicine A, University Medicine Greifswald, Greifswald, Germany

Søren Schou Olesen Department of Gastroenterology and Hepatology, Centre for Pancreatic Diseases, Mech-Sense, Clinical Institute, Aalborg University Hospital, Aalborg, Denmark

Sumit Paliwal Genome Research on Complex Diseases (GRC Group), CSIR-Centre for Cellular and Molecular Biology, Hyderabad, Telangana, India

Raffaele Pezzilli Department of Digestive System, Sant'Orsola-Malpighi Hospital, Bologna, Italy

Jakob Lykke Poulsen Department of Gastroenterology and Hepatology, Centre for Pancreatic Diseases, Mech-Sense, Clinical Institute, Aalborg University Hospital, Aalborg, Denmark

Yang-Yang Qian Department of Gastroenterology, Changhai Hospital, The Second Military Medical University, Shanghai, China

Matthias Sendler Department of Medicine A, University Medicine Greifswald, Greifswald, Germany

Tooru Shimosegawa Division of Gastroenterology, Tohoku University Graduate School of Medicine, Sendai, Japan

Song Su Department of Gastroenterology, The 307 Hospital of Academy of Military Medical Science, Beijing, China

Department of Internal Medicine, Changhai Hospital, The Second Military Medical University, Shanghai, China

Xin-Ying Tang Department of Gastroenterology, Changhai Hospital, The Second Military Medical University, Shanghai, China

Aliye Uc Division of Pediatric Gastroenterology, Stead Family Department of Pediatrics, University of Iowa Children's Hospital, Iowa City, IA, USA

Li Wang Department of Gastroenterology, Changhai Hospital, The Second Military Medical University, Shanghai, China

Luo-Wei Wang Department of Gastroenterology, Changhai Hospital, The Second Military Medical University, Shanghai, China

Shanghai Institute of Pancreatic Diseases, Shanghai, China

Ke-Ping Xie Departments of Gastroenterology, Hepatology and Nutrition, The University of Texas MD Anderson Cancer Center, Houston, TX, USA

Lei Xin Department of Gastroenterology, Changhai Hospital, The Second Military Medical University, Shanghai, China

Mao-Jin Xu Department of Internal Medicine, Changhai Hospital, The Second Military Medical University, Shanghai, China

Bo Ye Department of General Surgery, Jinling Hospital, Medical School of Nanjing University, Nanjing, China

Jin Yu Department of Gastroenterology, Changhai Hospital, The Second Military Medical University, Shanghai, China

Tibet Military General Hospital, Tibet, China

An-Jing Zhao Department of Gastroenterology, Changhai Hospital, The Second Military Medical University, Shanghai, China

Shanghai Institute of Pancreatic Diseases, Shanghai, China

Jian-Wei Zhu Department of Gastroenterology, Changhai Hospital, The Second Military Medical University, Shanghai, China

Qian-Qian Zhu Center for Clinical Epidemiology and Evidence-Based Medicine, Changhai Hospital of Second Military Medical University, Shanghai, China

Wen-Bin Zou Deputy editor of this book, Department of Gastroenterology, Changhai Hospital, The Second Military Medical University, Shanghai, China

Shanghai Institute of Pancreatic Diseases, Shanghai, China

A Short History of Research into Chronic Pancreatitis

1

Wen-Bin Zou, David N. Cooper, Zhuan Liao, Jian-Min Chen, and Zhao-Shen Li

1 Introduction

Chronic pancreatitis (CP) is an irreversible condition of the pancreas characterized by chronic progressive pancreatic inflammation and fibrosis, resulting in the failure of exocrine and endocrine function. Of all pancreatic diseases, CP is the most complicated, a condition with increasing incidence but a relatively short research history. Because of its uncertain and complicated pathogenesis, there is no effective diagnostic test or treatment measure. Thus, CP still exerts an adverse impact on the quality of life of those affected. Herein, we briefly review the history of basic and clinical research into chronic pancreatitis.

The first description of the pancreas has been attributed to Herophilus of Chalcedon (circa 300 B.C.), who named the organ "pancreas" (from the Greek Πάν (pan) meaning all and κρέας (kreas) meaning flesh or meat) (Fitzgerald 1980). In his *De Humani Corporis Fabrica* (1543), Andreas Vesalius described the pancreas as a "glandulous organ or kannelly body of substance growing in the near pannicle of the caule (omentum)" (Singer 1957). During the seventeenth century, the anatomy of the pancreas began to be explored when the pancreatic duct was discovered by J.C. Wirsung in 1642. The duodenal papilla was described both by J.K. Brunner in 1683 and A. Vater in 1750 (Sachs 1993). In the nineteenth century, W. Balser was the first to report the presence of fatty necrosis in acute pancreatitis in 1882, while pancreatic autodigestion ("the pancreas succumbs to its own digestive properties") was proposed by H. Chiari in 1896 (Chiari 1896).

2 Etiology and Pathogenesis

It is generally held that alcoholism is the most common cause of CP worldwide, accounting for 70–80% of cases. The risk of CP has been related to both the quantity and time of alcohol intake. In 1788, Thomas Cawley (Cawley 1788) first related

W.-B. Zou, M.D. • Z. Liao, M.D. (✉)
Z.-S. Li, M.D. (✉)
Department of Gastroenterology, Changhai Hospital, the Second Military Medical University, Shanghai, China

Shanghai Institute of Pancreatic Diseases, Shanghai, China
e-mail: liaozhuan@smmu.edu.cn; zhaoshenli@hotmail.com

D.N. Cooper, Ph.D.
Institute of Medical Genetics, School of Medicine, Cardiff University, Cardiff, UK

J.-M. Chen, Ph.D., M.D.
Institut National de la Santé et de la Recherche Médicale (INSERM), Brest U1078, France

Etablissement Français du Sang (EFS)—Bretagne, Brest, France

Faculté de Médecine et des Sciences de la Santé, Université de Bretagne Occidentale (UBO), Brest, France

Z.-S. Li et al. (eds.), *Chronic Pancreatitis*, DOI 10.1007/978-981-10-4515-8_1

alcohol to pancreatic disease by reference to the case of a male patient with chronic alcoholism who died of diabetes, and whose pancreas was widely calcified after autopsy. In 1878, Friedrich (Friedrich 1878) proposed that chronic inflammation of the pancreas might be associated with long-term excessive intake of alcohol, coining the phrase "Drunkard's pancreas". In 1946, Comfort, Gambill and Baggenstoss (Comfort et al. 1946) from America's Mayo Clinic described the clinical features of CP, including recurrent abdominal pain, and injury of pancreatic exocrine and endocrine function. These authors reported that 68% of patients belonged to the category of alcoholic CP. On the basis of their surgical specimens and autopsy pathological results, they put forward the theory that pancreatic tissue damage caused by repeated episodes of acute inflammation led to a process of pancreatic tissue necrosis and fibrosis, culminating in CP. This still forms the theoretical basis of research into the biological mechanism of CP.

Clinicians have in the past explained the pathogenesis of alcohol-induced CP in terms of alcohol stimulating the pancreas to produce more enzymes and proteins in the pancreatic juice, forming protein plugs in the small pancreatic duct, thereby causing calcification and pancreatic duct obstruction leading to inflammatory infiltration, acinar atrophy and fibrosis. Recent research suggests that activation of digestive zymogen in cells plays a key role in the pathogenesis of CP.

Apart from alcohol, genetic factors also constitute an important cause of CP. In 1952, Comfort and Steinberg (Comfort and Steinberg 1952) reported a family with hereditary CP. Over the past two decades, investigators have identified several susceptibility genes whose *modus operandi* involves the premature activation of trypsinogen or failure to inactivate trypsin during pancreatic inflammation; these susceptibility genes include four firmly established loci, namely *PRSS1*, *SPINK1*, *CTRC* and *CFTR*. In 1996, Whitcomb and colleagues (Whitcomb et al. 1996) reported the first gene predisposing to hereditary pancreatitis (*PRSS1*), encoding cationic trypsinogen and located on chromosome 7q34. In 1998, two simultaneous studies Sharer et al. (1998), Cohn et al. (1998) demonstrated that mutations of the *CFTR* (cystic fibrosis transmembrane conductance regulator) gene are also associated with CP. Two years later, Witt and coworkers (2000) reported another CP susceptibility gene, termed *SPINK1* (Kajal type 1 serine proteinase inhibitor), located on chromosome 5q32, and detected a missense mutation in codon 34 (p.Asn34Ser). Molecular biology research has helped us to greatly improve our understanding of the causes and pathogenesis of CP. In 2008, the *CTRC* gene encoding the trypsin-degrading enzyme chymotrypsin C, located on 1p36.21, was reported to be yet another pancreatitis susceptibility gene (Masson et al. 2008; Rosendahl et al. 2008).

In 1995, Yoshida et al. (Yoshida et al. 1995) proposed the concept of autoimmune pancreatitis (AIP), which had a good response to steroid therapy. In 2001, the high serum concentration of immunoglobulins G4 (IgG4) was reported as a diagnostic biomarker of AIP (Hamano et al. 2001). In recent years, the concept of AIP as a unique clinical entity has gained increasing recognition as a special cause of CP.

In 1955, Zuideman (Zuideman 1955) first proposed the concept of tropical pancreatitis, mainly encountered in the tropical regions of developing countries, a disease entity which might be associated with inadequate nutrition, involving low protein and fat intake. In 1989, it was shown that high cassava intake with its inherent cyanide toxicity, was involved in the pathogenesis of tropical pancreatitis (Narendranathan et al. 1989). Nowadays, a combination of malnutrition, oxidative stress and inherited genetic mutations are thought to be responsible for tropical pancreatitis.

3 Diagnosis

The variety and complexity of the pathogenic factors that underlie CP make its classification and diagnosis difficult. Over the past decades, no widely accepted classification system or established diagnostic criteria have emerged for CP. This is despite several meetings on the topic held in Marseilles (1963 and 1984), Cambridge (1984) and Rome (1985) which greatly improved our knowledge of the pathogenesis and diagnosis of CP (Buchler et al. 2009). The Marseilles symposium, organized by Henri Sarles, became a milestone of research into CP. In 1984, the Marseilles standard was revised, abandoning the concept of chronic recurrent pancreatitis, and constituting a relatively complete description of CP from the pathology, exocrine and endocrine function in spite of not being widely applicable in clinical practice. In 1988, the Marseille-Rome international conference classified CP into three types: chronic calcifying pancreatitis, chronic obstructive pancreatitis and chronic inflammatory pancreatitis, according to the specific pathological changes involved in CP. In 1998, the Zürich international classification system defined patient cohorts in patients undergoing surgery for CP (Ammann 1998).

The clinical evaluation of CP depends mainly on computed tomography (CT), magnetic resonance imaging (MRI), endoscopic retrograde cholangiopancreatography (ERCP) and endoscopic ultrasonography (EUS). With the development of X-ray investigation, McCune, Shorb and Moscovitz (1968) completed the first endoscopic cannulation of the ampulla of Vater in 1968, which made the diagnosis of CP much easier. In 1980, DiMagno and colleagues (DiMagno et al. 1980) proposed the concept of ultrasonic endoscopy, for the first time combining an ultrasonic probe with gastroscopy. Thereafter, Vilmann and colleagues (1993) developed a new method of endoscopic ultrasound (EUS)-guided fine needle aspiration using an ultrasonic endoscope with a curved array transducer mounted in front of the optic lens.

The early diagnosis of CP is still difficult today because of two problems: (1) the lack of a high sensitivity/specificity pancreatic exocrine function test, (2) the non-obviousness of the change in early chronic inflammation imaging. Recently, reports of EUS in the diagnosis of CP are increasing. EUS examination when the ultrasonic probe is close to the pancreas has the potential to obtain a clear image of the pancreas; tissue could be easily and safely obtained under EUS-guided biopsy. Therefore, the use of EUS for the early diagnosis of CP is quite promising.

4 Treatment

The management of CP could be divided into drug therapy, surgical or endoscopic intervention. The great French physiologist, Claude Bernard (1813–1878) demonstrated the role of pancreatic secretion in the digestion of protein, carbohydrate and fat by injecting mutton fat into the pancreatic ducts of dogs (DiMagno 1993), an experiment that helped to spawn research into pancreatic exocrine replacement therapy. In 1868, Alexander Fles used fresh pancreatic tissue homogenate to alleviate the symptoms of fat diarrhea (Modlin 2003). At the end of the nineteenth century and the beginning of the twentieth century, Langdon Down, von Noorden and Salomon extracted the fresh active ingredient in the pancreas to treat chronic diarrhea and steatorrhea successfully. Over the past few decades, the use of an enzyme mixture extracted from porcine pancreas (trypsin, lipase and amylase) has been widely accepted for the treatment of exocrine deficiency and steatorrhea in CP patients. Employing modern separation techniques, the current clinical application of pancreatic enzymes generally contains high concentrations of enzymes, can tolerate acid inactivation and release to be in sync with normal food digestion in the duodenum.

Surgical treatment is an effective and irreplaceable option for selected CP patients. Surgical treatment of CP can be divided into two types: pancreatectomy and decompression drainage. In 1935, Whipple, Parsons and Mullins (Whipple et al. 1935) began work on their procedure for resection of the pancreas (pancreaticoduodenectomy). In 1940, they shortened the procedure from a two-stage to a one-stage process. The key improvement lay in employing bile duct jejunum anastomosis instead of gallbladder stomach anastomosis, and this remains a landmark in pancreatic surgery. In 1954, to resolve the pancreatic hypertension problem in patients with CP, DuVal and Zollinger independently performed main pancreatic duct decompression (Duval 1954). In 1891, Alfred Pearce Gould became the first surgeon to remove pancreatic stones from the duct of Wirsung (Hess 1912), which was found to alleviate the pressure of pancreatic duct thereby ameliorating the disease process.

Stone extraction was widely applied as part of the surgical treatment of CP until the advent of endoscopy and shock-wave lithotripsy (ESWL). In 1973 and 1974, endoscopic sphincterotomy (EST) was reported by Kawai and colleagues (1974) and Classen and Demling (1974) respectively, and represents the basic technology underpinning pancreatic endoscopic treatment. In 1983, Seigel (Seigel 1983) successfully performed pancreatic duct stenting in patients with pancreatic duct stricture. In 1980, Chaussy (Chaussy et al. 1980) performed high-energy shock waves to disintegrate kidney stones in both dogs and human. Thereafter, Sauerbruch and collegues (1987) disintegrated a pancreatic duct stone with ESWL in a patient with chronic pancreatitis.

Over the past 20 years, with the development of endoscopic techniques, dilatation of the pancreatic duct, extraction of pancreatic duct stones, and drainage of pseudocysts are now widely used in pancreatic interventional therapy. With recent developments in pancreatic surgery and the use of endoscopic technology, the treatment of CP has made great strides. In the future, with the further elucidation of the etiology and pathogenesis of CP, patients with CP should receive earlier diagnosis, improved treatment with better prognosis.

References

Ammann RW. Zürich workshop on alcoholic chronic pancreatitis. Int J Pancreatol. 1998;23:81–2.

Buchler MW, Martignoni ME, Friess H, et al. A proposal for a new clinical classification of chronic pancreatitis. BMC Gastroenterol. 2009;9:93.

Cawley T. A singular case of diabetes, consisting entirely in the quantity of the urine with an enquiry into the different theories of that disease. Lond Med J. 1788;9:286.

Chaussy C, Brendel W, Schmiedt E. Extracorporeally induced destruction of kidney stones by shock waves. Lancet. 1980;2:1265–8.

Chiari H. Ueber Selbstverdauung des menschlichen Pankreas. Zeitschrift für Heilkunde. 1896;17:69–96.

Classen M, Demling L. Endoscopic sphincterotomy of the papilla of Vater and extraction of stones from the choledochal duct (author's transl). Dtsch Med Wochenschr. 1974;99:496–7.

Cohn JA, Friedman KJ, Noone PG, et al. Relation between mutations of the cystic fibrosis gene and idiopathic pancreatitis. N Engl J Med. 1998;339:653–8.

Comfort M, Steinberg A. Pedigree of a family with hereditary chronic replasing pancreatitis. Gastroenterology. 1952;21:54–63.

Comfort M, Gambill E, Baggenstoss AH. Chronic relapsing pancreatitis: a study of twenty-nine cases without associated disease of the biliary or gasto-intestinal tract. Gastroenterology. 1946;6:238–76.

DiMagno EP. A short, eclectic history of exocrine pancreatic insufficiency and chronic pancreatitis. Gastroenterology. 1993;104:1255–62.

DiMagno EP, Buxton JL, Regan PT, et al. Ultrasonic endoscope. Lancet. 1980;1:629–31.

Duval MK Jr. Caudal pancreatico-jejunostomy for chronic relapsing pancreatitis. Ann Surg. 1954;140:775–85.

Fitzgerald PJ. Medical anecdotes concerning some diseases of the pancreas. In: Fitzgerald PJ, Morrison AB, editors. The pancreas. Baltimore: Williams and Wilkins; 1980. p. 1–29.

Friedrich N. Diseases of the pancreas. In: Cyclopedia of the practice of medicine, vol. 8. New York: William Wood; 1878. p. 599.

Hamano H, Kawa S, Horiuchi A, et al. High serum IgG4 concentrations in patients with sclerosing pancreatitis. N Engl J Med. 2001;344:732–8.

Hess AF. A consideration of the pancreas and its ducts in congenital obliteration of the bile-ducts. Arch Intern Med. 1912;1:37–44.

Kawai K, Akasaka Y, Murakami K, et al. Endoscopic sphincterotomy of the ampulla of Vater. Gastrointest Endosc. 1974;20:148–51.

Masson E, Chen JM, Scotet V, et al. Association of rare chymotrypsinogen C (CTRC) gene variations in patients with idiopathic chronic pancreatitis. Hum Genet. 2008;123:83–91.

McCune WS, Shorb PE, Moscovitz H. Endoscopic cannulation of the ampulla of Vater: a preliminary report. Ann Surg. 1968;167:752–6.

Modlin IM. The paradox of the pancreas: from wirsüng to whipple. Hannover: Politzki Print Productions; 2003.

Narendranathan M, Sharma KN, Sosamma PI. Serum rhodanese in goitre and calcific pancreatitis of tropics. J Assoc Physicians India. 1989;37:648–9.

Rosendahl J, Witt H, Szmola R, et al. Chymotrypsin C (CTRC) variants that diminish activity or secretion are associated with chronic pancreatitis. Nat Genet. 2008;40:78–82.

Sachs M. Study of the pancreas and its inflammatory diseases from the 16th–19th century. Zentralbl Chir. 1993;118:702–11.

Sauerbruch T, Holl J, Sackmann M, et al. Disintegration of a pancreatic duct stone with extracorporeal shock waves in a patient with chronic pancreatitis. Endoscopy. 1987;19:207–8.

Seigel J. Evalution and treatment of acquired and congenital pancreatic disorders: endoscopic dilatation and insertion of endoprostheses. Am J Gastroenterol. 1983;78:A696.

Sharer N, Schwarz M, Malone G, et al. Mutations of the cystic fibrosis gene in patients with chronic pancreatitis. N Engl J Med. 1998;339:645–52.

Singer C. A short history of anatomy from the greeks to harvey. New York: Dover Publications; 1957. p. 111.

Vilmann P, Hancke S, Henriksen FW, et al. Endosonographically-guided fine needle aspiration biopsy of malignant lesions in the upper gastrointestinal tract. Endoscopy. 1993;25:523–7.

Whipple AO, Parsons WB, Mullins CR. Treatment of carcinoma of the ampulla of Vater. Ann Surg. 1935;102:763–79.

Whitcomb DC, Gorry MC, Preston RA, et al. Hereditary pancreatitis is caused by a mutation in the cationic trypsinogen gene. Nat Genet. 1996;14:141–5.

Witt H, Luck W, Hennies HC, et al. Mutations in the gene encoding the serine protease inhibitor, Kazal type 1 are associated with chronic pancreatitis. Nat Genet. 2000;25:213–6.

Yoshida K, Toki F, Takeuchi T, et al. Chronic pancreatitis caused by an autoimmune abnormality. Proposal of the concept of autoimmune pancreatitis. Dig Dis Sci. 1995;40:1561–8.

Zuideman P. Calcification and cirrhosis of the pancreas in patients with deficient nutrition. Doc Med Geograph Trop Amsterdam. 1955;5:229–31.

Definition and Classification of Chronic Pancreatitis

2

Xin-Ying Tang, Zhuan Liao, and Zhao-Shen Li

1 Definition

Chronic pancreatitis describes a wide range of irreversible progressive diseases of the pancreas in which recurrent inflammatory processes result in substitution of normal pancreatic parenchyma by fibrous connective tissue (Hoffmeister et al. 2015). Thus, the exocrine and endocrine functions of the pancreas are gradually lost. Patients with CP often have intricate symptoms, such as abdominal pain, steatorrhea, malnutrition, diabetes type 3c and gut dysmotility. Pain presents to be the main typical symptom of patients with CP. Besides, further characteristic complications may arise, such as pseudocysts, stenosis of pancreatic duct or bile ducts, duodenal obstruction, vascular complications, malnutrition and chronic pain. CP is one of the vital risk factors of pancreatic carcinoma. It significantly reduces the quality of life and the lifespan of relevant patients (Mayerle et al. 2013; Ito et al. 2016).

The definitions above only centers morphology. Advances in epidemiology, molecular genetics, biochemistry, modeling and other disciplines have new understandings of pathogenesis of CP, and allow the specialists reach an initial agreement on a mechanistic definition—"Chronic pancreatitis is a pathologic fibro-inflammatory syndrome of the pancreas in individuals with genetic, environmental and/or other risk factors who develop persistent pathologic responses to parenchymal injury or stress". In addition, 'Common features of established and advanced CP include pancreatic atrophy, fibrosis, pain syndromes, duct distortion and strictures, calcifications, pancreatic exocrine dysfunction, pancreatic endocrine dysfunction and dysplasia' (Whitcomb et al. 2016). The definition recognizes the complex character of CP and departs risk factors from disease activity markers and disease endpoints. If international consensus is reached after debates in rebuttals and indorsations among experts and pancreatic societies, the definition would be of great benefit to early diagnosis, classification and prognosis.

2 Classification

In 1963, the Marseilles classification first proposed the substances of acute and chronic pancreatitis, both with relapsing and non-relapsing variants (Sarles 1965). In the following years, Cambridge classification and M-ANNHEIM classification (Schneider et al. 2007) were proposed to depart obstructive CP from other types of CP (Sarner and Cotton 1984; Singer et al. 1985;

X.-Y. Tang, M.D. • Z. Liao, M.D. (✉)
Z.-S. Li, M.D.
Department of Gastroenterology, Changhai Hospital, the Second Military Medical University, Shanghai, China

Shanghai Institute of Pancreatic Diseases, Shanghai, China
e-mail: liaozhuan@smmu.edu.cn

Z.-S. Li et al. (eds.), *Chronic Pancreatitis*, DOI 10.1007/978-981-10-4515-8_2

Table 2.1 Previous classifications of chronic pancreatitis (Schneider et al. 2007)

Classifications of chronic pancreatitis	Major objectives, definitions, and criteria
Clinical description 1946	Description of the clinical presentation of chronic pancreatitis and its association with increased alcohol consumption
Marseille 1963	Description of morphologic characteristics and etiological factors of the disease; no discussion of the correlation between anatomic and functional changes; no categorization according to disease severity or clinical presentation; no inclusion of pancreatic imaging findings
Marseille 1984	Further description and subclassification of morphological changes; "obstructive chronic pancreatitis" listed as distinct form; no discussion of the correlation between anatomic and functional changes; no categorization according to disease severity or clinical presentation; no inclusion of pancreatic imaging findings
Marseille-Rome 1988	Further description of "chronic calcifying" and "chronic inflammatory" pancreatitis as distinct forms; description of etiological factors; no further elaboration of clinical, functional, or imaging criteria
Marseille 1984	Further description and subclassification of morphological changes; "obstructive chronic pancreatitis" listed as distinct form; no discussion of the correlation between anatomic and functional changes; no categorization according to disease severity or clinical presentation; no inclusion of pancreatic imaging findings
Marseille-Rome 1988	Further description of "chronic calcifying" and "chronic inflammatory" pancreatitis as distinct forms; description of etiological factors; no further elaboration of clinical, functional, or imaging criteria
Cambridge 1984	Further description and subclassification of morphological changes; "obstructive chronic pancreatitis" listed as distinct form; no discussion of the correlation between anatomic and functional changes; no categorization according to disease severity or clinical presentation; no inclusion of pancreatic imaging findings
Clinical stages 1994	Detailed subclassification of chronic pancreatitis with correlation of etiological factors with different morphological forms of the disease; differentiation of clinical stages of the disease; linkage of pancreatic imaging findings and functional testing with stages of the disease
Japan Pancreas Society 1997	Description of clinical presentation and classification of disease in "definite" and "probable" chronic pancreatitis according to imaging findings, functional testing, and histological examination
Zürich Workshop 1997	Description of clinical presentation and classification of disease in "definite" and "probable" chronic pancreatitis according to imaging findings, functional testing, and histological examination
Manchester system 2006	Disease grading according to clinical criteria, but limited separation of different disease severities; not all clinical presentations can be categorized

US ultrasonography, *CT* computed tomography, *ERCP* endoscopic retrograde cholangiopancreatography

Sarles 1991). Table 2.1 lists a variety of CP classification systems that have appeared in history.

The M-ANNHEIM classification which is most commonly used in clinical practice nowadays provides simultaneously a simple standardized system for the clinical classification of chronic pancreatitis according to etiology, clinical stage, and severity of the disease, and it is usually suitable for directing clinicians. On the whole, the classification is based on recent research of the mechanism of CP (Etemad and Whitcomb 2001; Lankisch and Banks 1998), epidemiological studies (Lin et al. 2000), recent genetic findings (Cohn et al. 2005; Bishop et al. 2005), insights gained from experimental studies.

3 M-ANNHEIM Multiple Risk Factors

Based on the assumption that the interaction of multiple risk factors results in most patients with CP, the M-ANNHEIM classification is established. Thus, it is named because the multiple (M) risk factors consist of several possible ones such as alcohol consumption (A), nicotine consumption

Table 2.2 The M-ANNHEIM multiple risk factor classification of chronic pancreatitis (Schneider et al. 2007)

M Pancreatitis with Multiple risk factors	
A	Alcohol consumption
	Excessive consumption (>80 g/day)
	Increased consumption (20–80 g/day)
	Moderate consumption (<20 g/day)
N	Nicotine consumption
	(In cigarette smokers: description of nicotine consumption by pack-years)
N	Nutritional factors
	Nutrition (e.g., high caloric proportion of fat and protein)
	Hyperlipidemia
H	Hereditary factors
	Hereditary pancreatitis (defined according to Whitcomb96)
	Familial pancreatitis (defined according to Whitcomb96)
	Early-onset idiopathic pancreatitis
	Late-onset idiopathic pancreatitis
	Tropical pancreatitis
	(possible mutations in the PRSS1, CFTR, or SPINK1 genes)
E	Efferent duct factors
	Pancreas divisum
	Annular pancreas and other congenital abnormalities of the pancreas
	Pancreatic duct obstruction (e.g., tumors)
	Posttraumatic pancreatic duct scars
	Sphincter of Oddi dysfunction
I	Immunological Factors
	Autoimmune pancreatitis
	Sjögren syndrome-associated chronic pancreatitis
	Inflammatory bowel disease-associated chronic pancreatitis
	Chronic pancreatitis with autoimmune diseases
	(e.g., primary sclerosing cholangitis, primary biliary cirrhosis)
M	Miscellaneous and rare metabolic factors
	Hypercalcemia and hyperparathyroidism
	Chronic renal failure
	Drugs
	Toxins

(N), nutritional factors (N), hereditary factors (H), efferent pancreatic duct factors (E), immunological factors (I), and various rare miscellaneous and metabolic (M) factors (Table 2.2).

4 M-ANNHEIM Clinical Staging of Chronic Pancreatitis

The M-ANNHEIM clinical staging system referred to a previous one (Chari and Singer 1994). It is subcategorized into an asymptomatic phase (stage 0) and a symptomatic phase (stages I, II, III, IV) of CP (Table 2.3). "Stage I is characterized by abdominal pain without pancreatic insufficiency" (Ammann et al. 1984, 1996; Lankisch et al. 1993; Layer et al. 1994; Ammann and Muellhaupt 1999). "Stage II is determined by the presence of partial pancreatic insufficiency with or without abdominal pain" (Lankisch et al. 1993; Layer et al. 1994; Ammann et al. 1996; Ammann and Muellhaupt 1999). In this stage, patients present with only one of exocrine and endocrine insufficiency, but not with both of them. "Stage III is characterized by the presence of both exocrine and endocrine insufficiency" (Lankisch et al. 1993; Layer et al. 1994;

Table 2.3 M-ANNHEIM clinical staging of chronic pancreatitis (modified from Chari and Singer 21) (Schneider et al. 2007)

Asymptomatic chronic pancreatitis	
(0)	Stage of subclinical chronic pancreatitis
	(a) Period without symptoms (determination by chance, e.g., autopsy)
	(b) Acute pancreatitis—single episode (possible onset of chronic pancreatitis)
	(c) Acute pancreatitis with severe complications
Symptomatic chronic pancreatitis	
(I)	Stage without pancreatic insufficiency
	(a) (Recurrent) acute pancreatitis (no pain between episodes of acute pancreatitis)
	(b) Recurrent or chronic abdominal pain (including pain between episodes of acute pancreatitis)
	(c) I a/b with severe complications
(II)	Stage of partial pancreatic insufficiency
	(a) Isolated exocrine (or endocrine) pancreatic insufficiency (without pain)
	(b) Isolated exocrine (or endocrine) pancreatic insufficiency (with pain)
	(c) II a/b with severe complications
(III)	Stage of painful complete pancreatic insufficiency
	(a) Exocrine and endocrine insufficiency (with pain, e.g., requiring pain medication)
	(b) III a with severe complications
(IV)	Stage of secondary painless disease (burnout)
	(a) Exocrine and endocrine insufficiency without pain and without severe complications
	(b) Exocrine and endocrine insufficiency without pain and with severe complications

Ammann et al. 1996; Ammann and Muellhaupt 1999). At last, in stage IV, abdominal pain may alleviate and almost more than 10 years later, permanent pain relief may typically occur. It is a natural course followed by fibrotic destruction, progressive functional insufficiency and burnout of the gland finally (Ammann and Muellhaupt 1999; Girdwood et al. 1981).

5 Proposed Staging/Classification of CP (Stages A)

In order to combine clinical experience in the field of CP with progress in diagnostic methods and new molecular technologies for the assessment of CP, it is important to propose a classification of CP based on key clinical aspects. In 2010, Milosavljevic T and his colleagues established a new classification for the definition and staging of CP.

5.1 Specific Definition of CP Stage A

Milosavljevic defined stage A as the early stage of CP where complications have not yet ocurred and the clinical exocrine and endocrine function is preserved. However, some subclinical signs such as impaired glucose tolerance, reduced exocrine function but without steatorrhea might already exist. Patients with pain of any type and degree and/or attacks of acute pancreatitis, no complications, no steatorrhea, no insulin-dependent diabetes mellitus may be divided as Stage A.

5.2 Specific Definition of CP Stage B

When specified complications (e.g. stage B, bile duct) have appeared without exocrine and endocrine insufficiency, patients with CP turn to stage B. Patients with complications but without steatorrhea or diabetes mellitus may be divided as Stage B.

5.3 Specific Definition of CP Stage C

When it comes to Stage C, the end stage of CP, pancreatic fibrosis has led to specified clinical exocrine and/or endocrine pancreatic function loss (e.g. stage C steatorrhea and/or diabetes mellitus) with/without complications. There are three sub-classified categories of Stage C: “C1-patients with endocrine function impairment; C2-patients with exocrine function impairment; C3-patients with exocrine/endocrine function impairment and/or complications”.

Patients with clinical manifestation of end-stage functional impairment with/without complications may be divided as Stage C (Milosavljevic et al. 2010).

6 TIGAR-O System

A new classification of CP, TIGAR-O system, recommending new insights of various risk factors is close to clinical practice and gradually applied. The recent TIGAR-O system consists of six groups categorized as (1) Toxic-metabolic, (2) Idiopathic, (3) Genetic, (4) Autoimmune, (5) Recurrent and severe acute pancreatitis, or (6) Obstructive (Milosavljevic et al. 2010) (Table 2.4).

Table 2.4 TIGAR-O system of classification of chronic pancreatitis [24]

Etiologic risk factors associated with chronic pancreatitis: TIGAR-O classification system
Toxic–metabolic
Alcoholic
Tobacco smoking
Hypercalcemia
Hyperparathyroidism
Hyperlipidemia (rare and controversial)
Chronic renal failure
Medications
Phenacetin abuse (possibly from chronic renal insufficiency)
Toxins
Organotin compounds (e.g. DBTC)
Idiopathic
Early onset
Late onset
Tropical
Tropical calcific pancreatitis
Fibrocalculous pancreatic diabetes
Other
Genetic
Autosomal dominant
Cationic trypsinogen (codon 29 and 122 mutations)
Autosomal recessive/modifier genes
CFTR mutations
SPINK1 mutations
Cationic trypsinogen (codon 16, 22, 23 mutations)
Antitrypsin deficiency (possible)
Autoimmune
Isolated autoimmune chronic pancreatitis
Syndromic autoimmune chronic pancreatitis
Sjogren syndrome associated chronic pancreatitis
Inflammatory bowel disease associated chronic pancreatitis
Primary biliary cirrhosis associated chronic pancreatitis

(continued)

Table 2.4 (continued)

Etiologic risk factors associated with chronic pancreatitis: TIGAR-O classification system
Recurrent and severe acute pancreatitis
Postnecrotic (severe acute pancreatitis)
Recurrent acute pancreatitis
Vascular diseases/ischemic
Postirradiation
Obstructive
Pancreatic divisum
Sphincter of Oddi disorders (controversial)
Duct obstruction (e.g. tumor)
Preampullary duodenal wall cysts
Posttraumatic pancreatic duct scars

References

Ammann RW, Muellhaupt B. The natural history of pain in alcoholic chronic pancreatitis. Gastroenterology. 1999;116:1132–40.

Ammann RW, Akovbiantz A, Largiader F, Schueler G. Course and outcome of chronic pancreatitis. Longitudinal study of a mixed medical–surgical series of 245 patients. Gastroenterology. 1984;86:820–8.

Ammann RW, Heitz PU, Klöppel G. Course of alcoholic chronic pancreatitis: a prospective clinicomorphological long-term study. Gastroenterology. 1996;111:224–31.

Bishop MD, Freedman SD, Zielenski J, Ahmed N, Dupuis A, Martin S, et al. The cystic fibrosis transmembrane conductance regulator gene and ion channel function in patients with idiopathic pancreatitis. Hum Genet. 2005;118:372–81.

Chari ST, Singer MV. The problem of classification and staging of chronic pancreatitis. Proposals based on current knowledge of its natural history. Scand J Gastroenterol. 1994;29:949–60.

Cohn JA, Neoptolemos JP, Feng J, Yan J, Jiang Z, Greenhalf W, et al. Increased risk of idiopathic chronic pancreatitis in cystic fibrosis carriers. Hum Mutat. 2005;26:303–7.

Etemad B, Whitcomb DC. Chronic pancreatitis: diagnosis, classification, and new genetic developments. Gastroenterology. 2001;120:682–707.

Girdwood AH, Marks IN, Bornman PC, Kottler RE, Cohen M. Does progressive pancreatic insuficiency limit pain in calcific pancreatitis with duct stricture or continued alcohol insult? J Clin Gastroenterol. 1981;3:241–5.

Hoffmeister A, et al. English language version of the S3-consensus guidelines on chronic pancreatitis: definition, aetiology, diagnostic examinations, medical, endoscopic and surgical management of chronic pancreatitis. Z Gastroenterol. 2015;53(12): 1447–95.

Ito T, et al. Evidence-based clinical practice guidelines for chronic pancreatitis 2015. J Gastroenterol. 2016;51(2):85–92.

Lankisch PG, Banks PA. Chronic pancreatitis: etiology. In: Lankisch PG, Banks PA, editors. Pancreatitis. Berlin: Springer; 1998. p. 199–208.

Lankisch PG, Lohr-Happe A, Otto J, Creutzfeldt W. Natural course in chronic pancreatitis. Digestion. 1993;54:148–55.

Layer P, Yamamoto H, Kalthoff L, Clain JE, Bakken LJ, DiMagno EP. The different courses of early and late onset idiopathic and alcoholic chronic pancreatitis. Gastroenterology. 1994;107:1481–7.

Lin Y, Tamakoshi A, Hayakawa T, Ogawa M, Ohno Y. Cigarette smoking as a risk factor for chronic pancreatitis: a case-control study in Japan. Research Committee on Intractable Pancreatic Diseases. Pancreas. 2000;21:109–14.

Mayerle J, et al. Chronic pancreatitis—definition, etiology, investigation and treatment. Dtsch Arztebl Int. 2013;110(22):387–93.

Milosavljevic T, Kostic Milosavljevic M, Krstic M, Jovanovic I. Classification of chronic pancreatitis. Dig Dis. 2010;28(2):330–3.

Sarles H. Pancreatitis symposium. Marseilles: Karger; 1965.

Sarles H. Definitions and classifications of pancreatitis. Pancreas. 1991;6:470–4.

Sarner M, Cotton PB. Classification of pancreatitis. Gut. 1984;25:756–9.

Schneider A, Lohr JM, Singer MV. The M-ANNHEIM classification of chronic pancreatitis: introduction of a unifying classification system based on a review of previous classifications of the disease. J Gastroenterol. 2007;42:101–19.

Singer MV, Gyr K, Sarles H. 2d symposium on the classification of pancreatitis. Marseilles, 28–30 March 1984. Acta Gastroenterol Belg. 1985;48:579–82.

Whitcomb DC, et al. Chronic pancreatitis: an international draft consensus proposal for a new mechanistic definition. Pancreatology. 2016;16(2):218–24.

The Epidemiology of Chronic Pancreatitis

3

Qian-Qian Zhu, Quan-Cai Cai, Luo-Wei Wang, Zhuan Liao, and Zhao-Shen Li

1 Descriptive Epidemiology

1.1 Incidence and Prevalence

The changing incidence and prevalence of CP over time worldwide is presented in Table 3.1 (Levy et al. 2014; Jupp et al. 2010). Reported incidence in the USA was 1.9, 4.2, and 3.5 cases per 100,000 people in 1940s, 1950s, and 1960s, respectively (Osullivan et al. 1972). A nationwide survey in England and Wales showed increasing incidence of CP from 0.83 cases per 100,000 people in the early 1960s to 3.18 cases per 100,000 people in the early 1980s (Johnson and Hosking 1991). Another study reported the incidence of CP in England was 4.3 cases per 100,000 people in the years between 1989 and 1990, and 8.6 cases per 100,000 people in the years between 1999 and 2000 (Tinto et al. 2002). The incidence and prevalence of CP was 4.0–4.2 cases per 100,000 people, and 13.0 to 14.4/100,000 persons in Denmark surveyed from 1978 to 1979, respectively (Andersen et al. 1982). CP is also widely prevalent in Asia. Both the incidence and the prevalence of CP increased during the 17 years from 1994 to 2011 in Japan (Hirota et al. 2012, 2014; Otsuki and Tashiro 2007). The annual incidence and prevalence was 5.4 and 28.5 per 100,000 in the third nationwide survey conducted in Japan in 1994, respectively. The incidence increased to 5.8 per 100,000 in the fourth nationwide survey conducted in 1999, while the prevalence was 32.9 per 100,000. The fifth survey reported the incidence and prevalence increased to 14.4 and 35.5 per 100,000 in 2002, respectively. The sixth nationwide survey in 2007 showed an incidence rate of 11.9 cases per 100,000 persons and a prevalence rate of 36.9 cases per 100,000 population. The estimated annual incidence and prevalence of CP in Japan from the seventh nationwide survey in 2011 was 14.0/100,000 and 52.4/100,000, respectively.

A multicenter survey was conducted in 22 hospitals in 6 urban health care regions of China to determine the nature and magnitude of chronic pancreatitis between May 1994 and April 2004 (Wang et al. 2009). The results showed the prevalence of CP was increasing year by year. It was 3.08, 3.91, 5.28, 7.61, 10.43, 11.92, 12.84, and 13.52 per 100,000 inhabitants respectively in the 8 years between 1996 and 2003. In addition,

Q.-Q. Zhu, M.D.
Department of Assisted Reproduction, Shanghai Ninth People's Hospital, Shanghai Jiaotong University School of Medicine, Shanghai, China

Q.-C. Cai, M.D.
Center for Clinical Epidemiology and Evidence-Based Medicine, Changhai Hospital, the Second Military Medical University, Shanghai, China

L.-W. Wang, M.D. • Z. Liao, M.D. (✉)
Z.-S. Li, M.D. (✉)
Department of Gastroenterology, Changhai Hospital, the Second Military Medical University, Shanghai Institute of Pancreatic Diseases, Shanghai, China
e-mail: liaozhuan@smmu.edu.cn; zhaoshenli@hotmail.com

Z.-S. Li et al. (eds.), *Chronic Pancreatitis*, DOI 10.1007/978-981-10-4515-8_3

Table 3.1 The changing worldwide incidence and prevalence of chronic pancreatitis over time (Levy et al. 2014; Jupp et al. 2010)

Country	Year(s)	Incidence (per 100,000)	Prevalence (per 100,000)
Europe and North America			
United States of America[a] (Osullivan et al. 1972)	1940–1949	1.9	N/A
	1950–1959	4.2	N/A
	1960–1969	3.5	N/A
United States of America[b] (Yang et al. 2008)	1988	7.0	N/A
	2004	8.1	N/A
United States of America[c] (Yadav et al. 2011)	1997–2006	4.05	41.76
Switzerland[c] (Capitaine 1991)	1958–1962	0.15	N/A
	1973–1982	1.64	N/A
England and Wales[b] (Johnson and Hosking 1991)	1960–1964	0.83	N/A
	1965–1969	1.02	N/A
	1970–1974	1.08	N/A
	1975–1979	1.77	N/A
	1980–1984	3.18	N/A
England[b] (Tinto et al. 2002)	1989–1990	4.3	N/A
	1999–2000	8.6	N/A
Denmark[d] (Andersen et al. 1982)	1970–1974	6.9	N/A
	1975–1979	10.0	N/A
Denmark[d] (The Copenhagen Pancreatitis Study Group 1981)	1978–1979	4.0–4.2	13.0–14.4
Finland[b] (Jaakkola and Nordback 1993)	1977	10.4	N/A
	1989	13.4	N/A
Poland[c] (Dzieniszewski et al. 1990a)	1982–1987	5.0	17.0
Germany[a] (Lankisch et al. 2002a)	1988–1995	6.4	N/A
Czech Republic[c] (Dite et al. 2001)	1999	7.9	N/A
France[c] (Levy et al. 2006)	2003	5.9–7.7	15.4–26.4
Asia			
Japan[c] (Hirota et al. 2012, 2014; Otsuki and Tashiro 2007)	1974	2.0	N/A
	1992–1993	5.0–5.9	N/A
	1994	5.4	28.5
	1999	5.8	32.9
	2002	14.4	35.5
	2007	11.9	36.9
	2011	14.0	52.4
China[c] (Wang et al. 2009)	1996	N/A	3.08
	2003	N/A	13.52
India[c] (Balaji et al. 1994)	1994	N/A	125

N/A data not available
[a]Single centre; all patients with chronic pancreatitis
[b]National statistics for admissions with chronic pancreatitis
[c]Multicentre or nationwide survey of all patients with chronic pancreatitis
[d]Single centre; all patients admitted with chronic pancreatitis

in the six health care areas, which were different in economy and life habits, the CP prevalence was increasing at different rates. The prevalence of the east, which was the most developed area, was growing the fastest. It was increasing from 3.27 per 100,000 inhabitants in 1996 to 13.73 per 100,000 inhabitants in 2003. From 1996 to 2003, the CP prevalence in the north of China was 2.93, 3.88, 4.99, 6.89, 9.95, 11.47, 12.78 and 13.05 per 100,000 inhabitants. The prevalence of CP was 2.97 per 100,000 inhabitants in the northeast of China, 2.94 per 100,000 inhabitants in the northwest of China, 2.67 per 100,000 inhabitants in the middle south of China, 2.55 per 100,000 inhabitants in the southwest of China in 1996. It increased to 13.12 per 100,000 inhabitants in the northeast of China, 12.92 per 100,000 inhabitants in the northwest of China, 11.62 per 100,000 inhabitants in the middle south of China, 12.61 per 100,000 inhabitants in the southwest of China in 2003.

1.2 Age and Gender

Gender differences exist in chronic pancreatitis, and the majority of patients were male. The seventh nationwide epidemiological study of CP in Japan reported the sex ratio (male/female) of the patients with CP was 4.6 (Hirota et al. 2014). James estimated between 73% and 91% of CP patients were male based on previous studies (Jupp et al. 2010; Wang et al. 2009; Levy et al. 2006; Lankisch et al. 2002b; Garg and Tandon 2004; Wehler et al. 2004). The gender distribution of CP is related with etiological factors. Men are more likely to have Alcohol-related pancreatitis than women, but the gender differences decrease with the rising alcohol consumption among women (Muniraj et al. 2014; Yadav and Lowenfels 2013). Pancreatitis is more associated with gallstones, endoscopic retrograde cholangiopancreatography (ERCP), autoimmune diseases, or to be idiopathic among women (Yadav and Lowenfels 2013).

Chronic pancreatitis is more common among persons who are between 40 and 60 years old. The mean age of the CP patients varied with geographical region and time based on the previous studies. A study in England and Wales described the hospital admissions for chronic pancreatitis peaked in those aged between 35 and 54 years (Tinto et al. 2002). A prospective nationwide survey among1086 subjects in India reported the mean age of patients was 39.7 years (Balakrishnan et al. 2008). The mean age of CP patients in a retrospective multicenter survey from 22 hospitals in China was 48.90 years (Wang et al. 2009). The average age of CP patients was 47.80 years for both men and women in the 1960s, and it increased to 57.6 years for men and 60.2 years for women in the 1990s in Japan (Jupp et al. 2010; Garg and Tandon 2004). The data from the sixth nationwide epidemiological survey in Japan in 2007 showed the mean age of males and females with definite and possible CP was 59.3 and 60.2 years, respectively (Hirota et al. 2012). In the seventh survey conducted in Japan in 2011, the mean age increased to 62.2 years in males and 63.3 years in females (Hirota et al. 2014).

1.3 Race

The racial disparity in chronic pancreatitis has been reported in some epidemiological studies. A study aiming to explore the importance of race as a risk factor for CP was carried out in America and Europe. The result showed that black males and females have a higher risk of chronic pancreatitis than the white (Lowenfels et al. 1999). The reason is unclear, and more research is needed to explore whether the difference is related with lifestyle, and dietary, genetic, or other factors. Data from both national and state hospitals in American revealed that black males and females have the higher hospitalization rates for CP than all other races (Jupp et al. 2010; Yang et al. 2008; Tao et al. 2003).

1.4 Mortality

Previous surveys exploring the survival of CP patients indicate the life expectancy of these patients is reduced significantly comparing with the general population. It is estimated that the median survival time is about 15–20 years since the onset of CP. A study was conducted among 174 CP patients (95% were smokers) to explore the survival rates and cause of death (Pedrazzoli et al. 2008). The result showed the mortality rate was increased from 15.3% for 5 years to 76.5% for 30 years, and the median survival time was 15.5 years. The death of CP patients is mainly caused (60%–75%) by the extrapancreatic consequences of alcohol and smoking over use rather than CP by itself (Levy et al. 2014).The survival time of patients with alcohol-related pancreatitis is significantly shorter than the general population, but the mortality risk was not different between those with hereditary pancreatitis and the general population (Pedrazzoli et al. 2008; Cavallini et al. 1998; Rebours et al. 2009).

2 Risk Factors

2.1 Alcohol

Alcohol plays an important role in chronic pancreatitis. The proportion of chronic pancreatitis caused by alcohol varied across geographical regions. Between 32.6% and 95% of CP can be ascribed to alcoholism in the Western or Industrialized Asia-pacific region, and the percentage is between 18.8% and 41% in the developing Asia-pacific region (Table 3.2). In China, the main etiology of CP in six health care areas of China was changed from biliary stone diseases to alcohol over 10 years (Wang et al. 2009). About 40% of CP was caused by alcohol in the six regions of China in the years between 2000 and 2003.

The incidence of alcohol chronic pancreatitis varied with gender. The results from the North American Pancreatitis Study-2 (NAPS-2) showed that men (59.4%) were more likely than women (28.1%) to develop alcohol CP (Coté et al. 2011). The genome-wide association study found the variants in the CLDN2 gene loci could be associated with alcohol-related pancreatitis (Whitcomb et al. 2012). The higher frequency of homozygosity for this genetic variant in males (0.26) than females (0.07) provided a possible explanation for the different gender distribution of CP.

Table 3.2 Percentage of patients with chronic pancreatitis in whom the cause is alcohol abuse (Reprint with permission from Jupp et al. 2010)

Geographical area	Percentage of chronic pancreatitis caused by alcohol
Northern Europe	42–84.8%
Southern Europe	43–80.4%
North and Central America	44–67%
South America	89.6%
Western/Industrialized Asia-pacific region	32.6–95%
Developing Asia-pacific region	18.8–41%
Africa	62–93%

Northern Europe comprises: Czech Republic, France, Germany, Poland, Switzerland, United Kingdom (Dite et al. 2001; Levy et al. 2006; Lankisch et al. 2002b; Wehler et al. 2004; Dzieniszewski et al. 1990b; Ammann et al. 1973; Gastard et al. 1973; James et al. 1974; Melia et al. 1992). Southern Europe comprises: Italy (Cavallini et al. 1998; Frulloni et al. 2009; Pezzilli et al. 2007)
North and Central America comprises: USA, Mexico (Thuluvath et al. 2003; Whitcomb et al. 2008; Robles-Diaz et al. 1990). South America comprises: Brazil (Dani et al. 1990)
Western/industrialised Asia-Pacific Region comprises: Australia, Japan, Singapore, South Korea (Otsuki and Tashiro 2007; Garg and Tandon 2004; Ishii et al. 1973; Ryu et al. 2005)
Developing Asia-Pacific Region comprises: China, India, Malaysia (Wang et al. 2009; Garg and Tandon 2004; Balakrishnan et al. 2008). Africa comprises: French speaking African Nations, South Africa (Marks et al. 1973; Moshal 1973; Uys et al. 1973)

Previous studies provide evidence supporting that there is a threshold effect and a dose-response relationship between alcohol and CP (Irving et al. 2009; Yadav et al. 2009). Compared with abstaining and light drinking, very heavy drinking was positively associated with CP (odds ratio, 3.10; 95% confidence interval, 1.87–5.14) after controlling for age, sex, smoking status, and body mass index in the North American Pancreatitis Study-2. This study demonstrated that the risk of CP could be significantly increased for those who had five alcoholic drinks or more per day. (Yadav et al. 2009). A systematic review and meta-analysis of epidemiologic studies on the relationship between alcohol and pancreatitis found that there is not differences in the risk of pancreatitis between those consumed two or fewer drinks on average per day and non-drinkers (RR = 1.0, 95% CI: 0.8–1.2; $P = 0.887$). Those who consumed three to four drinks per day had the higher risk of pancreatitis than the non-drinkers, but the difference was marginally slightly significant (RR = 1.2, 95% CI: 1.0–1.5, $P = 0.059$).Compared with non-drinkers, the risk of pancreatitis was higher than those who consumed more than four drinks per day (RR = 2.5, 95% CI: 2.0–3.1, $P < 0.001$) (Irving et al. 2009).

In addition, research found alcoholic CP was correlated with drinking age and daily consumption, but not the drinking frequency. The results from a survey conducted among male sobriety association members in Japan revealed that the drinking age was younger and the daily alcohol intake was greater among alcoholics with a history of pancreatitis than the alcoholics without pancreatitis (Maruyama and Otsuki 2007). A study aiming to explore the relationship between pancreatitis and alcohol drinking habits showed drinking frequency may be not independently associated with pancreatitis (Kristiansen et al. 2008). Currently, the pathological mechanism of alcoholic chronic pancreatitis is unclear, and it is probable that chronic alcohol consumption sensitizes the acinar cell to injury (Pandol et al. 2010).

2.2 Smoking

Smoking is an independent risk factor for CP. The research has demonstrated acinar cell alterations including cytoplasmic vacuolization and cellular edema could be induced by nicotine. In addition, it also could affect digestive enzymes in the pancreas (Luaces-Regueira et al. 2014). A meta-analysis about smoking and CP reported the pooled risk estimate of CP for smokers vs. never smokers was 2.5 (95%CI, 1.3–4.6), after adjustment for alcohol consumption (Andriulli et al. 2010). Moreover, it found there was a dose-response effect on smoking and pancreatic injury. The pooled risk for CP was 3.3 (95%CI, 1.4–7.9) among those who smoked one or more packs per day and 2.4 (95%CI, 0.9–6.6) among those who smoked less than one pack per day. The association between smoking and CP was found to be stronger among patients who also consume alcohol (Falk et al. 2006; Yadav et al. 2010). A study in experimental animal model provided evidence that smoking and drinking had the synergistic detrimental effects on pancreatitis (Hartwig et al. 2000).

Previous studies have shown smoking can accelerate the progression of pancreatic calcification, functional impairment and the progression of acute pancreatitis to CP (Lankisch et al. 2009; Imoto and DiMagno 2000; Maisonneuve et al. 2005, 2006). Moreover, smoking was correlated with many complications of CP, such as exocrine insufficiency, development of calcifications, and ductal changes (Luaces-Regueira et al. 2014). On the contrary, smoking cessation could slow the development and progression of CP. Result from a meta-analysis showed the risk of CP significantly dropped from 2.8 (95%CI, 1.8–4.2) in current smokers to 1.4 (95%CI, 1.1–1.9) in former smokers (Andriulli et al. 2010). The clinical study found smoking cessation in the first years after the clinical onset of CP reduced the risk of developing pancreatic calcifications (Talamini et al. 2007).

2.3 Diseases

Patients with celiac disease were nearly three times more likely to develop CP (Sadr-Azodi et al. 2012). The risk of CP is positively related with diseases such as inflammatory bowel disease, systemic lupus erythematosis, and other disorders.

References

Ammann RW, Hammer B, Fumagalli I. Chronic pancreatitis in Zurich, 1963–1972. Clinical findings and follow-up studies of 102 cases. Digestion. 1973;9:404–15.

Andersen BN, Pedersen NT, Scheel J, et al. Incidence of alcoholic chronic-pancreatitis in copenhagen. Scand J Gastroenterol. 1982;17:247–52.

Andriulli A, Botteri E, Almasio PL, et al. Smoking as a cofactor for causation of chronic pancreatitis: a meta-analysis. Pancreas. 2010;39:1205–10.

Balaji LN, Tandon RK, Tandon BN, et al. Prevalence and clinical-features of chronic-pancreatitis in southern India. Int J Pancreatol. 1994;15:29–34.

Balakrishnan V, Unnikrishnan AG, Thomas V, et al. Chronic pancreatitis. A prospective nationwide study of 1,086 subjects from India. JOP. 2008;9:593–600.

Capitaine Y. Epidemiology of chronic pancreatitis in Switzerland. In: Sarles H, Johnson C, Sauniere JF, editors. Pancreatitis; Oxford, Blackwell, 1991.

Cavallini G, Frulloni L, Pederzoli P, et al. Long-term follow-up of patients with chronic pancreatitis in Italy. Scand J Gastroenterol. 1998;33:880–9.

Coté GA, Yadav D, Slivka A, et al. Alcohol and smoking as risk factors in an epidemiology study of patients with chronic pancreatitis. Clin Gastroenterol Hepatol. 2011;9:266–73.

Dani R, Mott CB, Guarita DR, et al. Epidemiology and etiology of chronic pancreatitis in Brazil: a tale of two cities. Pancreas. 1990;5:474–8.

Dite P, Stary K, Novotny I, et al. Incidence of chronic pancreatitis in the Czech Republic. Eur J Gastroenterol Hepatol. 2001;13:749–50.

Dzieniszewski J, Jarosz M, Ciok J. Chronic pancreatitis in Warsaw. Mater Med Pol. 1990a;3:202–4.

Dzieniszewski J, Jarosz M, Ciok J. Chronic pancreatitis in Warsaw. Mater Med Pol. 1990b;22:202–4.

Falk DE, Yi HY, Hiller-Sturmhofel S. An epidemiologic analysis of co-occurring alcohol and tobacco use and disorders: findings from the National Epidemiologic Survey on Alcohol and Related Conditions. Alcohol Res Health. 2006;29:162–71.

Frulloni L, Gabbrielli A, Pezzilli R, et al. Chronic pancreatitis: report from a multicenter Italian survey (PanCroInfAISP) on 893 patients. Dig Liver Dis. 2009;41:311–7.

Garg PK, Tandon RK. Survey on chronic pancreatitis in the Asia-Pacific region. J Gastroenterol Hepatol. 2004;19:998–1004.

Gastard J, Joubaud F, Farbos T, et al. Etiology and course of primary chronic pancreatitis in Western France. Digestion. 1973;9:416–28.

Hartwig W, Werner J, Ryschich E, et al. Cigarette smoke enhances ethanol-induced pancreatic injury. Pancreas. 2000;21:272–8.

Hirota M, Shimosegawa T, Masamune A, et al. The sixth nationwide epidemiological survey of chronic pancreatitis in Japan. Pancreatology. 2012;12:79–84.

Hirota M, Shimosegawa T, Masamune A, et al. The seventh nationwide epidemiological survey for chronic pancreatitis in Japan: clinical significance of smoking habit in Japanese patients. Pancreatology. 2014;14(6):490.

Imoto M, DiMagno EP. Cigarette smoking increases the risk of pancreatic calcification in late-onset but not early-onset idiopathic chronic pancreatitis. Pancreas. 2000;21:115–9.

Irving HM, Samokhvalov AV, Rehm J. Alcohol as a risk factor for pancreatitis. A systematic review and meta-analysis. JOP. 2009;10:387–92.

Ishii K, Nakamura K, Takeuchi T, et al. Chronic calcifying pancreatitis and pancreatic carcinoma in Japan. Digestion. 1973;9:429–37.

Jaakkola M, Nordback I. Pancreatitis in finland between 1970 and 1989. Gut. 1993;34:1255–60.

James O, Agnew JE, Bouchier IA. Chronic pancreatitis in England: a changing picture? Br Med J. 1974;2:34–8.

Johnson CD, Hosking S. National statistics for diet, alcohol-consumption, and chronic-pancreatitis in england and wales, 1960–88. Gut. 1991;32:1401–5.

Jupp J, Fine D, Johnson CD. The epidemiology and socioeconomic impact of chronic pancreatitis. Best Pract Res Clin Gastroenterol. 2010;24:219–31.

Kristiansen L, Grønbæk M, Becker U, et al. Risk of pancreatitis according to alcohol drinking habits: a population-based cohort study. Am J Epidemiol. 2008;168:932–7.

Lankisch PG, Assmus C, Maisonneuve P, et al. Epidemiology of pancreatic diseases in Luneburg County. A study in a defined german population. Pancreatology. 2002a;5:469–77.

Lankisch PG, Assmus C, Maisonneuve P, et al. Epidemiology of pancreatic diseases in Luneburg County. A study in a defined german population. Pancreatology. 2002b;2:469–77.

Lankisch PG, Breuer N, Bruns A, et al. Natural history of acute pancreatitis: a long-term population-based study. Am J Gastroenterol. 2009;104:2797–805; quiz 2806

Levy P, Barthet M, Mollard BR, et al. Estimation of the prevalence and incidence of chronic pancreatitis and its complications—a prospective survey in adults attending gastroenterologists in France. Gastroenterol Clin Biol. 2006;30:838–44.

Levy P, Dominguez-Munoz E, Imrie C, et al. Epidemiology of chronic pancreatitis: burden of the disease and consequences. United European Gastroenterol J. 2014;2:345–54.

Lowenfels AB, Maisonneuve P, Grover H, et al. Racial factors and the risk of chronic pancreatitis. Am J Gastroenterol. 1999;94(3):790–4.

Luaces-Regueira M, Iglesias-Garcia J, Lindkvist B, et al. Smoking as a risk factor for complications in chronic pancreatitis. Pancreas. 2014;43:275–80.

Maisonneuve P, Lowenfels AB, Mullhaupt B, et al. Cigarette smoking accelerates progression of alcoholic chronic pancreatitis. Gut. 2005;54(4):510.

Maisonneuve P, Frulloni L, Mullhaupt B, et al. Impact of smoking on patients with idiopathic chronic pancreatitis. Pancreas. 2006;33:163–8.

Malka D, Hammel P, Sauvanet A, et al. Risk factors for diabetes mellitus in chronic pancreatitis. Gastroenterology. 2000;119:1324–32.

Marks IN, Bank S, Louw JH. Chronic pancreatitis in the Western Cape. Digestion. 1973;9:447–53.

Maruyama K, Otsuki M. Incidence of alcoholic pancreatitis in Japanese alcoholics—survey of male sobriety association members in Japan. Pancreas. 2007;34:63–5.

Melia WM, Sims MM, Whitehouse DP, et al. Chronic pancreatitis in the British Army 1978–1989. J R Army Med Corps. 1992;138:126–8.
Moshal MG. A study of chronic pancreatitis in Natal. Digestion. 1973;9:438–46.
Muniraj T, Aslanian HR, Farrell J, et al. Chronic pancreatitis, a comprehensive review and update. Part I: epidemiology, etiology, risk factors, genetics, pathophysiology, and clinical features. Dis Mon. 2014;60:530–50.
Osullivan JN, Nobrega FT, Brown AL, et al. Acute and chronic pancreatitis in rochester, minnesota, 1940–1969. Gastroenterology. 1972;62:373–9.
Otsuki M, Tashiro M. Chronic pancreatitis and pancreatic cancer, lifestyle-related diseases. Intern Med. 2007;46:109–13.
Pandol SJ, Gorelick FS, Gerloff A, et al. Alcohol abuse, endoplasmic reticulum stress and pancreatitis. Dig Dis. 2010;28:776–82.
Pedrazzoli S, Pasquali C, Guzzinati S, et al. Survival rates and cause of death in 174 patients with chronic pancreatitis. J Gastrointest Surg. 2008;12:1930.
Pezzilli R, Morselli-Labate AM, Fantini L, et al. Assessment of the quality of life in chronic pancreatitis using Sf-12 and EORTC Qlq-C30 questionnaires. Dig Liver Dis. 2007;39:1077–86.
Rebours V, Boutron-Ruault MC, Jooste V, et al. Mortality rate and risk factors in patients with hereditary pancreatitis: uni- and multidimensional analyses. Am J Gastroenterol. 2009;104:2312–7.
Robles-Diaz G, Vargas F, Uscanga L, et al. Chronic pancreatitis in Mexico City. Pancreas. 1990;5:479–83.
Ryu JK, Lee JK, Kim YT, et al. Clinical features of chronic pancreatitis in Korea: a multicenter nationwide study. Digestion. 2005;72:207–11.
Sadr-Azodi O, Sanders DS, Murray JA, et al. Patients with celiac disease have an increased risk for pancreatitis. Clin Gastroenterol Hepatol. 2012;10:1136–1142.e3.
Talamini G, Bassi C, Butturini G, et al. Outcome and quality of life in chronic pancreatitis. JOP. 2001;2:117–23.
Talamini G, Bassi C, Falconi M, et al. Smoking cessation at the clinical onset of chronic pancreatitis and risk of pancreatic calcifications. Pancreas. 2007;35:320–6.
Tao N, Sussman S, Nieto J, et al. Demographic characteristics of hospitalized patients with alcoholic liver disease and pancreatitis in los angeles county. Alcohol Clin Exp Res. 2003;27:1798–804.
The Copenhagen Pancreatitis Study Group. An interim report from a prospective epidemiological multicentre study. Scand J Gastroenterol. 1981;2:305–12.
Thuluvath PJ, Imperio D, Nair S, et al. Chronic pancreatitis. Long-term pain relief with or without surgery, cancer risk, and mortality. J Clin Gastroenterol. 2003;36:159–65.
Tinto A, Lloyd D, Kang JY, et al. Acute and chronic pancreatitis—diseases on the rise: a study of hospital admissions in England 1989/90-1999/2000. Aliment Pharmacol Ther. 2002;16:2097–105.
Uys CJ, Bank S, Marks IN. The pathology of chronic pancreatitis in Cape Town. Digestion. 1973;9:454–68.
Wang LW, Li ZS, Li SD, et al. Prevalence and clinical features of chronic pancreatitis in china a retrospective multicenter analysis over 10 years. Pancreas. 2009;38:248–54.
Wehler M, Nichterlein R, Fischer B, et al. Factors associated with health-related quality of life in chronic pancreatitis. Am J Gastroenterol. 2004;99:138–46.
Whitcomb DC, Yadav D, Adam S, et al. Multicenter approach to recurrent acute and chronic pancreatitis in the United States: the North American Pancreatitis Study 2 (NAPS2). Pancreatology. 2008;8:520–31.
Whitcomb DC, LaRusch J, Krasinskas AM, et al. Common genetic variants in the CLDN2 and PRSS1-PRSS2 loci alter risk for alcohol-related and sporadic pancreatitis. Nat Genet. 2012;44:1349–54.
Yadav D, Lowenfels AB. The epidemiology of pancreatitis and pancreatic cancer. Gastroenterology. 2013;144:1252–61.
Yadav D, Hawes RH, Brand RE, et al. Alcohol consumption, cigarette smoking, and the risk of recurrent acute and chronic pancreatitis. Arch Intern Med. 2009;169:1035–45.
Yadav D, Slivka A, Sherman S, et al. Smoking is underrecognized as a risk factor for chronic pancreatitis. Pancreatology. 2010;10:713–9.
Yadav D, Timmons L, Benson JT, et al. Incidence, prevalence, and survival of chronic pancreatitis: a population-based study. Am J Gastroenterol. 2011; 106:2192–9.
Yang AL, Vadhavkar S, Singh G, et al. Epidemiology of alcohol-related liver and pancreatic disease in the united states. Arch Intern Med. 2008;168:649–56.

Etiology of Chronic Pancreatitis 4

Raffaele Pezzilli

1 Why Etiology Is the Cornerstone of the Disease

A disease can be recognized only when its natural history is known. This old but fundamental concept implies that we must know the etiology of the disease in order to modify the consequence of an inappropriate lifestyle or environmental factors and to detect genetic predisposition. Moreover, etiology can be used to provide clues into methods of treatment and understanding the pathogenesis of a disease may lead to identify novel molecular targets and to develop new drugs for treating chronic pancreatitis. However, some aspects of chronic pancreatitis are presently not fully understood, such as the mechanisms which underlie the development of chronic pancreatitis, those which cause the pain which is the presenting symptom of the majority of chronic pancreatitis patients, and the factors capable of maintaining the inflammation and the progression of the disease. Finally and most importantly, only epidemiological data exist regarding the progression of chronic pancreatitis in pancreatic cancer. Etiology seems to be an important factor in all these cases.

2 How Many People Have This Disease Right Now?

It has been reported that the prevalence of chronic pancreatitis ranges from 3 to 10 per 100,000 people around the world (Lankisch and Banks 1998). Lankisch and Banks pointed out that abdominal pain, steatorrhea, and diabetes mellitus are the major problems in treating chronic pancreatitis patients and that chronic pancreatitis must be considered a premalignant disease (Lowenfels et al. 1993, 1997; Raimondi et al. 2010). If this is true for Western countries (Banks 2002), in Japan, the estimated annual prevalence and incidence of chronic pancreatitis in 2011 were 52.4/100,000 and 14.0/100,000, respectively (Hirota et al. 2014). Finally, the data from other countries are largely unknown and this represents a notable stumbling block for planning adequate health strategies, especially in low- and middle-income countries where economic resources are limited (Mills 2014).

There is also a newcomer to the scene of chronic pancreatitis, namely autoimmune pancreatitis (AIP) (Pezzilli and Pagano 2014) and its exact incidence is still unknown (Pezzilli et al. 2012). The only epidemiological data regarding

R. Pezzilli
Department of Digestive System, Sant'Orsola-Malpighi Hospital,
Via Massarenti 9, 40138 Bologna, Italy
e-mail: raffaele.pezzilli@aosp.bo.it

Z.-S. Li et al. (eds.), *Chronic Pancreatitis*, DOI 10.1007/978-981-10-4515-8_4

AIP is that, in patients having a Whipple resection for the suspicion of a pancreatic neoplasm, 2.5% have AIP (Abraham et al. 2003).

3 The Etiology of Chronic Pancreatitis in Western Countries and in Japan

Alcohol is considered the most frequent factor associated with chronic pancreatitis in Western countries, and alcoholic chronic pancreatitis develops mainly in young male adults of 30–40 years of age; the pathological lesions are chronic and, clinically, the disease is characterized by recurrent flares of abdominal pain. The frequency of alcohol as an associated factor of chronic pancreatitis increased from 19 (O'Sullivan et al. 1972) to 50% (James et al. 1974) and even up to 80% (Durbec and Sarles 1978; Sarles et al. 1979) in the period from 1940 to 2003 in Western countries. These results on the etiology of chronic pancreatitis have been subsequently confirmed in studies coming from Europe (Gullo et al. 1977; Thorsgaard Pedersen et al. 1982; Ammann et al. 1984; Dzieniszewski et al. 1990; Johnson and Hosking 1991; Jaakkola and Nordback 1993; Cavallini et al. 1998; Díte et al. 2001) as well as from Brazil (Dani et al. 1990), Australia (Garg and Tandon 2004) and South Africa (Marks et al. 1980). Four consecutive surveys carried out in Japan (from 1977 to 1979, from 1978 to 1984, in 1994, and in 1999, respectively) (Otsuki 2003) reported that alcohol in chronic pancreatitis accounted is an associated factor for fewer than 60% of chronic pancreatitis cases. Regarding Japan, the last survey on chronic pancreatitis reported an incidence of alcoholic chronic pancreatitis of 67.5% (Hirota et al. 2014). This latter study introduced a new insight into the etiology of chronic pancreatitis because it has been found that, among patients without a drinking habit, the incidences of diabetes mellitus and pancreatic calcifications were significantly higher in smokers than in non-smokers; however, smoking was not identified as an independent risk factor for the appearance of abdominal pain (Hirota et al. 2014).

The results of a study on chronic pancreatitis carried out recently in United States reported that alcohol accounted for 44.5% of the cases as an etiological factor of chronic pancreatitis (Coté et al. 2011).

The most important finding of the recent studies is the increase in the idiopathic form of chronic pancreatitis reaching 20%. How can this finding be explained? It is probable that the introduction of sophisticated and highly sensitive imaging techniques, such as magnetic resonance imaging (Pezzilli 2014) and endoscopic ultrasonography (Catalano et al. 2009) into clinical practice have allowed the diagnosis of chronic pancreatitis in patients without any symptoms and apparent risk factors, and these results in an increase of chronic pancreatitis of unknown origin.

4 The Etiology of Chronic Pancreatitis in Low- and Middle-Income Countries

French authors (Sarles et al. 1979) have reported a particular form of chronic pancreatitis in India found in malnourished in childhood having a low fat and low protein diet. This form of the disease was called "tropical pancreatitis" and it is defined as a form of chronic pancreatitis and it is clinically characterized by abdominal pain, intraductal calculi and diabetes mellitus in young non-alcoholic subjects. The first description of this disease included a series of 45 patients with pancreatic calcifications associated with diabetes mellitus who were of low economic class and consumed a protein- and calorie-deficient diet, and who were malnourished, emaciated, has an increase in size of parotids, and had hair and skin changes similar to that of Kwashiorkor (Zuidema 1959). Similar findings were then reported from various tropical countries in Asia (India, Bangladesh, Sri Lanka) (Chari et al. 1992; Tandon et al. 2002) and Africa (Uganda, Nigeria, Zambia, Madagascar, Ethiopia) (Lester 1993). Thus, tropical pancreatitis has been recognized as a distinct entity with unique clinical and epidemiological features different from that of alcoholic chronic pancreatitis. Subsequent studies coming from India and Africa confirmed these findings (Mohan et al. 2003). In these countries, recent data have also shown important changes in the etiology of chronic pancreatitis. In fact, idiopathic chronic pancreatitis was the predominant etiology accounting for 57.0–69.9% of all cases of chronic pancreatitis (Rajesh et al. 2014). However, an increase in the prevalence of alcoholic chronic pancreatitis (41%) was noted whereas hypertriglyceridemia and hyperparathyroidism were less common causes of non-alcoholic chronic pancreatitis and, finally, autoimmune pancreatitis remains a rare cause of the disease (Rajesh et al. 2014). Of course, the increase in alcoholic pancreatitis in India as an etiological factor of chronic pancreatitis represents the changing lifestyle in this country, but the increase in the idiopathic form of the disease has no explanation. In these countries, the clinical assessment of the etiology of chronic pancreatitis probably requires more effort, and the limit of 80 g of pure alcohol per day for at least 5 years should be revised according to the new international organization against the recommendations for alcohol use (Pezzilli 2015).

5 The Significance of Etiology in Chronic Pancreatitis

French authors (Durbec and Sarles 1978) have undoubtedly demonstrated that alcohol is a risk factor for chronic pancreatitis showing that the relative risk is multiplied by approximately a factor of 1.4 passing from 1 to 20-g of alcohol intake. In addition, the increase of risk to develop a chronic pancreatitis appears to be more rapid when passing from the class of non-drinkers to that of a 20-g alcohol intake per day. The mechanism which determines fibrosis of the pancreatic gland has been pointed out in a well-written paper by Talukdar et al. (2006). The oxidation of ethanol to acetaldehyde determines the activation of the quiescent pancreatic stellate cells without any pre-activation; determining the development of pancreatic fibrosis even in the absence of necroinflammation process. We have also reported using breath analysis that oxidative stress is an important process in chronic pancreatitis patients (Morselli-Labate et al. 2007). In fact, using a mass spectrometer to analyze breath samples obtained from patients with chronic pancreatitis, having mainly alcoholic pancreatitis without pancreatic pain, we found that the volatile compounds H_2S, NO and malononitrile were significantly higher in these chronic pancreatitis patients as compared to healthy subjects (Kuroda et al. 1998). We should underline that the above mentioned substances are the final products of ethanol and oxidative stress able to initiate fibrogenesis of the pancreas.

Thus, alcohol induces pancreatic fibrosis as has frequently been found in autoptic series of alcoholics without a clinical history of chronic pancreatitis (Kuroda et al. 1998; Martin and Bedossa 1989; Suda et al. 1996).

Unfortunately, in experimental animals the administration of alcohol is not able to induce pancreatic damage similar to that observed in human chronic pancreatitis because alcohol to damage the pancreas requires prior sensitization with other agents.

The etiology of tropical pancreatitis is different and several hypotheses have been proposed such as the malnutrition theory, the suggested role of Cassava metabolites in inducing chronic alterations of the pancreas and, finally, the oxidant stress hypothesis (Martin and Bedossa 1989). Thus, it is possible that unknown substances cause an activation of the pancreatic stellate cells. In addition, the occurrence of the SPINK-1 mutation in patients with tropical pancreatitis suggests a combined etiology of this disease (Bhatia et al. 2002; Schneider et al. 2002).

6 Other Etiologies of Chronic Pancreatitis

6.1 Genetic Disorders

The mutations of the cystic fibrosis transmembrane conductance regulator-gene (CFTR-gene)

(Rommens et al. 1989) and the identification of mutations of the cationic trypsinogen gene (protease-serine-1 gene, PRSS-1) (Whitcomb et al. 1996), the serine protease inhibitor and Kazal type 1 gene (SPINK-1) (Witt et al. 2000), has led to identifying the role of the familial/hereditary factors in the development of chronic pancreatitis in Western countries. Furthermore, also in tropical pancreatitis it has been noted that this disease is highly associated with the SPINK-1 N34S mutation (Bhatia et al. 2002; Schneider et al. 2002) whereas the frequency of CFTR mutations was lower than in white subjects (Bhatia et al. 2000). It is well-known that PRSS1 mutations are able to induce chronic pancreatitis and the same does not happen for CFTR and SPINK-1 mutations; thus the latter two genes seem to be modifiers able to induce chronic pancreatitis only when other risk factors such as alcohol are present (Schneider et al. 2002; Pezzilli et al. 2003).

Another mutation which seems to be related to chronic pancreatitis is the chymotrypsinogen C (CTRC) mutation; the gene protects the pancreas by prematurely degrading activated trypsinogen, and rare mutations are associated with CP in Europe and Asia (LaRusch et al. 2015).

Finally, the regulation of calcium levels (intra-acinar) is critical for preventing trypsinogen activation and pancreatic injury, and the calcium-sensing receptor gene (CASR) plays a major role in maintaining the calcium homeostasis by means of its effect on the renal tubules and the parathyroid gland. The first report on CASR gene mutations and chronic pancreatitis is that regarding a family comprising five individuals who were all heterozygous for the N34S SPINK1 polymorphism. Two of these five heterozygous individuals developed chronic pancreatitis and both these individuals presented with a T > C mutation at position 518 in the CASR gene, which is a leucine to proline amino acid change in the extracellular domain of the CASR protein (Felderbauer et al. 2003); this suggests that CASR mutations may be a predisposing genetic factor which increases susceptibility for chronic pancreatitis.

Hereditary chronic pancreatitis is highly related to the development of cancer and the risk of developing pancreatic cancer in these subjects appears to be highest in those patients who have an early onset of hereditary chronic pancreatitis (Raimondi et al. 2010).

6.2 Autoimmune Diseases

In the last 10 years it has been reported an increasing number of cases of autoimmune pancreatitis (AIP) in all countries around the world (Pearson et al. 2003); the frequency of autoimmune pancreatitis will probably increase in the next few years. Autoimmune pancreatitis is clinically characterized by obstructive jaundice and, histologically, by a lymphoplasmacytic infiltrate with fibrosis; from a therapeutic point of view, there is a dramatic response to corticosteroid therapy. Several classifications of autoimmune pancreatitis have been proposed (Fantini et al. 2007). Recently, two distinct diseases have been identified: one is called type 1 and the other one, type 2 AIP (Hart et al. 2015). Type 1 AIP is the pancreatic manifestation of immunoglobulin G4-related disease whereas type 2 AIP is less commonly recognized has no biomarker and may be associated with inflammatory bowel disease in about ¼ of patients (Hart et al. 2015).

7 The Changes in Lifestyle

The changes in lifestyle may contribute to modify the etiology of chronic pancreatitis. An example is that happens in developing countries where alcohol consumption is increased (Das et al. 2006); this has changed the etiology of chronic pancreatitis in these countries. On the other hand, in Europe there was a progressive reduction in alcohol consumption from 1961 to 1991 (WHO 2004) and this may explain the incidence of chronic pancreatitis in the Western countries. In addition, suggesting a change in the lifestyle of chronic pancreatitis patients, even if the pancreatic functional changes caused by alcohol progress after cessation of alcohol abuse, the progression of the disease slows and becomes less severe when alcohol intake is abolished (Gullo et al. 1988).

8 The Frequency of Change in Etiology

The discovery of new factors able to induce chronic pancreatitis, new forms of chronic pancreatitis and changes in lifestyle of patients having chronic pancreatitis contribute to the changes in frequencies of the etiologies of chronic pancreatitis. Thus, from 2004 various studies carried out around the world have claimed that the etiological features of chronic pancreatitis are different to those reported in the past. For example, in Korea (Ryu et al. 2005), even if the main etiological factor of chronic pancreatitis remains alcohol (64.3%) the frequency of idiopathic chronic pancreatitis is increased (20.8%), followed by obstructive (8.6%) and autoimmune pancreatitis (2.0%). On the other hand, in the Asian-Pacific region (Garg and Tandon 2004), the frequency of alcoholic pancreatitis is highly variable, ranging from 19% of chronic pancreatitis cases in China to 95% in Australia. Finally, tropical pancreatitis is 46.4% in China and it is not present in Australia. Also in Italy has been observed that chronic pancreatitis associated with alcohol abuse accounted for less than 50% of cases (Frulloni et al. 2009), and this figure is lower than that reported by Gullo et al. in 1977 (Gullo et al. 1977). However, it is important to note that in Italy there are regional differences regarding the frequency of alcoholic chronic pancreatitis; in Northern Italy, alcohol is the main etiological factor (80.4%) (Pezzilli et al. 2007), whereas in Southern Italy, the percentage of alcoholic chronic pancreatitis dropped to 60% (Montalto et al. 1990). In addition, after alcohol abuse, obstruction (27%), pancreatitis of unknown origin (17%), autoimmunity (4%) and hereditary/genetic factors (4%) are the other associated factors of chronic pancreatitis in Italy (Frulloni et al. 2009). Surprisingly, in a prospective nationwide study carried out in India (Balakrishnan et al. 2008), the authors found that the majority of patients had pancreatitis of unknown origin (60% of the cases); alcoholic chronic pancreatitis accounted for a third of the cases whereas tropical pancreatitis was present in only 3.8% of the cases. However, these data need to be re-evaluated because the frequency of chronic pancreatitis of unknown origin was 17% in the Italian survey (Frulloni et al. 2009) ranging from 12% in Northern Italy (Pezzilli et al. 2007) to 38% in Southern Italy (Montalto et al. 1990).

Conclusions

The results coming from recent surveys on chronic pancreatitis around the world show that alcohol remains the main factor associated with chronic pancreatitis and that alcohol abuse and smoking habits are independent risk factors for chronic pancreatitis (Yadav et al. 2009).

Autoimmune pancreatitis having a frequency of 2–4% of all case of chronic pancreatitis will probably increase in frequency over the next years. Hereditary chronic pancreatitis has a low impact on the etiology of acute pancreatitis but it is highly related to the development of cancer (Raimondi et al. 2010). The rise in idiopathic chronic pancreatitis probably indicates our poor clinical confidence in the definition and quantification of risk factors in our patients or, especially in Africa and Asia, the misleading classification of tropical pancreatitis as idiopathic chronic pancreatitis.

References

Abraham SC, Wilentz RE, Yeo CJ, Sohn TA, Cameron JL, Boitnott JK, Hruban RH. Pancreaticoduodenectomy (Whipple resections) in patients without malignancy: are they all 'chronic pancreatitis'? Am J Surg Pathol. 2003;27(1):110–20.

Ammann RW, Akovbiantz A, Largiader F, Schueler G. Course and outcome of chronic pancreatitis.

Longitudinal study of a mixed medical-surgical series of 245 patients. Gastroenterology. 1984;86:820–8.

Balakrishnan V, Unnikrishnan AG, Thomas V, Choudhuri G, Veeraraju P, Singh SP, et al. Chronic pancreatitis. A prospective nationwide study of 1,086 Subjects from India. JOP. 2008;9:593–600.

Banks PA. Epidemiology, natural history, and predictors of disease outcome in acute and chronic pancreatitis. Gastrointest Endosc. 2002;56:S226–30.

Bhatia E, Durie P, Zielenski J, Lam D, Sikora SS, Choudhuri G, Tsui LC. Mutations in the cystic fibrosis transmembrane regulator gene in patients with tropical calcific pancreatitis. Am J Gastroenterol. 2000;95:3658–9.

Bhatia E, Choudhuri G, Sikora SS, Landt O, Kage A, Becker M, Witt H. Tropical calcific pancreatitis: strong association with SPINK1 trypsin inhibitor mutations. Gastroenterology. 2002;123:1020–5.

Catalano MF, Sahai A, Levy M, et al. EUS-based criteria for the diagnosis of chronic pancreatitis: the Rosemont classification. Gastrointest Endosc. 2009;69: 1251–61.

Cavallini G, Frulloni L, Pederzoli P, Talamini G, Bovo P, Bassi C, et al. Long-term follow-up of patients with chronic pancreatitis in Italy. Scand J Gastroenterol. 1998;33:880–9.

Chari ST, Mohan V, Jayanthi V, Snehalatha C, Malathi S, Viswanathan M, Madanagopalan N. Comparative study of the clinical profiles of alcoholic chronic pancreatitis and tropical chronic pancreatitis in Tamil Nadu, South India. Pancreas. 1992;7:52–8.

Coté GA, Yadav D, Slivka A, Hawes RH, Anderson MA, Burton FR, Brand RE, Banks PA, Lewis MD, Disario JA, Gardner TB, Gelrud A, Amann ST, Baillie J, Money ME, O'Connell M, Whitcomb DC, Sherman S, North American Pancreatitis Study Group. Alcohol and smoking as risk factors in an epidemiology study of patients with chronic pancreatitis. Clin Gastroenterol Hepatol. 2011;9:266–73.

Dani R, Mott CB, Guarita DR, Nogueira CE. Epidemiology and etiology of chronic pancreatitis in Brazil: a tale of two cities. Pancreas. 1990;5:474–8.

Das SK, Balakrishnan V, Vasudevan DM. Alcohol: its health and social impact in India. Natl Med J India. 2006;19:94–9.

Díte P, Starý K, Novotný I, Precechtelová M, Dolina J, Lata J, Zboril V. Incidence of chronic pancreatitis in the Czech Republic. Eur J Gastroenterol Hepatol. 2001;13:749–50.

Durbec JP, Sarles H. Multicenter survey of the etiology of pancreatic diseases. Relationship between the relative risk of developing chronic pancreatitis and alcohol, protein and lipid consumption. Digestion. 1978;18:337–50.

Dzieniszewski J, Jarosz M, Ciok J. Chronic pancreatitis in Warsaw. Mater Med Pol. 1990;22:202–4.

Fantini L, Zanini N, Fiscaletti M, Calculli L, Casadei R, Campana D, Pezzilli R. Autoimmune pancreatitis: the classification puzzle. Adv Med Sci. 2007;52:71–5.

Felderbauer P, Hoffmann P, Einwächter H, Bulut K, Ansorge N, Schmitz F, Schmidt WE. A novel mutation of the calcium sensing receptor gene is associated with chronic pancreatitis in a family with heterozygous SPINK1 mutations. BMC Gastroenterol. 2003;3:34.

Frulloni L, Gabbrielli A, Pezzilli R, Zerbi A, Cavestro GM, Marotta F, et al. Chronic pancreatitis: report from a multicenter Italian survey (PancroInfAISP) on 893 patients. Dig Liver Dis. 2009;41:311–7.

Garg PK, Tandon RK. Survey on chronic pancreatitis in the Asia-Pacific region. J Gastroenterol Hepatol. 2004;19:998–1004.

Gullo L, Costa PL, Labò G. Chronic pancreatitis in Italy. Aetiological, clinical and histological observations based on 253 cases. Rendic Gastroenterol. 1977;9:97–104.

Gullo L, Barbara L, Labò G. Effect of cessation of alcohol use on the course of pancreatic dysfunction in alcoholic pancreatitis. Gastroenterology. 1988;95:1063–8.

Hart PA, Zen Y, Chari ST. Recent advances in autoimmune pancreatitis. Gastroenterology. 2015;149:39–51.

Hirota M, Shimosegawa T, Masamune A, Kikuta K, Kume K, Hamada S, Kanno A, Kimura K, Tsuji I, Kuriyama S. Research committee of intractable pancreatic diseases. The seventh nationwide epidemiological survey for chronic pancreatitis in Japan: clinical significance of smoking habit in Japanese patients. Pancreatology. 2014;14:490–6.

Jaakkola M, Nordback I. Pancreatitis in Finland between 1970 and 1989. Gut. 1993;34:1255–60.

James O, Agnew JE, Bouchier IA. Chronic pancreatitis in England: a changing picture. Br Med J. 1974;2:34–8.

Johnson CD, Hosking S. National statistics for diet, alcohol consumption, and chronic pancreatitis in England and Wales, 1960–88. Gut. 1991;32:1401–5.

Kuroda J, Suda K, Hosokawa Y. Periacinar collagenization in patients with chronic alcoholism. Pathol Int. 1998;48:857–68.

Lankisch PG, Banks PA. Pancreatitis. New York: Springer; 1998.

LaRusch J, Lozano-Leon A, Stello K, Moore A, Muddana V, O'Connell M, Diergaarde B, Yadav D, Whitcomb DC. The common Chymotrypsinogen C (CTRC) Variant G60G (C.180T) increases risk of chronic pancreatitis but not recurrent acute pancreatitis in a North American population. Clin Transl Gastroenterol. 2015;6:e68.

Lester FT. A search for malnutrition-related diabetes mellitus among Ethiopian patients. Diabetes Care. 1993;16:187–92.

Lowenfels AB, Maisonneuve P, Cavallini G, Ammann RW, Lankisch PG, Andersen JR, et al. Pancreatitis and the risk of pancreatic cancer. International Pancreatitis Study Group. N Engl J Med. 1993;328:1433–7.

Lowenfels AB, Maisonneuve P, DiMagno EP, Elitsur Y, Gates LK Jr, Perrault J, Whitcomb DC. Hereditary pancreatitis and the risk of pancreatic cancer. International Hereditary Pancreatitis Study Group. J Natl Cancer Inst. 1997;89(6):442.

Marks IN, Girdwood AH, Bank S, Louw JH. The prognosis of alcohol-induced calcific pancreatitis. S Afr Med J. 1980;57:640–3.

Martin E, Bedossa P. Diffuse fibrosis of the pancreas: a peculiar pattern of pancreatitis in alcoholic cirrhosis. Gastroenterol Clin Biol. 1989;13:579–84.

Mills A. Reflections on the development of health economics in low- and middle-income countries. Proc Biol Sci. 2014;281(1789):20140451.

Mohan V, Premalatha G, Pitchumoni CS. Tropical chronic pancreatitis: an update. J Clin Gastroenterol. 2003;36:337–46.

Montalto G, Carroccio A, Soresi M, Ficano L, Notarbartolo A. Chronic pancreatitis in Sicily. Preliminary reports. Ital J Gastroenterol. 1990;22:33–5.

Morselli-Labate AM, Fantini L, Pezzilli R. Hydrogen sulfide, nitric oxide and a molecular mass 66 u substance in the exhaled breath of chronic pancreatitis patients. Pancreatology. 2007;7:497–504.

O'Sullivan JN, Nobrega FT, Morlock CG, Brown AL Jr, Bartholomew LG. Acute and chronic pancreatitis in Rochester, Minnesota, 1940–1969. Gastroenterology. 1972;62:373–9.

Otsuki M. Chronic pancreatitis in Japan: epidemiology, prognosis, diagnostic criteria, and future problems. J Gastroenterol. 2003;38:315–26.

Pearson RK, Longnecker DS, Chari ST, Smyrk TC, Okazaki K, Frulloni L, Cavallini G. Controversies in clinical pancreatology: autoimmune pancreatitis: does it exist. Pancreas. 2003;27:1–13.

Pezzilli R. Pancreatitis. Secretin increases the diagnostic yield of MRCP. Nat Rev Gastroenterol Hepatol. 2014;11:519–20.

Pezzilli R. Alcohol abuse and pancreatic diseases: an overview. Recent Patents Inflamm Allergy Drug Discov. 2015;9(2):102–6.

Pezzilli R, Pagano N. Pathophysiology of autoimmune pancreatitis. World J Gastrointest Pathophysiol. 2014;5(1):11–7.

Pezzilli R, Morselli-Labate AM, Mantovani V, Romboli E, Selva P, Migliori M, Corinaldesi R, Gullo L. Mutations of the CFTR gene in pancreatic disease. Pancreas. 2003;27:332–6.

Pezzilli R, Morselli-Labate AM, Fantini L, Campana D, Corinaldesi R. Assessment of the quality of life in chronic pancreatitis using Sf-12 and EORTC Qlq-C30 questionnaires. Dig Liver Dis. 2007;39:1077–86.

Pezzilli R, Imbrogno A, Fabbri D. Autoimmune pancreatitis management: reflections on the past decade and the decade to come. Expert Rev Clin Immunol. 2012;8(2):115–7.

Raimondi S, Lowenfels AB, Morselli-Labate AM, Maisonneuve P, Pezzilli R. Pancreatic cancer in chronic pancreatitis; aetiology, incidence, and early detection. Best Pract Res Clin Gastroenterol. 2010;24:349–58.

Rajesh G, Girish BN, Panicker S, Balakrishnan V. Time trends in the etiology of chronic pancreatitis in South India. Trop Gastroenterol. 2014;35(3):164–7.

Rommens JM, Iannuzzi MC, Kerem B, Drumm ML, Melmer G, Dean M, et al. Identification of the cystic fibrosis gene: chromosome walking and jumping. Science. 1989;245:1059–65.

Ryu JK, Lee JK, Kim YT, Lee DK, Seo DW, Lee KT, et al. Clinical features of chronic pancreatitis in Korea: a multicenter nationwide study. Digestion. 2005;72:207–11.

Sarles H, Cros RC, Bidart JM. A multicenter inquiry into the etiology of pancreatic diseases. Digestion. 1979;19:110–25.

Schneider A, Suman A, Rossi L, Barmada MM, Beglinger C, Parvin S, et al. SPINK1/PSTI mutations are associated with tropical pancreatitis and type II diabetes mellitus in Bangladesh. Gastroenterology. 2002;123:1026–30.

Suda K, Takase M, Takei K, Nakamura T, Akai J, Nakamura T. Histopathologic study of coexistent pathologic states in pancreatic fibrosis in patients with chronic alcohol abuse: two distinct pathologic fibrosis entities with different mechanisms. Pancreas. 1996;12:369–72.

Talukdar R, Saikia N, Singal DK, Tandon R. Chronic pancreatitis: evolving paradigms. Pancreatology. 2006;6:440–9.

Tandon RK, Sato N, Garg PK, Consensus Study Group. Chronic pancreatitis: Asia-Pacific consensus report. J Gastroenterol Hepatol. 2002;17:508–18.

Thorsgaard Pedersen N, Nyboe Andersen B, Pedersen G, Worning H. Chronic pancreatitis in Copenhagen. A retrospective study of 64 consecutive patients. Scand J Gastroenterol. 1982;17:925–31.

Whitcomb DC, Gorry MC, Preston RA, Furey W, Sossenheimer MJ, Ulrich CD, et al. Hereditary pancreatitis is caused by a mutation in the cationic trypsinogen gene. Nat Genet. 1996;14:141–5.

WHO. WHO global status report on alcohol 2004. World Health Organization. Department of Mental Health and Substance Abuse, Geneva 2004.

Witt H, Luck W, Hennies HC, Classen M, Kage A, Lass U, Landt O, Becker M. Mutations in the gene encoding the serine protease inhibitor, Kazal type 1 are associated with chronic pancreatitis. Nat Genet. 2000;25:213–6.

Yadav D, Hawes RH, Brand RE, Anderson MA, Money ME, Banks PA, Bishop MD, Baillie J, Sherman S, DiSario J, Burton FR, Gardner TB, Amann ST, Gelrud A, Lawrence C, Elinoff B, Greer JB, O'Connell M, Barmada MM, Slivka A, Whitcomb DC, North American Pancreatic Study Group. Alcohol consumption, cigarette smoking, and the risk of recurrent acute and chronic pancreatitis. Arch Intern Med. 2009;169:1035–45.

Zuidema PJ. Cirrhosis and disseminated calcification of the pancreas in patients with malnutrition. Trop Geogr Med. 1959;11:70–4.

The Pathogenesis of Chronic Pancreatitis

5

Jakob Lykke Poulsen, Søren Schou Olesen, Asbjørn Mohr Drewes, Bo Ye, Wei-Qin Li, Ali A. Aghdassi, Matthias Sendler, Julia Mayerle, and Markus M. Lerch

1 Pain Mechanisms in Chronic Pancreatitis

Jakob Lykke Poulsen, Søren Schou Olesen, and Asbjørn Mohr Drewes

Abstract Chronic abdominal pain remains a major clinical challenge in chronic pancreatitis (CP) and is present in up to 90% of the patients. It is associated with a poor life quality, an increased health resource utilization and is the primary cause of hospitalization Lieb et al. (Aliment Pharmacol Ther 29:706–19, 2009). The etiologies of pain in CP are increasingly better understood and likely involve multiple mechanisms. The focus of this chapter is to provide an overview of the mechanisms involved in chronic pancreatic pain. First, the traditional view of pain in CP is discussed where pain is thought to arise due to mechanical problems such as obstruction of the pancreatic gland. Although this theory is widely accepted and forms the theoretical background for invasive treatments of pain it is largely undocumented and has been challenged by recent research where no uniform associations between morphological changes and pain exist. The next section provides an overview of a novel neurobiological understanding of pain in CP, which is shifting the focus of pain from mechanical problems towards changes in peripheral and central pain processing. This has substantial consequences for treatment and may result in a paradigm shift of pain management of CP in a foreseeable future. Finally, we briefly discuss extra-pancreatic causes of pain in associated with CP, which are important to diagnose, as they are often easy to treat.

J.L. Poulsen • S.S. Olesen • A.M. Drewes (✉)
Mech-Sense, Department of Gastroenterology and Hepatology, Clinical Institute, Centre for Pancreatic Diseases, Aalborg University Hospital, Aalborg, Denmark
e-mail: amd@rn.dk

B. Ye, M.D. • W.-Q. Li, M.D. (✉)
Department of General Surgery, Jinling Hospital, Medical School of Nanjing University, Nanjing, China
e-mail: liweiqindr@vip.163.com

A.A. Aghdassi • M. Sendler • J. Mayerle
M.M. Lerch, M.D., F.R.C.P. (✉)
Department of Medicine A, University Medicine Greifswald, Ferdinand-Sauerbruch-Straße, 17475 Greifswald, Germany
e-mail: lerch@uni-greifswald.de

1.1 "Plumbing" Problems

Traditionally, it is generally accepted that pain is generated by increased pressure in the pancreatic ductal system or in the pancreatic parenchyma due to duct obstruction, stricture and/or peri-pancreatic fibrosis (Lieb et al. 2009; Anderson et al. 2015). Thus the "the plumbing theory" has been the theoretical background for most interventions with the common purpose to alleviate

Z.-S. Li et al. (eds.), *Chronic Pancreatitis*, DOI 10.1007/978-981-10-4515-8_5

the increased pressure through different surgical and endoscopic drainage procedures (Anaparthy and Pasricha 2008).

1.1.1 Ductal Pressure and Pain

White and co-workers described the first case report of a relationship between pancreatic duct pressure and pain in 1970 (White and Bourde 1970). Following acute necrotizing pancreatitis, a patient underwent open necrosectomy and with a drainage catheter communicating the pancreatic duct, he reproducibly reported pain with increased ductal pressure (White and Bourde 1970). Later studies attempted to verify the consumptiocccccn while most of them were flawed by inappropriate methodology (Fasanella et al. 2007). In a study by Sato and co-workers reported that compared to patients with gastric cancer, intraoperative measured pancreatic ductal pressure significantly increased in CP patients (Sato et al. 1986). Moreover, another study reconfirmed the ductal hypertension during endoscopic management (Okazaki et al. 1986). However other studies with the same manometry reported no ductal hypertension (Laugier 1994; Rolny et al. 1986; Ugljesić et al. 1996; Vestergaard et al. 1994), and demonstrated no difference in pressure levels referring to pain (Novis et al. 1985), which was supported by another study with the finding that ductal pressure did not precisely predict the ductal decompression (Renou et al. 2000). Furthermore, the link between ductal hypertension and pain in CP remains speculative as the mechanism was unclear.

1.1.2 Parenchymal Pressure and Pain

Increased parenchymal pressure measurement of the pancreas has also been suggested as a cause of pancreatic pain. A pioneer study was done by Ebbehøj and co-workers, which depicted a novel needle probe inserted directly into the pancreatic parenchyma to measure parenchymal pressure (Ebbehøj et al. 1984). In a cohort of 39 CP patients, patients with pain resulted in higher intrapancreatic pressure and pain was relieved after surgical drainage (Ebbehøj et al. 1990a). In a 1-year study, it was reported that recurrent pain can cause rebound of increased intrapancreatic pressure (Ebbehøj et al. 1990b). However, these findings were flawed by inclusion of patients without pain and not reproduced in a more recent study using a similar technique (Manes et al. 1994).

The pathophysiological link between increased intrapancreatic pressure and pain has been described as a "compartment-like syndrome" (Fasanella et al. 2007). In an animal model of CP, increased interstitial pressures, diminished blood flow and ensuing tissue acidosis were documented after stimulation with cholecystokinin and secretin (Patel et al. 1995). A human controlled experiment reported in the same paper drew a conclusion that the CP patients demonstrated significantly more acidotic tissue, which was suggested to be the result of secondary ischemia mimicking the pathophysiology underlying muscular compartment syndrome (Zhu et al. 2011; Schwartz et al. 2013) (described further below). Nonetheless, it must be underlined that these findings have never been reproduced.

1.1.3 Pancreatic Morphology and Pain

As measurement of pancreatic pressure can be invasive and potentially harmful, most decisions regarding surgery or endotherapy to relieve pain in the clinic rely on morphological abnormalities of the pancreas, such as pancreatic duct stricture, obstruction or pseudocysts (Lieb et al. 2009; Fasanella et al. 2007; Warshaw et al. 1998). Yet the correlation between morphological changes and pain have been challenged by a number of studies demonstrating no obvious morphological difference referring to pain, and even severe pain (Bornman et al. 1980; Lankisch et al. 1993; Malfertheiner et al. 1987; Jensen et al. 1984). The largest study examining the association between abdominal imaging features and pancreatic pain was done by Wilcox and co-workers (2015). Of the 518 CP patients examined, 427 reported abdominal pain from CP during the year before enrolment and the pattern (i.e. constant vs. intermittent pain) and severity of pain were independent of morphological changes.

Diffusion weighted imaging with MR imaging, which can provide information of atrophy, ductal pathology and microstructure of the tissue, was applied in a study by Frøkjær et al. In this study, the association between pathological imaging and pain came to the same result in agreement with the aforementioned study but morphological changes were associated with pancreatic function (Balci et al. 2009; Frokjaer et al. 2013).

Taken together, pancreatic morphology is not associated with pain in CP and, as such, the rationale for invasive treatment solely based on the results of imaging is questionable.

1.2 "Wiring" Problems

In patients with CP, inflammation and progressive replacement of the normal pancreatic tissue with fibrosis can lead to changes in the function and morphology of intrapancreatic nerves. Collectively these processes have been referred to as "wiring problems" (Moran et al. 2015) and represents a wide spectrum of changes in peripheral nociception and central pain processing which is discussed in detail below.

1.2.1 Peripheral Changes

To understand the neurobiological perspective on pain in CP, a basic knowledge about pain perception and processing is required Depending on the excitability of the neural membrane, the stimulus sensed by a variety of nociceptors may lead to generation of an action potential, which travels along afferent nerves to the spinal end of the nerves in the dorsal horn to trigger the release of neurotransmitters, which cross the synapse and activate secondary neurons that transmit the noxious stimulus to the brain through different pathways, ultimately resulting in the sensation of pain (Anaparthy and Pasricha 2008).

Peripheral Sensitization

Nerve growth factor, normally expressed by islets in the pancreas, is amongst the most important and well-characterized neuropeptides involved in growth, regulation and proliferation of certain neurons (Woolf et al. 1994). In rats with CP, it is upregulated. Nerve growth factor can not only significantly increase nociceptor excitability, pancreatic hyperalgesia and referred pain to somatic structures but also upregulate the nociceptor transient receptor potential vanilloid-1 in animal model of CP, as well as in humans with CP (Xu et al. 2007; Toma et al. 2000; Hartel et al. 2006). Thus, in preliminary studies, antagonists for transient receptor potential vanilloid-1 have been developed and proved to be effective in humans with neuropathic pain. However, hyperthermia, is still a concern of transient receptor potential vanilloid-1 antagonism (Wong and Gavva 2009).

Release of cytokines and chemokines, such as IL-8 and fractalkine, from immune cells infiltrating the pancreas during CP has been associated with pancreatic pain (Ceyhan et al. 2009a; Di Sebastiano et al. 1997). Specifically, compared to patients with painless CP, the number of mast cells can reach a 3.5 fold increase in those with pain (Hoogerwerf et al. 2005; Esposito et al. 2001). A proposed mechanism is increased activation of protease-activated receptor 2, triggered by tryptase released from the mast cells (Hoogerwerf et al. 2005). Other upregulated, proinflammatory cytokines have also been suspected to play a role in the pain generation in CP, and in some cases this upregulation and resulting pancreatic neuritis may increase pain intensity and/or frequency (Bockman et al. 1988; Keith et al. 1985; Ceyhan et al. 2009b) (for a thorough review see (Fasanella et al. 2007)).

Additionally, upregulation of neurotransmitters involved in pain signalling at the central end of the nociceptor, such as calcitonin gene-related peptide, substance P and brain-derived neurotrophic factor, has been demonstrated in animals with CP along with increased sensory nerve excitability, and pharmacological blockade of these receptors has likewise been shown to reduce pain (Hughes et al. 2011; Liu et al. 2011; Büchler et al. 1992).

These functional alterations render the nociceptors more sensitive to further stimulation (Gebhart 2000; Anand et al. 2007). This so called *peripheral sensitization*, results in an increased barrage of pain signals to the spinal cord (Woolf and Salter 2000), which is believed to increase clinical pain intensity, can be an important factor in the pathogenesis of pain in CP (Bockman et al. 1988; Keith et al. 1985; Ceyhan et al. 2009c).

Peripheral Neuropathy

Besides the changes on the molecular level, CP is also associated with prominent morphological and/or functional alterations of pancreatic nerves (Bockman et al. 1988; Ceyhan et al. 2009c). These changes are collectively referred to as "neural plasticity" at the cellular (neuronal) level. The characteristic features of pancreatic nerves in human CP are increased neural density (neural sprouting), increased neural size (neural hypertrophy), and perineural inflammations (neuritis) (Ceyhan et al. 2009c; Friess et al. 2002; Demir et al. 2015). In addition to the morphological alterations it has been demonstrated that nerves in patients with CP contain fewer sympathetic or adrenergic nerve fibres than normal pancreatic tissue—a phenomenon referred to as neural remodelling (Ceyhan et al. 2009b). Although these changes in many cases have been shown to relate to sensation in CP, the mechanisms and interactions with the functional neural changes are not fully understood (Demir et al. 2015) (Table 5.1).

Table 5.1 Peripheral pain mechanisms in chronic pancreatitis and its associated experimental evidence

Mechanism	Experimental evidence
Enhanced nociception	Upregulated transient receptor potential vanilloid-1
	Increased activation of protease-activated receptor 2
Upregulated neurotransmitter expression	Increased nerve growth factor and expression of calcitonin gene-related peptide, substance P and brain-derived neurotrophic factor
Pancreatic neuritis	Increased number of immune cells e.g. pancreatic mast cells, increased IL-8 and fractalkine level
Pancreatic neuropathy	Neural sprouting, neural hypertrophy

1.2.2 Central Changes

Central Sensitization

An augmented signalling of noxious stimuli to the spinal cord induces increased responsiveness of central pain transmitting neurons and thereby increases the gain in the whole pain system. This phenomenon is known as *central sensitization* leading to intense peripheral noxious stimuli, tissue injury, or nerve damage (Woolf 2011; Latremoliere and Woolf 2009). The process it typically characterised by increased excitability, expansion of the dorsal horn neurons receptive field and by sprouting of non-nociceptive afferents into "pain-specific" areas of the spinal cord. These functional and structural changes explain the clinical and experimental findings associated with central sensitization:

- primary hyperalgesia: increased sensitiveness to painful stimuli of the diseased organ (e.g. increased sensitiveness to stimulation of the pancreas)
- secondary hyperalgesia: a receptive field expansion that enables input from non-injured tissue to produce pain (e.g. increased sensitiveness to stimulation of visceral organs remote to the pancreas such as the rectosigmoid or somatic structures)
- allodynia: pain in response to a non-noxious stimulus (e.g. postprandial pain reported by patients with CP)

Several experimental human pain studies have reported increased areas of referred pain and augmented pain sensitiveness was seen in CP patients corresponding to primary and secondary hyperalgesia as discussed above (Dimcevski et al. 2007). Along this line, additional studies reported decreased pain thresholds to somatic stimulation of muscle and bone as well as stimulation of the rectosigmoid (Olesen et al. 2010a; Buscher et al. 2006). The latter reflects a special form of secondary hyperalgesia (viscero-visceral hyperalgesia) seen in visceral pain disorders accompanied by central sensitization.

Many patients with CP report postprandial pain, which, in addition to changes in ductal or parenchymal pressure mediated by humeral mechanisms, may also reflect allodynia triggered by non-noxious mechanical stimuli when the food passes the upper segments of the gastrointestinal tract in close proximity to the pancreas. In a sensitized pain-system, food passage may activate previous non-nociceptive neurons that now covey noxious information due to e.g., sprouting into pain signalling areas of the spinal cord. This again leads to allodynia perceived as postprandial pain by the patient.

One of the best characterised mechanisms involved in central sensitization is activation of the N-methyl-D-aspartic acid (NMDA) receptor, thus revealing a key involvement of glutamate in this process (Willert et al. 2004). Blocking of the NMDA receptor by ketamine has been shown to reverse hyperalgesia associated with CP in an experimental study (Bouwense et al. 2011a) and ketamine is currently under investigation in a randomised placebo controlled-trial of painful CP (Juel et al. 2015). Also, changes in ion channel properties have been shown to play a key role in the process of central sensitization. These can be modulated by gabapentoids, such as gabapentin and pregabalin, which target the pre-synaptic voltage-dependent calcium channels. In patients with CP, pregabalin is effective as an adjuvant treatment of pain in patients with CP and reverse associated primary and secondary hyperalgesia. Interestingly its effect can be predicted by segmental hyperalgesia of the pancreatic viscerotome (the upper abdominal skin area sharing spinal innervation with the pancreatic gland) and, as such, pregabalin treatment can be tailored to the individual patients pain profile (Olesen et al. 2013a).

Taken together, these clinical, experimental, and pharmacological findings characterise a generalised hyperalgesic state of the pain system in patients with CP and likely mirrors widespread sensitization of central pain pathways. The abnormalities seem to be linked to disease severity and at some point may become independent of the peripheral nociceptive input (see discussion later) (Bouwense et al. 2013).

Abnormal Patterns of Cortical Activity

Several studies have indicated that deafferentation, chronic pain, and hyperalgesia, as seen in CP patients, are associated with a functional reorganisation of the brain areas involved in sensory processing (Flor et al. 2006). Accordingly, people with arm or hand amputations show a shift of the mouth into the hand representation in the primary somatosensory cortex, with the quantity of cortical reorganisation being correlated with subjective pain ratings (Flor et al. 1995). In patients with CP, pancreatic nerve damage and modulation may to some degree mimic the peripheral nerve pathology seen in patients following amputations. Along this line, experimental pain studies have indicated that chronic pain and hyperalgesia is associated with functional reorganisation of the visceral sensory cortex (Dimcevski et al. 2007; Olesen et al. 2010b; Lelic et al. 2014). Hence, CP patients show reorganisation of the brain areas involved in visceral sensory processing. In addition, the evidence of impaired habituation to noxious stimuli in CP patients possibly reflecting a cortical neuronal hyperexcitability (Olesen et al. 2013b). Functional reorganization and hyperexcitability may be reversed by transcranial magnetic stimulation and a sham-controlled randomised trial has documented the effectiveness of this technique for pain alleviation in patients with CP.

The thalamus, as a critical relay site in the sensory system, has been implicated in chronic pain. Hence, a disturbance of the thalamocortical interplay evidenced by global changes in the rhythmicity of the cerebral cortex was observed in patients with neuropathic pain of mixed origin (Sarnthein et al. 2006). Parallel findings were observed in CP patients in studies based on spectral analysis of visceral evoked brain potentials and resting state electroencephalography (Olesen et al. 2011; Drewes 2008). Remarkably, changes in brain oscillations following pregabalin treatment have been associated with its analgesic efficacy (Graversen et al. 2012). Thus, in addition to a spinal effect on central sensitization, the analgesic effect of pregabalin may also be mediated by supraspinal mechanisms.

Structural Cortical Alterations

With advanced imaging technology, the correlation of structural cortical alterations and hyperexcitability was found. In one study, diffusion weighted MRI demonstrate the link between microstructural changes in the insular and frontal brain areas and clinical pain intensity and functional scores (Frøkjær et al. 2011). Pain intensity was proportional to the severity of microstructural abnormalities (Mullady et al. 2011). In another MRI based cortical volumetry study, a reduced brain areas involved in visceral pain processing suggested a central neurodegenerative response to severe and chronic pain (Frøkjær et al. 2012). Whether such structural changes represent specific signatures of pancreatic pain has yet to be determined, but evidence from other chronic pain diseases suggest that morphological changes of brain structure may be unique for different pain conditions and, as such, it suggests the possibility of unique therapies by targeting the underlying specific pathways for each type of chronic pain (Apkarian et al. 2011).

Changes in Spinal Interneurons and Pain Modulation

The pain system has several inherent mechanisms whereby inflowing pain signals are modulated. Among many mechanisms, inhibitory spinal interneurons and descending modulatory pathways from the brain stem and higher cortical structures plays a key role. Such endogenous pain modulation control the afferent input of nociceptive signals at the spinal level and the process can lead to either facilitate or inhibit the spinal transmission of pain to brain (Heinricher et al. 2009). Facilitation have been implicated in the form of chronic pain and several studies have documented the involvement of brainstem structures in the generation and maintenance of central sensitization and hyperalgesia (Zambreanu et al. 2005; Gebhart 2004). Impaired inhibitory modulation was reported in painful CP patients base on human model (Olesen et al. 2010a; Bouwense et al. 2013). In addition, brainstem facilitation was reported to maintain pancreatic pain in an animal model of CP (Vera-Portocarrero et al. 2006). Until today, no studies have attempted to modulate pain modulation in patients with CP, but emerging evidence from other chronic pain conditions suggest that selective serotonin–noradrenaline reuptake inhibitors (SNRIs) may be useful to augment descending inhibitory modulation and thereby to relieve pain (Yarnitsky et al. 2012). In Fig. 5.1 a schematic illustration of the different mechanisms is shown.

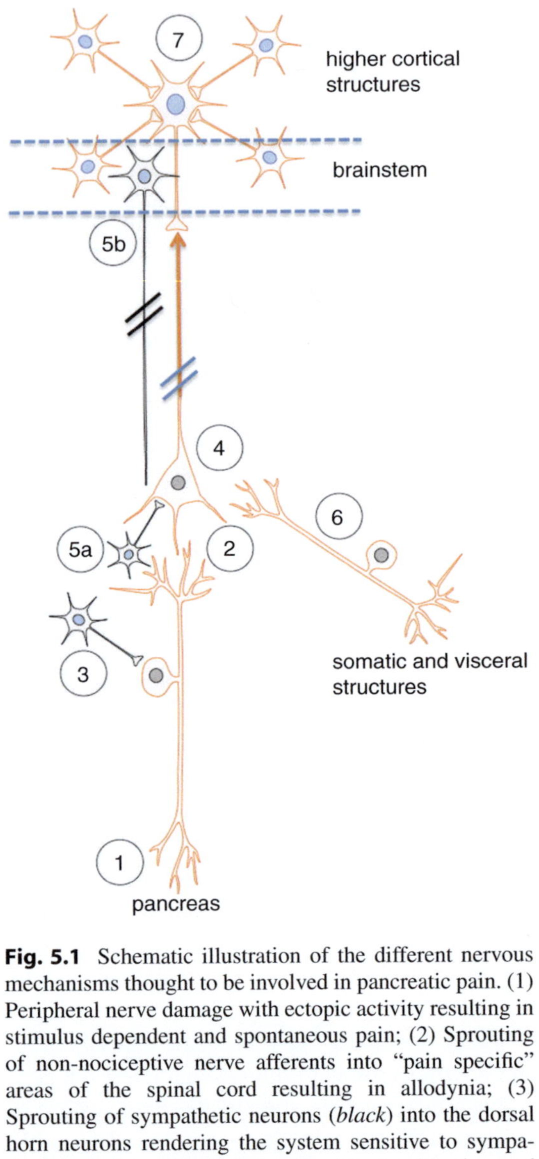

Fig. 5.1 Schematic illustration of the different nervous mechanisms thought to be involved in pancreatic pain. (1) Peripheral nerve damage with ectopic activity resulting in stimulus dependent and spontaneous pain; (2) Sprouting of non-nociceptive nerve afferents into "pain specific" areas of the spinal cord resulting in allodynia; (3) Sprouting of sympathetic neurons (*black*) into the dorsal horn neurons rendering the system sensitive to sympathetic activity and catecholamine; (4) Sensitization and phenotypic changes of spinal neurons due to the increased afferent barrage; (5) Defects in the normal inhibition from (a) interneurons and (b) descending tracts arising in the brainstem (*black*); (6) Abnormal coding of the afferent input from somatic areas and other viscera resulting in increased referred pain and viscero-visceral hyperalgesia; (7) Reorganisation and structural changes in the brain that encodes complex sensations such as affective, evaluative and cognitive responses to pain

Are Changes in Central Pain Processing Depending on a Nociceptive Input from the Pancreatic Nerves?

As can be seen from the above sections, several lines of evidence indicate that central pain processing is abnormal in CP. However, from the current evidence it is difficult to determine whether these central abnormalities depend on a nociceptive input from the pancreatic nerves (Gebhart 2007). There is support from other diseases such as in peripheral nerve injury and painful polyneuropathy that regardless of signs of central sensitization, primary afferent input is critical for maintaining on going and evoked neuropathic pain (Haroutounian et al. 2014; Vaso et al. 2014). The efficacy of topically applied drugs in these conditions also supports peripheral pain-generating mechanisms (Backonja et al. 2008; Meier et al. 2003). A small cross-sectional study in CP patients found that in hyperalgesic patients the generation of pain was independent of the pancreatic nociceptive drive and consequently denervation of pancreatic nerves was ineffective (Bouwense et al. 2011b). However, larger and longer-term studies that include systematic evaluation of the pain system prior and after intervention are still needed for confirmation (Table 5.2).

Table 5.2 Central pain mechanisms in chronic pancreatitis and associated experimental and clinical manifestations

Mechanism	Experimental evidence and clinical manifestations
Central sensitization	Hyperalgesia
	Allodynia
	Expansion of referred pain area (pancreatic viscerotome—Th10)
Abnormal patterns of brain activity	Functional reorganization of the visceral pain matrix
	Increased cortical excitability
	Abnormal brain rhythmicity (increased theta activity)
Structural alterations of brain morphology	Changes in microstructure of the brain
	Cortical thinning
Impaired descending pain modulation	Blunted CPM response

1.3 Pancreatic and Extra-Pancreatic Complications

In addition to the "plumbing" and "wiring" problems discussed above, many patients with CP experience pain due to intra- and extra-pancreatic complications of the disease. These are often easy to diagnose and treat and should always be considered when the patient is experiencing an exacerbation in pain symptoms. Among many, the most common are listed below.

1.3.1 Pseudocysts

As a relatively common complication, the estimated incidence of pancreatic pseudocysts is 20–40% (Boerma et al. 2000; Andrén-Sandberg and Dervenis 2004). Although lacking of long term follow-up studies, due to the chronic nature course of the disease, CP patients are at high risk of developing pseudocyst (Ammann et al. 1984). However, it is important to identify whether pseudocysts are asymptomatic or not according to the etiology, localization and size, the most influential factor of pain (Aghdassi et al. 2008; Gouyon et al. 1997).

1.3.2 Duodenal and Bile Duct Obstruction

The clinical presentation of duodenal and bile duct obstruction secondary to CP can be from asymptomatic to variable as postprandial/upper abdominal pain, early satiety, nausea and potential vomiting, fever, jaundice (Vijungco and Prinz 2003; Kalvaria et al. 1989; Prinz et al. 1985). It is reported that without cholangitis bile duct obstruction does not cause pain and the relationship between "obstructive pain" and pain in patients with CP is still unclear (Kahl et al. 2004).

1.3.3 Peptic Ulcer

Previous studies have demonstrated that the prevalence of duodenal ulcer is high in patients with CP (ranges from 3.6 to 37.5%) and upper abdominal pain due to peptic ulcer can be mistaken as pancreatic pain (Lankisch et al. 1993; Chebli et al. 2002; Schulze et al. 1983). It is suggested that the high prevalence of peptic ulcer can be attributed to higher infection rate of *Helicobacter pylori* (Kalvaria et al. 1989), increased gastric acid secretion (Saunders et al. 1978; Piubello et al. 1982), and decreased bicarbonate secretion and duodenal pH due to pancreatic exocrine insufficiency (Brock et al. 2012). Moreover, recurrent acute pancreatic attack may redistribute gastric and intestinal blood flow.

As peptic ulcer can also be asymptomatic and patients with CP are more likely to undergo an diagnostic or therapeutic upper gastrointestinal endoscopy, the high prevalence may also can be a result of a "detection bias" (Schulze et al. 1983).

1.4 Side Effects to Treatment

While strong opioids are effective to relieve pain in CP patients, opioids frequently result in gastrointestinal side effects, including constipation, reflux, nausea and abdominal pain (Brock et al. 2012). Chronic abdominal pain was reported to be 58% in patients treated with opioids for non-cancerous diseases (Tuteja et al. 2010). Other medications that affect bowel motility and disturbed GI motor function due to exocrine pancreatic insufficiency may also indirectly contribute to the bacterial overgrowth that is reported in up to 40% of the patients and may result in abdominal distension and pain (Layer 1995; Casellas et al. 1998).

Complications to surgical and endoscopic therapy can also result in abdominal pain. However, no studies have examined the relative contribution to abdominal pain due to surgical complications in CP.

1.5 Conclusion

The pain mechanisms in chronic pancreatitis are heterogeneous and multifaceted, and likely often overlap and co-exist in the individual patient. Whereas the focus of pain treatment previously targeted abnormal anatomical findings such as strictures and stones in the main pancreatic duct there is little evidence to support that this is the reason for pain. Rather, neuronal changes in the peripheral and central nervous system are the main reasons for pain in most patients and often complicated further by cognitive and emotional distress. Therefore, the treatment should be multidisciplinary and based on a thorough workup of the pain system and in some cases combined with a psychological evaluation. It is mandatory to exclude secondary causes of pain, including side effects to treatment, as they are often reversible and easy to treat. As the combination of pain mechanisms in each patient is unique with distinct causes of pain and response to treatment, personalised treatment based on biomarkers that reflects the pain processing is an unmet need that invariably will be the focus for future studies.

2 The Mechanism of Pancreatic Stone Formation

Bo Ye and Wei-Qin Li

2.1 Introduction

Pancreatic stone is one of the features of chronic pancreatitis (CP) (Figs. 5.2 and 5.3), and almost 90% patients had pancreatic stones in the course

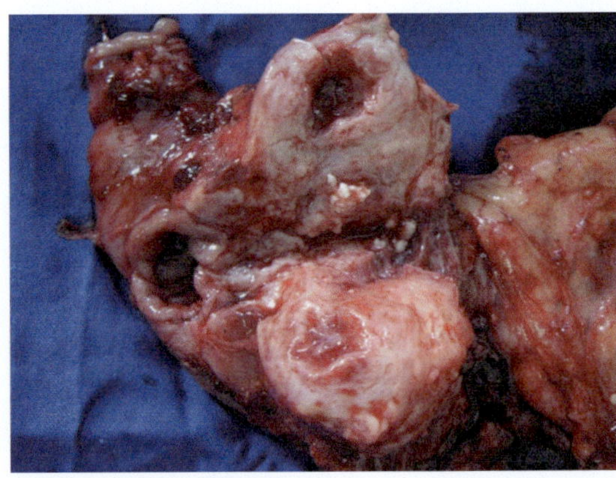

Fig. 5.2 Pancreatic stones in human surgical specimens. Reprint with permission from shanghai science & technology press

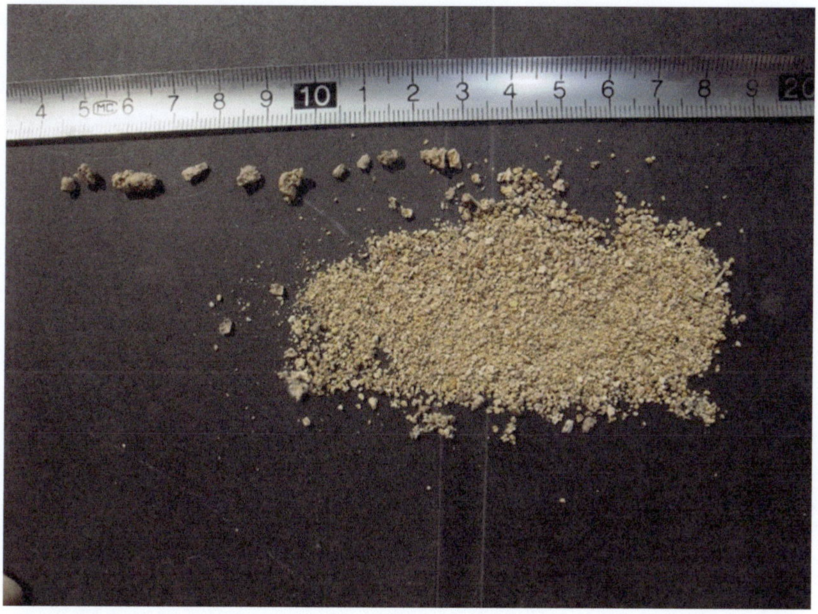

Fig. 5.3 Pancreatic stones in human fecal. Reprint with permission from shanghai science & technology press

of CP (Mariani et al. 1991). Researches on the composition and formation of pancreatic stones will help to understand the pathophysiological process of CP.

The composition of pancreatic stone is almost clear. Outer region of pancreatic stones consists of calcium carbonate as a major component, while the inner part (nidus) is comprised of a very fine network of fibers which are composed of proteins and glycosaminoglycans. The possible related mechanisms included the decreasing secretion of pancreatic stone protein, much greater concentration of lactoferrin in pancreatic juice, precipitating of trypsin in early stage, overexpressing of osteopontin and GP-2 in human pancreatic juice.

2.2 Analysis of Chemical Composition in Pancreatic Stones

2.2.1 Chemical Elements in Pancreatic Stones

Calcium is the most abundant chemical element in pancreatic stones (almost 90%). Other elements such as P, S, K, Fe, Cr, Ni were also found. Pitchumoni et al. (1987) studied the major, minor, and trace elements present in pancreatic stones by DC-plasma emission (DCP) spectroscopy and found that pancreatic stones were made up of calcite and contained, in addition to calcium, 17 other elements. They also studied the morphology, nature, and elements in human pancreatic stones by scanning electron microscopy (SEM) and energy dispersive X-ray fluorescence (EDXRF) and found that the amorphous nidus only contained iron, chromium, and nickel, whereas the outer shell was made up of calcium and 17 other elements.

2.2.2 Composition of Human Pancreatic Stones

It is important to know how the organic and inorganic components interact with each other during pancreatic stone formation. Calcium carbonate was the major inorganic component in pancreatic stones. The organic matrix of pancreatic stones includes proteins and glycosaminoglycans (mucopolysaccharides and mucosubstances). Comparing pancreatic stones before and after decalcification, Bockman et al. (1986) found carbonate more common on rounded, lamellar, or otherwise modified surfaces by scanning electron microscopy. They were embedded in a gel-like matrix. Histochemical studies found that the gel-like matrix was made up of acid glycosaminoglycans, acid glycoprotein, and neutral glycoprotein. Farnbacher et al. (2005) found that clogging material in pancreatic stents contained mucopolysaccharides, crystals, and plant material, as well as visible calcium carbonate calculi.

2.3 Mechanisms of Pancreatic Stones Formation

Pancreatic stones are, in fact, intraductal calculi. According to the locations of stones, pancreatic stones mainly divided into main pancreatic duct and branch duct stones. Calculi in main pancreatic ducts is more common in the tropical chronic pancreatitis (TCP), while alcoholic chronic pancreatitis (ACP) is mostly characterized by the formation in pancreatic branch ducts of calculi (Pitchumoni 1984). Pancreatic stone also includes the precalcified forms and the calcified forms. However, the mechanisms of different forms of pancreatic stone formation are almost the same, including protein precipitation and increased $CaCO_3$ crystal growth in pancreatic juice. Nevertheless, it is still not clear that which protein is secreted abnormally causing protein precipitation. Current theories or hypothesis involved mainly were as follows.

2.3.1 Pancreatic Stone Protein

Human pancreatic stone protein (PSP) is one of the regeneration (reg) gene proteins, which is located on the short arm of chromosome 2 in 2p12 spans. There are five immunoreactive forms PSP S1-5 detected in pancreatic juice. PSP S2-5 corresponds to the four isoforms distinguishable by SDS-PAGE (Stewart 1989). It was believed to inhibit spontaneous calcium carbonate precipitation from highly supersaturated solutions and was called "lithostathine" by some. PSP was detectable in almost all pancreatic stones, ranging widely from only a trace amount to 1.21% as a percentage of the stone weight. A wide range of percentages (ranging from 0.01 to 41.9%) of pancreatic stone protein in the total protein suggests that the mechanisms and protein components involved in the stone formation are multifactorial (Jin et al. 2002). Current hypothesis about PSP included stabilizing pancreatic juice hypothesis, calcium binding hypothesis and adsorption hypothesis.

Stabilizing Pancreatic Juice Hypothesis

Sarles and Bernard (1991) suggested that PSP would inhibit calcite crystal nucleation and growth in the pancreatic juice to prevent pancreatic stone formation. Bimmler et al. (1997) produced rat PSP in a baculovirus expression system and confirmed its calcite crystal inhibitor activity. They also found several organic and inorganic components of pancreatic juice (trypsinogen, phosphate) which had inhibitory activity on calcium carbonate crystal formation. Addadi and Weiner (1985) also reported PSP had an unspecific inhibition of calcite crystal growth. However, De Reggi et al. (1998) proposed that the inhibitory property was dut to a high concentration of Tris buffer. Therefore, PSP might affect stone formation, but the debate on lithostathine function remains.

Calcium Binding Hypothesis

Lohse and Kraemer (1984) found PSP had four equivalent and independent calcium binding sites by using radioactive ^{45}Ca in equilibrium dialysis experiments. They thought that calcium binding can modify the physico-chemical characteristics of PSP, result in the formation of protein plugs, which could illustrate the presence of the protein in pancreatic stones. However, Multigner et al. (1986) observed the absence of calcium in the proteic core of some stones. Therefore, calcium binding sites on PSP may explain its inhibition of calcite nucleation, precipitation and crystal growth.

Adsorption Hypothesis

Gross and Caro (Gross et al. 1985; De Caro et al. 1979) found that PSP had a greater affinity for the crystal. Sarles and Bernard (1991) thought that PSP can adsorb on crystal surface. Geider et al. (1996) proposed that the adsorption of PSP to the crystal resulted in the modification of the crystal shape. De Reggi et al. (1998) observed that the quantities of adsorbed PSP and albumin per unit of surface were in the same range and the adsorption of PSP on calcite was not much higher than for an amorphous phase (glass). Therefore, the adsorption of PSP on calcite does not interact specifically.

2.3.2 Lactoferrin

Lactoferrin (LF) is a globular glycoprotein 80 kDa, which is widely represented in tears, saliva, nasal secretions and other secretory fluids. Which is also present in PMN. And some acinar cells also secret it. It also has many immunoregulatory effects including antimicrobial activity (bacteriocide, fungicide) and innate defense.

The concentration of Lactoferrin tends to increase in CP. Hayakawa et al. (1983) found the concentration of LF was much higher the protein plugs by analyzing the pancreatic stones obtained from the 13 patients with chronic calcified pancreatitis (Nagai and Ohtsubo 1984). This suggested that lactoferrin may play an important role in early stage of protein plug formation in the pancreatic duct.

2.3.3 Trypsinogen

Trypsinogen is found in pancreatic juice, which is the precursor form or zymogen of trypsin. Once it is activated by enteropeptidase, the trypsin can activate more trypsinogen into trypsin. Allan and White (1974) found intraductal pancreatic zymogens were activated in some patients with CP. Hayakawa et al. (1994) observed the immunoreactivity of human cationic trypsin in protein extracts from pancreatic stones in CP patients ranged from 0 to 42.3 ng/μg protein. They also observed that more densely immunoreactivity was presented in the center of the stones than in the concentric laminar layer of the periphery by using an immunogold technic SEM. Tympner (1981) found trypsin activity increased in pure pancreatic juice aspirated from CP patients. Renner et al. (1980) also found trypsinogen increased highly in in the pure pancreatic secretions in ACP patients. Therefore, we can concluded that hyperconcentration of pancreatic zymogens and proteins and activation of the trypsinogen were associated with pancreatic stone formation in early stage.

2.3.4 Osteopontin

Osteopontin is a 44-kDa glycosylated phosphoprotein, which is one of a group of noncollagenous bone matrix components. Recently, it has been reported that there is a relation between osteopontin expression and several diseases associated with calcification, such as atherosclerosis, breast cancer, meningioma and urinary stone formation.

Nakamura et al. (2002) found that osteopontin mRNA was detected in CP but not in normal pancreas specimens. In situ RT-PCR, they revealed that osteopontin was expressed in acinar or ductal cells in all 11 CCP patients, whereas in 5 of 9 CP cases without pancreatic stones osteopontin was not expressed in acinar or ductal cells. Therefore, acinar cells and ductal cells may secrete osteopontin, which can bind to protein plague and may play a crucial role in in pancreatic stone formation.

2.3.5 GP-2

GP-2 (glycoprotein-2) is the most abundant protein of the zymogen granule membrane of the exocrine pancreas, which is linked to the membrane through a glycophophatidyl inositol (GPI) bond (Colomer et al. 1994). GP-2 was also shown to be homologous to Tamm-Horsfall protein, a GPI linked protein produced in kidney and excreted in urine, which is the major component of hyaline casts found in urine.

GP-2 is present in pancreatic juice and makes up 5–8% of unstimulated juice protein in the rat and pig. Stimulation with secretin has no effect on GP-2 output in pancreatic juice while stimulation with caerulein or carbachol increases secretion, but with a slower time course than the secretion of digestive enzymes. GP-2 is also present in ductal proteinaceous plugs found in chronic pancreatitis Freedman et al. (1994) examined the protein composition of intraductal plugs from patients with noncalcific chronic pancreatitis by SDS-PAGE and found GP-2 were both a reproducible constituent and enriched within intraductal plugs. Therefore, GP2 may play a role in pancreatic plug formation, which is an important step in pancreatic stone formation.

2.4 Conclusion

Study on pancreatic stone composition and its formation mechanism is ultimately able to give more intervention and treatment in early stage of CP. Noda and Tsujimoto et al. (Noda et al. 1997; Tsujimoto et al. 2005) found that bromhexine hydrochloride had a high affinity for the pancreas, acting directly on the mucus-producing cells and causing them to produce low-viscosity mucus. Lohse et al. (Lohse et al. 1981; Noda et al. 1984) observed that organic acids dissolved pancreatic stones by chelating with calcium ions. Therefore, further work is needed to identify agents that dissolve protein plugs and pancreatic stones, which may have potential to eliminate pancreatic duct obstruction to relieve pancreatitis attacks and pancreatic pain.

In conclusion, the mechanisms of pancreatic stone formation are complicated, and many proteins may play a role in the protein precipitation. So far, protein plugs formation and precipitation of $CaCO_3$ crystal are the most important two factors in pancreatic stone formation.

3 Experimental Models of Chronic Pancreatitis

Ali A. Aghdassi, Matthias Sendler, Julia Mayerle, and Markus M. Lerch

Chronic pancreatitis is an inflammatory disorder of the pancreatic gland. In western countries its incidence is reported to be between 4 and 13/100,000, which is somewhat lower compared to acute pancreatitis with an estimated incidence of 13–45/100,000 persons (Levy et al. 2014; Yadav and Lowenfels 2013). However, according to recent population based studies incidence rates of chronic pancreatitis have steadily increased during the last decades and showed regional differences (Yadav and Lowenfels 2013; Yadav et al. 2011).

From epidemiological data and clinical experience we know that chronic pancreatitis can develop from either recurrent bouts of acute pancreatitis in which the pancreas does not recover completely from the injury to the organ. About 20–30% of patients with acute pancreatitis suffer from recurrences and about 10% develop chronic pancreatitis. The presence of continuous environmental exposure (alcohol, tobacco) or genetic risk factors favor progression to chronic pancreatitis (Yadav and Lowenfels 2013; Yadav et al. 2012). To a much lesser extent chronic pancreatitis can develop as a result of one severe attack of acute pancreatitis that leads to necrosis and fibrosis directly (Lankisch et al. 2009).

3.1 Features of Chronic Pancreatitis

Both morphological changes and clinical symptoms characterize chronic pancreatitis and their knowledge is of importance for a comprehensive understanding of the available experimental models with their strengths and limitations. So far there is no animal model that incorporates *all* features of chronic pancreatitis that are seen in humans. Secondly, a variety of animal models exist that, although mimicking chronic pancreatitis, differ among each other regarding their morphologic and clinical characteristics. Choosing the right models is of importance and depends on the scientific question that is addressed by the investigator.

From a histopathologic point of view chronic pancreatitis is a progressive and destructive inflammatory process of the pancreatic parenchyma that finally involves ductal changes as well. In some cases the kind of histologic damage allows a deduction of the etiology of chronic pancreatitis, as some causative factors show typical histologic features (Klöppel 2013; Kloppel et al. 2004). Generally chronic pancreatitis starts with focal necrosis and inflammatory cell invasion. When pancreatic stellate cells are activated collagen deposition occurs leading to fibrosis of the organ. In early stages and particularly in alcoholic chronic pancreatitis fibrosis is mainly localized in a perilobular pattern that later affects the parenchyma (intralobular fibrosis) (Klöppel 2013). In late stages ductal changes with irregularities of the lumen width and strictures are seen that are the result of tissue traction due to fibrosis and scarring. Ductal changes ultimately predispose to precipitation of calculi and protein plugs (Ammann et al. 1996; Detlefsen et al. 2006; Klöppel 2007).

Typical clinical manifestations are pancreatic pain, steatorrhoea with weight loss and maldigestion due to exocrine insufficiency and impaired glucose tolerance up to manifest diabetes mellitus (Muniraj et al. 2014; Schütte et al. 2013). Continuous maldigestion without medical intervention leads to malnutrition with additional complications such as osteoporosis and vitamin deficiency (Gupte and Forsmark 2014). Signs of exocrine insufficiency occur late when secretory function is reduced to less than 10% of normal (Keller et al. 2009).

3.2 Animal Models for Chronic Pancreatitis

Experimental models for chronic pancreatitis have been established in many animal species using various techniques (Fig. 5.4). Most of them were adapted to rodents. Chronic pancreatitis models can be classified either according to their mechanism of induction, that are meant to resemble the pathophysiology in humans or based on a completely different mechanism (Aghdassi et al. 2011; Lerch and Gorelick 2013), or, alternatively, according to their morphological and clinico-biochemical characteristics. The aim of this section is to introduce frequently used animal models for experimental chronic pancreatitis including their strengths and shortcomings. We also want to point out recent developments in genetic models of chronic pancreatitis that attracted increasing attention. Furthermore, we specify what kind of pathology is seen in each model and whether it can be used for assessment of either morphological or clinical characteristics of chronic pancreatitis or both.

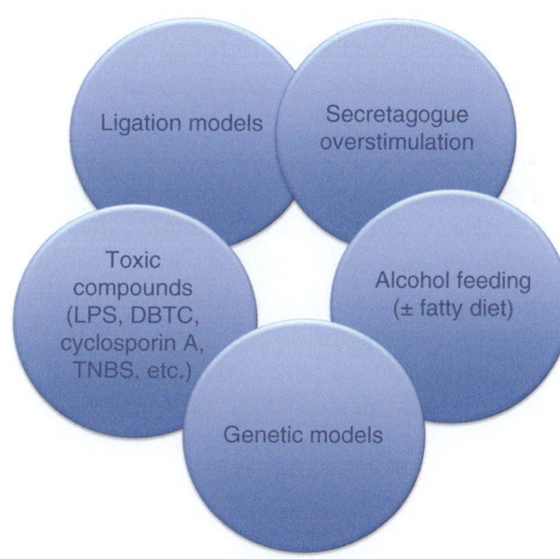

Fig. 5.4 In-vivo experimental models for chronic pancreatitis. Techniques have been applied alone or in combination

3.3 Duct Obstruction Models

Many studies have demonstrated that obstruction of the pancreatic duct, either partial or complete, leads to morphological changes compatible with chronic pancreatitis. Proximal to the stenosis intraductal pressure increases and favors duct dilation with atrophy of acinar cells and replacement by fibrous tissue. In humans possible causes for a blockage of the duct are tumors (either adenocarcinoma or cystic or endocrine neoplasms) or more rarely cystic fibrosis that plugs the ductal lumen by its viscous mucin (Kloppel et al. 2004). Humans have one main pancreatic duct that enters the duodenum at the major duodenal papilla after joining the bile duct. Early in embryonic development two efferent pancreatic ducts, which origin form the ventral and dorsal part of the organ, fuse together to form one main duct. If this fusion fails to occur (in up to 9% of autopsy studies) two separate pancreatic ducts are preserved, a condition known as pancreas divisum (Brock et al. 2013).

3.3.1 Pancreatic Anatomy in Rodents

Currently the majority of pancreatic duct obstruction models are performed in rodents. However, the anatomy of the pancreas differs among species. Since most studies are carried out in mice or rats we want to give more detailed information regarding anatomy of the pancreas in these two species. Compared to the human pancreas in which gross anatomy shows a more compact or cohesive pattern the mouse pancreas is more loose as it consists of three separate lobes, the gastric, duodenal and the splenic lobe and is frequently interspersed with fatty, connective or lymphoid tissue (Treuting et al. 2012). Each lobe is drained by a separate pancreatic duct. Duct anatomy of the mouse pancreas shows variations that make ligation procedures more complex. Usually the ducts from the splenic and gastric lobe converge and will be completed by the duct from the duodenal lobe to form one common channel before opening into the common bile duct. In about 10% the splenic and the gastric duct join the duodenum separately with an accessory papilla (Watanabe et al. 1995). Like in mice the rat pancreas also consists of three lobes, two smaller ones (the biliary and the duodenal lobe) and a larger gastrosplenic lobe (Kara 2005). The pancreatic duct system consists of two main ducts, the anterior and the posterior pancreatic duct. Both finally open into the biliopancreatic duct. In addition minor ducts of all three lobes are petering out separately to the biliopancreatic duct (Kara 2005).

The size of pancreatic duct varies naturally between species. Magnetic resonance imaging (MRI) and autopsy studies revealed that the mouse pancreatic duct has an approximate diameter of 88 μm and a total tractable length of 5850 μm (Grippo et al. 2011). Caliber of the rat biliopancreatic duct is larger with around 1 mm and a length of ca. 29 mm (Kara 2005) so that ligation procedures are technically easier.

Selective obstruction of one branch of the pancreatic duct and not of the whole biliopancreatic duct uncouples only one part of the pancreas that will be injured. For this reason induction of chronic pancreatitis can be locally controlled within the pancreas. Since the unobstructed part remains unaffected it can serve as an internal control (Kishi et al. 2003; Sendler et al. 2015). Technique of (selective) ductal ligation forms a big advantage over other models of chronic pancreatitis as a "negative" control is created within the same animal ruling out confounding variables.

3.3.2 Ligation Models in Rodents

Ligation models belong to the best experimental models for mimicking chronic pancreatitis and are well established for mice and rats. In general first changes start within the first 7–10 days after the intervention with necrosis, an inflammatory cell infiltrate and first signs of acinar cell atrophy, ductal cell proliferation and initiation of fibrosis that is often visible with periductal and intralobular arrangement (Watanabe et al. 1995; Sendler et al. 2015; Churg and Richter 1971; Miyauchi et al. 2007; Scoggins et al. 2000; Yamamoto et al.

2006). Emergence of fibrosis is associated with activation of pancreatic stellate cells (PSCs) that transform from a quiescent to an active state by increased expression of alpha smooth muscle actin (αSMA) and deposition of extracellular matrix components (Apte et al. 1999). Later (≥14 days) changes include more extensive fibrosis with upregulation of collagen I and III production and a more perilobular distribution. In addition a fatty tissue replacement occurs (Watanabe et al. 1995; Sendler et al. 2015; Yamamoto et al. 2006).

Notably, exocrine insufficiency is hardly seen in the ligation models unless a high fat diet is fed. On the one hand this is caused by the incomplete obstruction of the pancreatic ductal system so that one part of the pancreas remains unaffected and keeps up secretory enzyme production. Secondly very early after ligation a subgroup of pancreatic cells, intermediate cells, start a transdifferentiation and display both exocrine and endocrine phenotypes as indicated by co-expression of insulin and amylase (Bertelli and Bendayan 1997). These cells are detectable within the islets of Langerhans and within exocrine tissue and indicate a high degree of plasticity of the organ within the first days after the insult to maintain exocrine and endocrine function.

The lack of endocrine insufficiency might be also explained by an increased islet beta-cell proliferation in duct-ligated rats. The Beta cell population nearly doubled within the first week after the ligation and small islets and islet-cell clusters developed (Wang et al. 1995). Interestingly, glucose transporter type 2 (GLUT-2), the major glucose transporter isoform, was expressed in ductal cells, besides its primary location on insulin secreting beta cells. Obviously ligation-stimulated ductal cells reach a metaplastic state and acquire properties of endocrine cells with higher glucose sensitivity (Wang et al. 1995).

3.3.3 Variations of Classical Ligation Procedures

A continuous pancreatic duct hypertension was induced by double-ligation of the bilio-pancreatic duct at its proximal and distal end in rats. Both pancreatic juice and bile were selective collected and diverted into the duodenum. Two weeks after the procedure mucoprotein concentration of the pancreatic juice was increased despite a decrease of digestive enzyme contents indicating that non-enzymatic protein secretion starts on sustained pancreatic duct hypertension (Yamamoto et al. 2006). Previous studies in humans already showed that non-enzymatic protein secretion leads to enhanced viscosity of the pancreatic juice and formation of intraluminal protein plugs (Harada et al. 1981). First histomorphologic changes were observed earlier, i.e. at already 7 days, with intralobular and perilobular fibrosis and a peak of acinar cell apoptosis.

Possibly the observation time needs to be much longer for studying effects on exocrine function. In a model established by Isaksson and collaborators the rat pancreatic duct was obstructed with a glue-like substance consisting of either acrylate or prolamine and animals were monitored for 5 months in total. Exocrine insufficiency was present as evidenced by reduced secretory enzyme levels whereas endocrine function was not impaired (Isaksson et al. 1983). These results also tell us that the investigation of long-term effects on the pancreas is technically possible when using duct occlusion models but an observation time of months will be required.

3.3.4 Ligation Models in Non-rodents

There are fewer studies dealing with mammals whose pancreatic anatomy looks more similar to the human one. In dogs ligation procedures were studied that led to typical morphological characteristics of chronic pancreatitis. These changes developed within 3–6 months. Pancreatic excretory capacity was diminished, too (Tanaka et al. 1988, 1998). Compared to rats connective tissue replacement was stronger, however acinar atrophy was less marked (Churg and Richter 1971). The degree of pancreatic damage was much more distinct, when ligation was performed in conjunction with chronic ischemia or ethanol administration to these dogs (Tanaka et al. 1988).

3.3.5 Limiting Factors of Ligation Models

Comparison of ligation models is limited as the location of ligation differs among studies. In addition other stimuli were applied to animals such as caerulein (Sendler et al. 2015), ischemia (Tanaka et al. 1988) or ethanol feeding (Tanaka et al. 1988) that affect severity of the disease. Knowledge of the exact location of pancreatic duct ligation is of high importance when comparing the extent of changes of chronic pancreatitis.

Ligation procedures are rather invasive procedure and demand surgical skills and exact knowledge on the anatomy of abdominal organs. Moreover technical equipment has to be available for doing the operation. These factors set limitations on general application of duct-ligations models. A learning curve when doing the procedure is inevitable and has to be taken into account when analyzing the results.

3.4 Repeated Caerulein Models

The secretagogue hyperstimulation model is by far the most frequently used technique for induction of acute pancreatitis. This method was first used by Lampel and Kern who intravenously applied caerulein, an ortholog of the intestinal hormone cholecystokinin, to rats and observed signs of acute interstitial pancreatitis (Lampel and Kern 1977). Pancreatitis usually resolves spontaneously. This model was broadly adopted and modified to secretagogue application given intraperitoneally which is as effective but less technically challenging. Usually the required dose exceeds tenfold the concentration needed for maximal physiological secretion from the exocrine pancreas. Later caerulein-injection models were modified again to establish experimental chronic pancreatitis following the idea that multiple bouts of acute pancreatitis finally lead to chronic disease (Lerch and Gorelick 2013). Normally pro-fibrogenic cytokines peak within 3 or 4 days after acute pancreatitis and normalize within 1 week but reinjury before normalization of the profibrogenic milieu favors chronic pancreatic injury. TGF-beta is believed to regulate extracellular matrix deposition as it is elevated during the vulnerable phase of acute pancreatitis and, when inhibited, collagen and fibronectin production are reduced (Gress et al. 1994; Menke et al. 1997). Increase of TGF-beta was not only observed in caerulein-induced acute pancreatitis but also in an obstruction model (duodenal loop closure) underlining its general importance during acute pancreatitis (Kimura et al. 1995).

Supraphysiologic concentrations of caerulein given two or three times a week for up to 6–10 weeks showed substantial pancreatic fibrosis in line with a strong increase of procollagen I expression (Neuschwander-Tetri et al. 2000a, b). Longer intervals of caerulein applications seemed to be no more effective. No or hardly any fibrosis was observed during weekly applications unless recombinant TGF-beta was given additionally (Van Laethem et al. 1996). When intervals were extended up to 20 days no sustainable signs of fibrosis were seen (Elsasser et al. 1992).

Although chronic fibrotic changes can be generated successfully by repeated caerulein applications it remains unclear whether exocrine or endocrine insufficiency can be achieved. Diabetes was observed in an experimental model in rats using caerulein injections plus water-immersion stress (Goto et al. 1995; Miyahara et al. 1999). Stress or caerulein alone did not cause endocrine insufficiency. The intrapancreatic protein content, reflecting exocrine function, was nearly halved when mice were treated with caerulein (three times a week) and lipolysaccharide for 6 weeks (Ohashi et al. 2006).

There are several other noxious agents that have been combined with caerulein hyperstimulation to induce experimental chronic pancreatitis. Some of them will be introduced in the following sections.

3.5 Alcohol Feeding Models

Undoubtedly alcohol consumption increases the risk of acute and recurrent acute pancreatitis and it is the single most frequent cause for chronic pancreatitis in humans (Yadav and Lowenfels 2013; Aghdassi et al. 2015). Although there is no clear threshold of an alcohol amount that inevitably leads to pancreatic fibrosis heavy alcohol consumption is associated with a higher risk of developing chronic pancreatitis (Frulloni et al. 2009; Irving et al. 2009). The harmful effects of alcohol have been explored in several studies using whole animal or ex-vivo models and there are plausible data on the pathophysiologic way in which ethanol injures the pancreas (Gukovskaya et al. 2006; Pfutzer et al. 2002). Alcohol is metabolized either in an oxidative pathway by the successive action of alcohol-dehydrogenases (ADHs) and aldehyde-dehydrogenases (ALDHs) into its metabolites acetaldehyde and acetate. In the non-oxidative pathway ethanol is combined with fatty acids to fatty ethyl esters (FAEEs) (Criddle 2015). Both pathways occur in the pancreas and both ethanol and its catabolic end-products are toxic to pancreatic cells. On acinar cells they directly induce cellular and organellar (zymogen granules, mitochondria) injury that leads to intracellular protease activation and cell death. As a consequence cytokines are released and inflammatory cells are attracted aggravating the damage. Besides the effect on acinar cells ethanol and metabolites effect on pancreatic stellate cells (PSCs) causing synthesis of extracellular matrix components (Apte et al. 2000; Lugea et al. 2003).

It has attempted to translate the clinical features associated with alcohol consumption into experimental animal models for chronic pancreatitis. Unfortunately the results are very disappointing and so far there is no satisfactory model for chronic pancreatitis using ethanol application alone. Besides the pancreas other organs such as lung and liver are injured by alcohol exposure and animals don't develop proper chronic pancreatitis (Li et al. 2008; McIlwrath and Westlund 2015; Schneider et al. 2009).

3.5.1 Duration of Alcohol Application

Technically it is possible to induce chronic pancreatitis in animals with alcohol. Usually alcohol is given together with their daily diet via an oral route often as a Lieber-DeCarli liquid diet. The concentration of ingested ethanol can vary (see below). In more uncommon experimental setups alcohol is applied by other ways, i.e. via a gastrostomy or directly into the pancreatic duct.

Features of chronic pancreatitis such as acinar cell atrophy and fibrous tissue replacement were achieved by long-term ethanol feeding (up to 30 months) in rats. Pattern of fibrosis resembled those of human chronic pancreatitis (segmental or perilobular distribution) and intraductal protein plugs with partial calcifications were seen as known from humans. Signs of chronic pancreatitis appeared very late when only alcohol is applied and were noticed between the 20th and 30th month of alcohol exposure. By that time already half of the animals died of old age (Sarles et al. 1971). It is quite clear that application of alcohol alone imposes limitations, as long-term treatment and a high death rate are not only time consuming but also questionable from an ethical pathophysiology point of view.

In more recently developed experimental models shorter treatment periods (up to 6 months) were used. However, morphologic changes were less distinct. Secretory enzyme levels behaved differently under chronic ethanol exposure: Amylase secretion was impaired but levels of zymogens such as pro-elastase and (chymo-)trypsinogen were enhanced something normally observed during acute pancreatitis (Li et al. 2008; Perkins et al. 1995). When ethanol was injected directly into the pancreatic duct of rats histologic features of chronic disease like interstitial fibrosis, loss of exocrine acinar cells and ductal dilation were observed at quite early time points (7 days). Limiting factors are the invasive technique and the unphysiologic route of alcohol administration to the animals (Unal et al. 2015).

3.5.2 Techniques of Alcohol Application to Animals

Alcohol supplementation in nutrition needs to exceed a minimum amount so that blood alcohol reaches toxic concentrations in the pancreas. Charles Lieber and Elonore DeCarli contributed much to the development of optimal nutrition formulas for scientific use when they investigated different liquid diets containing ethanol and their effects on organs. The natural aversion of rats against alcohol has been overcome by incorporation of alcohol in a fluid. Usually liquid diets can be prepared more easily than solid foods and are more flexible to adjust depending on the experimental design and the investigator's need. Controls can be generated by replacement of alcohol with other macronutrients such as carbohydrates (Lieber and DeCarli 1989; Lieber et al. 1965). Alcohol concentration in liquids can be calculated according to their proportion of energy supply for total energy intake. In rats an ethanol amount of 5 g/dL or 36% of total energy supply was found to achieve a reasonable blood concentration of at least 20 mM or 100 mg/dL. Lower blood alcohol levels would be ineffective and would not fit to real clinical condition. Higher alcohol concentrations usually will not be consumed by the rat because they dislike its taste (Lieber and DeCarli 1989). Meanwhile Lieber-DeCarli diets have gained wide acceptance as a standard for scientific use when studying effects of chronic alcohol abuse (Perkins et al. 1995).

There are alternative routes such as an application via a gastrostomy or gavage or directly into the ductal system after laparotomy that allows ingestion of high-percentage ethanol diets (Tsukamoto et al. 1988) but it remains debatable whether this type of application interferes too much with physiologic intrinsic or extrinsic stimulation of the pancreas. In addition unphysiologic application routes won't mimic human situation and pancreatic injury can arise due to other factors rather than ethanol (Lugea et al. 2010).

Gender of animals affects severity of alcohol-induced injury and therefore should be considered when designing an experiment. Alcohol induced liver injury is greater in females than in males demonstrated by histology and levels of serum transaminases (Iimuro et al. 1997). No direct comparative studies have been performed for evaluation of pancreatic damage so far. When using female rats for experiments pancreatic damage under high-dose ethanol and fat diet occurs earlier at already 8 weeks observation time, indicating that female animals might be more susceptible to pancreatic damage (Kono et al. 2001).

3.5.3 Alcohol Application and Fat

Only a minority of alcoholics (around 5%) ultimately develops chronic pancreatitis so that other co-factors need to be present for manifestation of overt disease. A majority of patients suffered from recurrent acute pancreatitis (RAP) before they come down with chronic pancreatitis. Time to progression varies and lies between 1 and 19 years (median 5.7 years) (Ammann et al. 1994). Alcohol is regarded to be a kind of *predisposing* or *sensitizing* agent to the pancreas but other triggers need to be present so that chronic pancreatic will develop (Aghdassi et al. 2015; Pandol et al. 2011).

One of them is fat. Dietary fat is an important contributor to alcohol-induced pancreatic injury. In the Tsukamoto-French enteral alcohol feeding model rats were fed by a liquid diet containing ethanol and different concentrations of fat. Fat was prepared from corn oil, that is mainly composed of (poly-)unsaturated fatty acids. Diets were classified as low-fat (4–5% of total calory intake), high-fat (22–25%) or extra high-fat (30–35%) diet (Tsukamoto et al. 1988). With increase of dietary fat content there was a potentiation of pancreatic injury: Histopathologic changes included acinar atrophy, a patchy distribution of interstitial fibrosis, fatty replacement and some fat necrosis starting at 4 weeks of diet. Exocrine and endocrine function seemed to be not substantially altered, as plasma trypsinogen and glucose of the "high-fat" dietary group were comparable to controls. Results of high-fat diet were confirmed by further studies and some of them could even show impairment of endocrine function (McIlwrath and Westlund 2015).

Other routes of combined ethanol and fat administration have been tried. Direct intraperitoenal application of fatty acids and ethanol induced acute pancreatitis in a mouse model. Conversely, co-application of 3-benzyl-6-chloro-2-pyrone (3-BCP), an inhibitor of carboxy ester lipase (CEL), inhibited FAEE production and ameliorated pancreatic damage (Huang et al. 2014).

These results first indicate that a balance of oxidative and non-oxidative metabolization is critical for prevention of pancreatic damage. Preponderance of non-oxidative ethanol metabolism produces FAEEs and both ethanol and fatty acids exert toxic effects on the pancreas. An exogenous administration of fatty acids increases FAEE amounts and thus pancreatic damage. Secondly carboxy ester lipase (CEL) was identified to be one of the enzymes responsible for the damage. Notably, long-term ethanol feeding even increases pancreatic CEL activity (Pfutzer et al. 2002; Criddle 2015). On a cellular level FAEEs induced sustained high Ca^{2+} elevations that lead to uncontrolled trypsinogen activation (Gerasimenko et al. 2009). Moreover there is a loss of mitochondrial function by opening the mitochondrial transition pore leading to a fall of intracellular ATP levels that is a prerequisite for the emergence of necrosis (Criddle et al. 2006).

Pancreatic injury that is caused by high doses of ethanol and a fatty diet is less severe when medium-chain triglycerides, i.e. saturated fatty acids, are used instead of unsaturated fats (Kono et al. 2001). Less steatosis of the pancreas as well as reduced inflammatory infiltration and necrosis were observed. One of the underlying mechanisms might be a reduction of lipid peroxidation and consecutively a prevention of free radical formation in presence of MCT-fats.

3.5.4 Ethanol, Cholecystokinin and Chronic Pancreatitis

From ex-vivo experiments with isolated acinar cells and animal models it is well known that acute pancreatitis can be induced by repetitive applications of supraphysiologic doses of cholinergic and cholecystokinin (CCK) agonists in rodents (Lugea et al. 2010; Halangk et al. 2000). Therefore combinations of alcohol feeding with caerulein injections either as a single shot or by repetitive applications were thought to be an attractive way for induction of chronic pancreatitis (Lugea et al. 2010; Deng et al. 2005; Gukovsky et al. 2008; Perides et al. 2005). Usually ethanol feeding is performed prior to caerulein applications and lasts for approximately 2–8 weeks. Results consistently showed histopathologic changes compatible with chronic pancreatitis such as activation of pancreatic stellate cells with an increase of collagen content and fibrosis. Combination of alcohol and caerulein clearly enhanced fibrosis formation whereas alcohol alone only led to an inflammatory reaction (Deng et al. 2005; Perides et al. 2005). Exocrine insufficiency was not observed.

Usually a concentration of 50 μg/kg body weight is used for induction of acute pancreatitis but this dose can be markedly reduced (up to 0.5 μg/kg) when animals have been fed with an ethanol-diet before. This drastic reduction again underlines the ethanol sensitizing effect for other harmful stimuli.

3.5.5 Combination of Ethanol and Other Agents

Further agents have been used in combination with ethanol with promising results. Lipopolysaccharides (LPS) are known as endotoxins, cause activation of pancreatic stellate cells and inhibit apoptosis of PSCs so that extracellular matrix proteins will be increasingly synthesized and released. Mice fed with ethanol and subjected to (intraperitoneal) LPS injections showed morphological signs of chronic pancreatitis whereas ethanol alone was ineffective (Nakayama et al. 2014). Changes were detectable after 6 weeks of LPS treatment. Intraductal bile salt infusions to rats that received both a Lieber DeCarli diet and caerulein injections developed severe necrotizing pancreatitis with concomitant lung injury (Schneider et al. 2009).

Cyclosporin A is an immunosuppressant that is clinically used for suppression of organ transplant rejection. Simultaneous treatment of rats with caerulein and daily cyclosporin led to acute pancreatitis without any regeneration of the organ. This distortion of the repair mechanism caused myofibroblast proliferation, collagen production and fibrosis as seen in chronic pancreatitis (Vaquero et al. 1999). In a modified experimental model when rats were pre-fed with an ethanol containing Lieber DeCarli diet (36% of total calorie intake) pancreatic damage was aggravated with enhanced fibrosis formation, acinar tissue loss and sustained inflammatory infiltration (Gukovsky et al. 2008). It is still unclear whether these models will be useful for investigation of exocrine or endocrine deficiencies, as well.

In other experimental settings alcohol feeding was performed *after* preceding interventions. Trinitrobenzene sulfonic acid (TNBS) is a chemical hapten that binds to tissue proteins capable of inducing T-cell mediated immunity and generation of oxygen radicals and other inflammatory mediators (Tatsumi and Lichtenberger 1996). This compound has already been used in rats for experimental models of colitis and cholangitis. A retrograde instillation of TNBS into the pancreatic ductal system causes fibrotic change of the organ and continuous weight loss. Endocrine insufficiency was not observed (Puig-Divi et al. 1996). When rats were fed with ethanol for another 2–4 weeks fibrosis and glandular atrophy were more pronounced and animals now showed an impaired glucose tolerance indicating beginning of endocrine insufficiency (Puig-Divi et al. 1999).

3.6 Genetic Models

From human studies there is increasing evidence that genetics plays an important role in the susceptibility to recurrent acute or chronic pancreatitis. Linkage and candidate gene analysis have discovered six major genes that target either acinar cells in a trypsin-dependent pathway (PRSS1, PRSS2, CTRC, CASR, SPINK1) or ductal cells (CFTR) and their mutations finally lead to loss or gain of function of the proteins (Aghdassi et al. 2015; Whitcomb 2012). In a much broader approach recent studies investigated genetic variants using genomewide association studies (GWAS) that discovered polymorphism in genes, which have not been associated with pancreatitis yet (Derikx et al. 2015; Weiss et al. 2015; Whitcomb et al. 2012).

3.6.1 Trypsinogen

PRSS1 gain of function mutations, such as p.R122H, are known to increase the risk of recurrent acute and chronic pancreatitis in humans (Whitcomb et al. 1996). This amino acid exchange renders trypsin to be more resistant to degradation. Meanwhile more PRSS1 mutations were identified in association with hereditary pancreatitis. For these reasons a transfer of clinical findings from bedside to bench, i.e. an animal model became attractive: Indeed, a transgenic mouse carrying the PRSS1 mutant R122H, placed under the control of an elastase promoter showed signs of chronic pancreatic disease. Fibrosis and acinar cell degeneration were observed. Changes started at 7 weeks of age and progressed with older age resembling morphology in humans (Archer et al. 2006). This model has two strengths: First it represents an experimental system that shows histologic characteristics similar to those from human disease. Secondly, it is based on pathophysiologic mechanisms that are known from hereditary chronic pancreatitis in humans. It therefore might be a model that most closely mimics the human pathophysiology. Moreover, R122H_mPRSS1 mice displayed an enhanced reaction upon serial caerulein injections: while in wildtype animals the inflammatory reaction is largely resolved during the post-injection phase PRSS1 transgenic mice showed a chronic inflammatory response with extensive collagen deposition. Unfortunately, the findings have never been replicated in other laboratories and the model and the mouse are no longer available.

3.6.2 CFTR

Cystic fibrosis transmembrane conductance regulator (CFTR) is expressed on epithelial cells such as ductal cells and functions as a low conductance chloride ion selective channel (Wang et al. 2014). Its major function is believed to dilute and alkalinize the protein-rich acinar secretions, thereby preventing the formation of protein plugs (Chen and Ferec 2012). Various loss-of-function CFTR variants have been reported in patients with chronic pancreatitis, occurring in up to 37% in idiopathic and 15% in alcoholic chronic pancreatitis (Cohn et al. 1998; Sharer et al. 1998; Weiss et al. 2005).

Snouwaert and collaborators developed a murine model of cystic fibrosis by targeted disruption of the CFTR gene (cftr^{m1UNC}; UNC: University of North Carolina). Homozygous knockout mice displayed many features common to young human cystic fibrosis patients. Life expectancy of these mice was often no longer than 40 days resulting from intestinal obstruction causing death (Snouwaert et al. 1992). Although overt signs of chronic pancreatitis were absent in young mice pancreata of CFTR−/− mice showed at least mild features of early cystic fibrosis such as a dilation of the apical acinar lumen (Durie et al. 2004), impaired acinar endocytosis or acidification of the pancreatic juice (Freedman et al. 2001). In older animals (9–24 months) more severe changes were visible including a higher proportion of connective tissue areas, clogging of the pancreatic duct with mucus and concomitant duct dilation with loss of exocrine tissue, highly resembling human morphology (Durie et al. 2004; Dimagno et al. 2005). Untreated CFTR−/− mice showed a reduction of constitutive expression of pancreatic digestive proteins, lipase, pro-elastase and trypsinogen by around 20–25%. Upon caerulein hyperstimulation CFTR−/− mice developed more severe acute pancreatitis but displayed only a blunted increase of pancreatic digestive enzymes, which might suggest mild pancreatic exocrine insufficiency (Dimagno et al. 2005). Cell death was shifted from an apoptotic to a non-apoptotic form.

Limiting factors of this model imply the necessity of longer breeding periods to reach an older stage. In addition, other organs will be involved besides the pancreas because cystic fibrosis is a systemic disease affecting many organs. This means that this experimental model might not be an ideal system for studying pancreatic injury alone and its effects. Moreover life-threatening complications independent of pancreatic insufficiency can occur, such as respiratory airway obstruction due to defective mucociliary clearance or intestinal obstruction that cause early death of mice (Durie et al. 2004).

3.6.3 Cytokines/Chemokines

Many other genes are involved in acute and chronic inflammation and immune response in humans. Whether they affect human chronic pancreatitis as well is still a matter of debate and they will be good candidates for prospective genetic linkage analysis. During inflammation pro-inflammatory cytokines such as interleukin-6 (IL-6), interleukin-1β (IL-1β) or TNFα and chemokines, e.g. CXCL1 and CXCL2 are released causing an influx of immune cells (Steele et al. 2015). Invading inflammatory cells themselves augment local damage, perpetuate protease activation and further release of cytokines (Sendler et al. 2013).

Transgenic mice with overexpression of human IL-1β (sshIL-1β) were followed up for 2 years. The pancreas showed typical histologic features of chronic pancreatitis, i.e. organ atrophy, dilatation of the pancreatic and biliary tract, secondary to proximal fibrotic stenosis (Marrache et al. 2008). Overt sign of exocrine or endocrine insufficiency were not observed in elastase sshIL-1β mice.

This model also addressed the question of malignant transformation in the setting of chronic inflammation. Pancreatic adenocarcinoma can arise on the basis of chronic pancreatitis and p53 mutations are frequently seen in pancreatic cancer (Hingorani et al. 2005; Tuveson and Hingorani 2005). When crossed with heterozygous $p53^{R172H/+}$ mice to create a double transgenic mouse an increased frequency of tubular complexes including some evidence of acinar-ductal metaplasia, that are considered to be preneoplastic lesions, were detected. However pancreatic ductal adenocarcinoma was hardly seen.

CXCR−/− mice were protected from pancreatic damage when chronic pancreatitis was induced by serial caerulein injections (Steele et al. 2015). In particular pancreata showed less organ atrophy and a reduced leukocyte infiltration. Although neutrophil infiltration significantly increases during acute and chronic pancreatitis selective neutrophil depletion (by anti-Ly6G antibody) was less effective suggesting that CXCR2 on non-neutrophils contributes to the development of chronic pancreatitis. Extension of fibrosis was comparable to wildtypes indicating that activation of stellate cells is still maintained despite CXCR2 knockout.

Monocyte chemoattractant protein 1 (MCP-1) is classified as a CC-chemokine. Rats were treated with dibutyltin dichloride (DBTC) and received intramuscular injections of mutant MCP-1 (mMCP-1) plasmids for several days. Pancreatic fibrosis induced by DBTC was attenuated by transgenic expression of mutant MCP-1. Concomitantly a decrease of serum MCP-1 concentrations and less inflammation were seen. Rats carrying mMCP-1 were heavier than controls suggesting that exocrine insufficiency is abrogated in these animals (Zhao et al. 2005).

3.6.4 Autoimmune Mediated

MRL/MpJ mice bearing a mutated lymphoproliferative gene, *lymphoproliferation* (*lpr*), (MRL/MpJ-lpr/lpr) spontenously develop autoimmune disorders such as glomerulonephritis, arthritis and sialadenitis. Mice lacking the *lpr*-gene also develop autoimmune diseases, but at later stage of life (Andrews et al. 1978; Kanno et al. 1992). Inflammatory lesions with acinar destruction and fatty tissue replacement were found in up to 74% of female mice at 34–38 weeks. Endocrine function was preserved, as pancreatic islets remained unaffected. Interestingly male mice later developed pancreatitis that was less intense and only present in less than 40% of 46–50 week old mice. Sex-related factors are discussed to cause the attenuated form, since administration of androgens retarded autoimmune disease in female mice as well (Steinberg et al. 1980). Histology of MRL/Mp mice, in particular their inflammatory infiltrate and fibrosis pattern was comparable with autoimmune pancreatitis type I as seen in humans. Characteristic signs including periductal lymphoplasmocytic infiltration, storiform fibrosis or elevated antibody levels (lactoferrin, carboanhydrase) were present (Schwaiger et al. 2014). Application of polyinosinic:polycytidylic acid (poly I:C) accelerated and enhanced disease progression. Blockage of cytotoxic T-lymphocyte associated protein 4 (CTLA-4), one of the most potent modulators of T-cell response, increased the severity of autoimmune pancreatitis as well (Schwaiger et al. 2014).

Lymphotoxin receptors are membrane proteins of the TNF superfamily and are involved in intracellular signaling. Pleiotropic functions including control of an adequate immune response are maintained lymphotoxins (Wolf et al. 2010). Mice with transgenic expression of lymphotoxin α and β (Ela1-LTαβ) resembled features of autoimmune pancreatitis. When lymphocytes were depleted (Ela1-LTab/Rag1(−/−)) autoimmunity was lost whereas deletion of monocytes (Ela1-LTab/Ccr2(−/−)) preserved autoimmune disease but prevented early pancreatic tissue damage (Seleznik et al. 2012).

C5 is a factor of the complement system and complement activation drives many inflammatory responses. Cleavage of the C5 molecule generates C5a and b. C5a exerts a predominant pro-inflammatory activity mediating leukocyte chemotaxis and release of proinflammatory cytokines. An increased vascular permeability facilitates neutrophil transmigration (Kohl 2001). C5b holds cytolytic functions through the formation of the membrane attack complex (MAC) but also possess a multitude of non-cytolytic immune functions as well (Woodruff et al. 2011). Trypsin is known to act as a complement activator, and is able to cleave both C3 and C5 (Acioli et al. 1997).

C5 is functionally linked to liver fibrogenesis, as its receptor (C5R1) is expressed on endothelial and Kupffer cells and activates myofibroblasts. Deletion of C5, either genetically or pharmacologically resulted in reduced liver fibrosis upon CCL4 treatment (Hillebrandt et al. 2005). C5 exerts pro-fibrogenic effects in chronic pancreatitis as well. Sendler and coworkers subjected C5 deficient mice to either pancreatic duct ligation for up to 3 weeks or serial caerulein injections for 10 weeks. In both models pancreatic fibrosis was reduced in C5−/− animals and most predominant at later time points. Pharmacological anti-C5 treatment using a C5-receptor antagonist or a peptide inhibitor achieved comparable results to the knockout mouse model. Isolated pancreatic stellate cells were activated by C5a and synthesized massive amounts of extracellular proteins (Sendler et al. 2015).

3.6.5 WBN/Kob Rats

An example of a rat model mimicking chronic pancreatitis is given by the WBN/Kob (Wistar-Bonn/Kobori) strain. This strain is derived from Wistar rats and was originally generated as a model susceptible to gastric tumors. Starting with an age of 3–6 months male WBN/Kob rats show progressive fibrosis around the pancreatic ducts and vessels. A degradation of Langerhans islets leads to a reduction of number and size of the islets (Mori et al. 2009; Ohashi et al. 1990). At 9–12 months of age full manifestation of diabetes mellitus occurs with impaired glucose tolerance, hyperglycemia and glycosuria. Exocrine function measured by BT-PABA (n-benzoyl-l-tyrosyl-p-aminobenzoic acid) urinary excretion was diminished as well. Chromosomal mapping revealed two potentially responsible loci at chromosome 7 and X, Pdwk1 and 2 (pancreatitis and diabetes mellitus in WBN/Kob locus 1 and 2). Candidate genes were found in the Pdwk1 locus that makes a genetic origin of this phenotype likely (Mori et al. 2009).

More genetically engineered animals models exist describing chronic fibrotic disease in the pancreas. Good examples are a pancreas specific Kif3a knockout model that resulted in cyst formation and pancreatic fibrosis in aged mice. The Kif3a gene encodes a subunit of the kinesin-2 complex that is essential in cilia formation and its defect is associated with several human genetic diseases, including polycystic kidney disease (PCKD) Bardet-Biedl syndrome and primary ciliary dyskinesia (Cano et al. 2006). Perk−/− mice experienced a rapid loss of their endocrine and exocrine function accompanied with increasing cell death (Harding et al. 2001). Absence of PERK (Protein kinase R-line endoplasmic reticulum kinase), a transmembrane protein of the endoplasmic reticulum and usually highly expressed in the pancreas, renders cells to be more susceptible to ER stress and protein misfolding. For further information on genetic animal models for chronic pancreatitis please see Table 5.3.

Apparently the majority of studies using mouse models employ the C57BL/6 strain for their experiments. This strain is most frequently used in biomedical research. Moreover genetically modified mouse models are often derived from a C57BL/6 background. Meanwhile due to existence of various mouse breeding facilities and separate inbred colonies a high number of C57BL/6 substrains exist that have important genetic and phenotypic differences (Bourdi et al. 2011; Ulmasov et al. 2013; Watkins-Chow and Pavan 2008). In a recent study it could be shown that substrains of C57BL/6 mice show different disease severities of chronic pancreatitis

Table 5.3 Overview of genetic animal models for chronic pancreatitis (adapted from Lerch and Gorelick, 2013)

Gene	Function	Genetic manipulation (ko/tg)	Induction of CP	Morphology	Species	Author
Proteases/cellular components						
PRSS1 p.R122H	Cationic trypsinogen	tg (elastase promotor)	Spontaneous	Acinar cell necrosis, inflammatory cell infiltration, fibrosis, acinar dedifferentation	Mouse	Archer H, Gastroenterology 2006
CFTR	Chloride ion channel	ko	Spontaneous	Acinar cell atrophy, ductal dilatation, ductal clogging, fibrosis (at older age), no endocrine dysfunction	Mouse	Snouwaert JN, Science 1992
						Durie PR, Am J Pathol 2004
						DiMagno MJ, Gastroenterology 2005
KIf3a	Subunit of kinesin complex, cilia formation	ko (conditional)	Spontaneous	Fibrosis, acinar-ductal-metaplasia, lipomatosis, cysts	Mouse	Cano DA, Gastroenterology 2006
PERK	Prevents ER stress and protein misfolding	ko	Spontaneous	Cell death, exocrine and endocrine insufficiency	Mouse	Harding HP, Mol Cell 2001
Cytokines/chemokines						
Human IL-1β	Pro-inflammatory cytokine	tg (elastase promotor)	Spontaneous	Organ atrophy, dilatation of the pancreatic/biliary tract, no exocrine or endocrine insufficiency	Mouse	Marrache F, Gastroenterology 2008
Cxcr2	Chemokine receptor, neutrophil migration	ko	Caerulein	Less organ atrophy, less inflammation, no gross changes of fibrosis	Mouse	Steele CW, J Pathol 2015
MCP-1	Chemotaxis factor	tg (mutant MCP-1)	DBTC	Less fibrosis, less inflammation, less weight loss	Rat	Zhao HF, Gut 2005
C5	Complement factor, pro-inflammatory, chemotactic function	ko	Duct ligation, caerulein	Less fibrosis, reduced stellate cell activation, less collagen I synthesis	Mouse	Sendler M, Gastroenterology 2015

Autoimmune mediated						
MRL/MpJ	Lymphoproliferative gene	tg (mutant lpr)	Spontaneous	Signs of autoimmune pancreatitis, no endocrine insufficiency	Mouse	Kanno H, Clin Exp Immunol 1992
						Andrews BS, J Exp Med 1978
						Schwaiger T, Gut 2014
Lymphotoxin α and β	Intracellular signalling, immune response	Double tg (elastase promotor)	Spontaneous	Signs of autoimmune pancreatitis (type 2), no endocrine insufficiency	Mouse	Seleznik GM, Gastroenterology 2012
Other						
WBN/Kob	Pdwk1 and 2 (chromosome 7 and x), unknown function	Crossbreeding of Bonn (DE) and Kobori (Tokyo, JP) rats	Spontanous	Fibrosis, inflammatory infiltration, diabetes mellitus, reduced exocrine function	Rat	Ohashi K, Int J Pancreatol 1990
						Mori M, Exp Anim 2009

ko knockout, *tg* transgenic, + yes, – no, *n.a.* no information available upon repetitive caerulein injections. Fibrosis, acinar atrophy and inflammatory infiltrate were markedly more in B6J than in B6N substrains (Ulmasov et al. 2013). Knowledge of the exact background of genetically engineered animals and their control is of high importance, as an erroneous choice of the wrong genetic substrain most probably produces misleading results.

3.7 Concluding Remarks

Studies consistently showed that the available experimental models satisfactorily mimic histopathologic features of chronic pancreatitis whilst rodents (mice and rats) are investigated most thoroughly. There are different techniques that can be used to create pancreatic fibrosis and the most frequently used ones are ligation models and repetitive caerulein applications. Manifold combinations of techniques, often with additional dietary modifications (alcohol, fat) are practiced. There is increasing data on genetic animal models for chronic pancreatitis and some of them seem to imitate pathophysiology of humans quite well. Diabetes as the result of endocrine insufficiency was seen in only some models, however mostly after a long disease course and when the entire organ is affected.

In our opinion there is still a lack of usable models mimicking exocrine insufficiency. A small functioning part of the pancreas is sufficient to produce secretory digestive enzymes to avert clinically overt exocrine malfunction unless combined with a high fat diet. Probably exocrine function can only be impaired when using a model of very severe form of chronic pancreatitis. Secondly, other tools for measurement of exocrine function should be considered. In humans direct function tests are the gold standard that assess the secretion of enzymes and bicarbonate into the small intestine after stimulation. These enzymes are usually collected by an oro- or nasoduodenal tube and then quantitated. Definitely this procedure is invasive and time consuming and would be even more complicated in animals. Here further developments on indirect tests in animals will be necessary to overcome this problem.

References

Acioli JM, Isobe M, Kawasaki S. Early complement system activation and neutrophil priming in acute pancreatitis: participation of trypsin. Surgery. 1997;122(5):909–17.

Addadi L, Weiner S. Interaction between acidic proteins and crystals: stereochemical requirements in biomineralization. PNAS. 1985;82:4110–4.

Aghdassi A, Mayerle J, Kraft M, Sielenkämper AW, Heidecke C-DD, Lerch MM. Diagnosis and treatment of pancreatic pseudocysts in chronic pancreatitis. Pancreas. 2008;36:105–12.

Aghdassi AA, Mayerle J, Christochowitz S, Weiss FU, Sendler M, Lerch MM. Animal models for investigating chronic pancreatitis. Fibrogenesis Tissue Repair. 2011;4(1):26. doi:10.1186/1755-1536-4-26.

Aghdassi AA, Weiss FU, Mayerle J, Lerch MM, Simon P. Genetic susceptibility factors for alcohol-induced chronic pancreatitis. Pancreatology. 2015;15(4 Suppl):S23–31. doi:10.1016/j.pan.2015.05.476.

Allan J, White TT. An alternate mechanism for the formation of protein plugs in chronic calcifying pancreatitis. Digestion. 1974;11:428–31.

Ammann RW, Akovbiantz A, Largiader F, Schueler G. Course and outcome of chronic pancreatitis. Longitudinal study of a mixed medical-surgical series of 245 patients. Gastroenterology. 1984;86:820–8.

Ammann RW, Muellhaupt B, Meyenberger C, Heitz PU. Alcoholic nonprogressive chronic pancreatitis: prospective long-term study of a large cohort with alcoholic acute pancreatitis (1976-1992). Pancreas. 1994;9(3):365–73.

Ammann RW, Heitz PU, Kloppel G. Course of alcoholic chronic pancreatitis: a prospective clinicomorphological long-term study. Gastroenterology. 1996;111(1):224–31.

Anand P, Aziz Q, Willert R, van Oudenhove L. Peripheral and central mechanisms of visceral sensitization in man. Neurogastroenterol Motil. 2007;19:29–46.

Anaparthy R, Pasricha PJ. Pain and chronic pancreatitis: is it the plumbing or the wiring? Curr Gastroenterol Rep. 2008;10:101–6.

Anderson MA, Akshintala V, Albers KM, et al. Mechanism, assessment and management of pain in chronic pancreatitis: recommendations of a multidisciplinary study group. Pancreatology. 2015;16:83–94.

Andrén-Sandberg A, Dervenis C. Pancreatic pseudocysts in the 21st century. Part I: classification, pathophysiology, anatomic considerations and treatment. JOP. 2004;5:8–24.

Andrews BS, Eisenberg RA, Theofilopoulos AN, et al. Spontaneous murine lupus-like syndromes. Clinical and immunopathological manifestations in several strains. J Exp Med. 1978;148(5):1198–215.

Apkarian AV, Hashmi JA, Baliki MN. Pain and the brain: specificity and plasticity of the brain in clinical chronic pain. Pain. 2011;152:S49–64.

Apte MV, Haber PS, Darby SJ, et al. Pancreatic stellate cells are activated by proinflammatory cytokines:

implications for pancreatic fibrogenesis. Gut. 1999;44(4):534–41.
Apte MV, Phillips PA, Fahmy RG, et al. Does alcohol directly stimulate pancreatic fibrogenesis? Studies with rat pancreatic stellate cells. Gastroenterology. 2000;118(4):780–94.
Archer H, Jura N, Keller J, Jacobson M, Bar-Sagi D. A mouse model of hereditary pancreatitis generated by transgenic expression of R122H trypsinogen. Gastroenterology. 2006;131(6):1844–55. doi:10.1053/j.gastro.2006.09.049.
Backonja M, Wallace MS, Blonsky ER, Cutler BJ, Malan P Jr, Rauck R, Tobias J. NGX-4010, a high-concentration capsaicin patch, for the treatment of postherpetic neuralgia: a randomised, double-blind study. Lancet Neurol. 2008;7:1106–12.
Balci NC, Perman WH, Saglam S, Akisik F, Fattahi R, Bilgin M. Diffusion-weighted magnetic resonance imaging of the pancreas. Top Magn Reson Imaging. 2009;20:43–7.
Bertelli E, Bendayan M. Intermediate endocrine-acinar pancreatic cells in duct ligation conditions. Am J Phys. 1997;273(5 Pt 1):C1641–9.
Bimmler D, Graf R, Scheele GA, et al. Pancreatic stone protein (lithostathine), a physiologically relevant pancreatic calcium carbonate crystal inhibitor? J Biol Chem. 1997;272:3073–82.
Bockman DE, Kennedy RH, Multigner L, et al. Fine structure of the organic matrix of human pancreatic stones. Pancreas. 1986;1:204–10.
Bockman DE, Buchler M, Malfertheiner P, Beger HG. Analysis of nerves in chronic pancreatitis. Gastroenterology. 1988;94:1459–69.
Boerma D, Obertop H, Gouma DJ. Pancreatic pseudocysts in chronic pancreatitis. Surgical or interventional drainage? Ann Ital Chir. 2000;71:43–50.
Bornman PC, Marks IN, Girdwood AH, Clain JE, Narunsky L, Clain DJ, Wright JP. Is pancreatic duct obstruction or stricture a major cause of pain in calcific pancreatitis? Br J Surg. 1980;67:425–8.
Bourdi M, Davies JS, Pohl LR. Mispairing C57BL/6 substrains of genetically engineered mice and wild-type controls can lead to confounding results as it did in studies of JNK2 in acetaminophen and concanavalin A liver injury. Chem Res Toxicol. 2011;24(6):794–6. doi:10.1021/tx200143x.
Bouwense SA, Buscher HC, van Goor H, Wilder-Smith OH. S-ketamine modulates hyperalgesia in patients with chronic pancreatitis pain. Reg Anesth Pain Med. 2011a;36:303–7.
Bouwense SA, Buscher HC, van Goor H, Wilder-Smith OH. Has central sensitization become independent of nociceptive input in chronic pancreatitis patients who fail thoracoscopic splanchnicectomy? Reg Anesth Pain Med. 2011b;36:531–6.
Bouwense SA, Olesen SS, Drewes AM, Frøkjær JB, van Goor H, Wilder-Smith OH. Is altered central pain processing related to disease stage in chronic pancreatitis patients with pain? An exploratory study. PLoS One. 2013;8:e55460.
Brock C, Olesen SS, Olesen AE, Frokjaer JB, Andresen T, Drewes AM, Frøkjaer JB, Andresen T, Drewes AM. Opioid-induced bowel dysfunction: pathophysiology and management. Drugs. 2012;72:1847–65.
Brock C, Nielsen LM, Lelic D, Drewes AM. Pathophysiology of chronic pancreatitis. World J Gastroenterol. 2013;19(42):7231–40. doi:10.3748/wjg.v19.i42.7231.
Büchler M, Weihe E, Friess H, Malfertheiner P, Bockman E, Müller S, Nohr D, Beger HG. Changes in peptidergic innervation in chronic pancreatitis. Pancreas. 1992;7:183–92.
Buscher HC, Wilder-Smith OH, van Goor H. Chronic pancreatitis patients show hyperalgesia of central origin: a pilot study. Eur J Pain. 2006;10:363–70.
Cano DA, Sekine S, Hebrok M. Primary cilia deletion in pancreatic epithelial cells results in cyst formation and pancreatitis. Gastroenterology. 2006;131(6):1856–69. doi:10.1053/j.gastro.2006.10.050.
Casellas F, Guarner L, Vaquero E, Antolin M, de Gracia X, Malagelada JR. Hydrogen breath test with glucose in exocrine pancreatic insufficiency. Pancreas. 1998;16:481–6.
Ceyhan GO, Deucker S, Demir IE, et al. Neural fractalkine expression is closely linked to pain and pancreatic neuritis in human chronic pancreatitis. Lab Invest. 2009a;89:347–61.
Ceyhan GO, Demir IE, Rauch U, Bergmann F, Müller MW, Büchler MW, Friess H, Schäfer K-H. Pancreatic neuropathy results in "neural remodeling" and altered pancreatic innervation in chronic pancreatitis and pancreatic cancer. Am J Gastroenterol. 2009b;104:2555–65.
Ceyhan GO, Bergmann F, Kadihasanoglu M, et al. Pancreatic neuropathy and neuropathic pain—a comprehensive pathomorphological study of 546 cases. Gastroenterology. 2009c;136:177–186.e1.
Chebli JM, de Souza AF, Gaburri PD, Bastos KV, Ribeiro TC, Filho RJ, Chebli LA, Castro Ferreira LE. Prevalence and pathogenesis of duodenal ulcer in chronic alcoholic pancreatitis. J Clin Gastroenterol. 2002;35:71–4.
Chen JM, Ferec C. Genetics and pathogenesis of chronic pancreatitis: the 2012 update. Clin Res Hepatol Gastroenterol. 2012;36(4):334–40. doi:10.1016/j.clinre.2012.05.003.
Churg A, Richter WR. Early changes in the exocrine pancreas of the dog and rat after ligation of the pancreatic duct. A light and electron microscopic study. Am J Pathol. 1971;63(3):521–46.
Cohn JA, Friedman KJ, Noone PG, Knowles MR, Silverman LM, Jowell PS. Relation between mutations of the cystic fibrosis gene and idiopathic pancreatitis. N Engl J Med. 1998;339(10):653–8. doi:10.1056/NEJM199809033391002.
Colomer V, Lal K, Hoops TC, et al. Exocrine granule specific packaging signals are present in the polypeptide moiety of the pancreatic granule membrane protein GP2 and in amylase: implications for protein targeting to secretory granules. EMBO J. 1994;13(16):3711–9.

Criddle DN. The role of fat and alcohol in acute pancreatitis: a dangerous liaison. Pancreatology. 2015;15(4 Suppl):S6–12. doi:10.1016/j.pan.2015.02.009.

Criddle DN, Murphy J, Fistetto G, et al. Fatty acid ethyl esters cause pancreatic calcium toxicity via inositol trisphosphate receptors and loss of ATP synthesis. Gastroenterology. 2006;130(3):781–93. doi:10.1053/j.gastro.2005.12.031.

De Caro A, Lohse J, Sarles H. Characterization of a protein isolated from pancreatic calculi of men suffering from chronic calcifying pancreatitis. Biochem Biophys Res Commun. 1979;87:1176–82.

De Reggi M, Gharib B, Patard L, et al. Lithostathine, the presumed pancreatic stone inhibitor, does not interact specifically with calcium carbonate crystals. J Biol Chem. 1998;273:4967–71.

Demir IE, Friess H, Ceyhan GO. Neural plasticity in pancreatitis and pancreatic cancer. Nat Rev Gastroenterol Hepatol. 2015;12:649–59.

Deng X, Wang L, Elm MS, et al. Chronic alcohol consumption accelerates fibrosis in response to cerulein-induced pancreatitis in rats. Am J Pathol. 2005;166(1):93–106. doi:10.1016/S0002-9440(10)62235-3.

Derikx MH, Kovacs P, Scholz M, et al. Polymorphisms at PRSS1-PRSS2 and CLDN2-MORC4 loci associate with alcoholic and non-alcoholic chronic pancreatitis in a European replication study. Gut. 2015;64(9):1426–33. doi:10.1136/gutjnl-2014-307453.

Detlefsen S, Sipos B, Feyerabend B, Kloppel G. Fibrogenesis in alcoholic chronic pancreatitis: the role of tissue necrosis, macrophages, myofibroblasts and cytokines. Mod Pathol. 2006;19(8):1019–26. doi:10.1038/modpathol.3800613.

Di Sebastiano P, Fink T, Weihe E, Friess H, Innocenti P, Beger HG, Büchler MW. Immune cell infiltration and growth-associated protein 43 expression correlate with pain in chronic pancreatitis. Gastroenterology. 1997;112:1648–55.

Dimagno MJ, Lee SH, Hao Y, Zhou SY, McKenna BJ, Owyang C. A proinflammatory, antiapoptotic phenotype underlies the susceptibility to acute pancreatitis in cystic fibrosis transmembrane regulator (-/-) mice. Gastroenterology. 2005;129(2):665–81. doi:10.1016/j.gastro.2005.05.059.

Dimcevski G, Sami SA, Funch-Jensen P, Le Pera D, Valeriani M, Arendt-Nielsen L, Drewes AM. Pain in chronic pancreatitis: the role of reorganization in the central nervous system. Gastroenterology. 2007;132:1546–56.

Drewes A-M. Is the pain in chronic pancreatitis of neuropathic origin? Support from EEG studies during experimental pain. World J Gastroenterol. 2008;14:4020.

Durie PR, Kent G, Phillips MJ, Ackerley CA. Characteristic multiorgan pathology of cystic fibrosis in a long-living cystic fibrosis transmembrane regulator knockout murine model. Am J Pathol. 2004;164(4):1481–93. doi:10.1016/S0002-9440(10)63234-8.

Ebbehøj N, Svendsen LB, Madsen P. Pancreatic tissue pressure: techniques and pathophysiological aspects. Scand J Gastroenterol. 1984;19:1066–8.

Ebbehøj N, Borly L, Bülow J, Rasmussen SG, Madsen P, Matzen P, Owre A. Pancreatic tissue fluid pressure in chronic pancreatitis. Relation to pain, morphology, and function. Scand J Gastroenterol. 1990a;25:1046–51.

Ebbehøj N, Borly L, Bülow J, Rasmussen SG, Madsen P. Evaluation of pancreatic tissue fluid pressure and pain in chronic pancreatitis. A longitudinal study. Scand J Gastroenterol. 1990b;25:462–6.

Elsasser HP, Haake T, Grimmig M, Adler G, Kern HF. Repetitive cerulein-induced pancreatitis and pancreatic fibrosis in the rat. Pancreas. 1992;7(3):385–90.

Esposito I, Friess H, Kappeler A, Shrikhande S, Kleeff J, Ramesh H, Zimmermann A, Büchler MW. Mast cell distribution and activation in chronic pancreatitis. Hum Pathol. 2001;32:1174–83.

Farnbacher MJ, Voll RE, Faissner R, et al. Composition of clogging material in pancreatic endoprostheses. Gastrointest Endosc. 2005;61:862–6.

Fasanella KE, Davis B, Lyons J, Chen Z, Lee KK, Slivka A, Whitcomb DC. Pain in chronic pancreatitis and pancreatic cancer. Gastroenterol Clin North Am. 2007;36:335–64, ix.

Flor H, Elbert T, Knecht S, Wienbruch C, Pantev C, Birbaumer N, Larbig W, Taub E. Phantom-limb pain as a perceptual correlate of cortical reorganization following arm amputation. Nature. 1995;375:482–4.

Flor H, Nikolajsen L, Jensen TS. Phantom limb pain: a case of maladaptive CNS plasticity? Nat Rev Neurosci. 2006;7:873–81.

Freedman SD, Kern HF, Scheele GA. Apical membrane trafficking during regulated pancreatic exocrine secretion—role of alkaline pH in the acinar lumen and enzymatic cleavage of GP2, a GPI-linked protein. Eur J Cell Biol. 1994;65:354–65.

Freedman SD, Kern HF, Scheele GA. Pancreatic acinar cell dysfunction in CFTR(-/-) mice is associated with impairments in luminal pH and endocytosis. Gastroenterology. 2001;121(4):950–7.

Friess H, Shrikhande S, Shrikhande M, Martignoni M, Kulli C, Zimmermann A, Kappeler A, Ramesh H, Büchler M. Neural alterations in surgical stage chronic pancreatitis are independent of the underlying aetiology. Gut. 2002;50:682–6.

Frokjaer JB, Drewes AM, Olesen SS, Frøkjær JB, Olesen SS, Drewes AM. Fibrosis, atrophy, and ductal pathology in chronic pancreatitis are associated with pancreatic function but independent of symptoms. Pancreas. 2013;42:1182–7.

Frøkjær JB, Olesen SS, Gram M, Yavarian Y, Bouwense SA, Wilder-Smith OH, Drewes AM. Altered brain microstructure assessed by diffusion tensor imaging in patients with chronic pancreatitis. Gut. 2011;60:1554–62.

Frøkjær JB, Bouwense SA, Olesen SS, Lundager FH, Eskildsen SF, van Goor H, Wilder-Smith OH, Drewes AM. Reduced cortical thickness of brain areas involved in pain processing in patients with chronic pancreatitis. Clin Gastroenterol Hepatol. 2012;10:434–8.e1.

Frulloni L, Gabbrielli A, Pezzilli R, et al. Chronic pancreatitis: report from a multicenter Italian survey

(PanCroInfAISP) on 893 patients. Dig Liver Dis. 2009;41(4):311–7. doi:10.1016/j.dld.2008.07.316.

Gebhart GF. Visceral pain-peripheral sensitisation. Gut. 2000;47(Suppl 4):iv54–5, discussion iv58.

Gebhart GF. Descending modulation of pain. Neurosci Biobehav Rev. 2004;27:729–37.

Gebhart GF. It's chickens and eggs all over again: is central reorganization the result or cause of persistent visceral pain? Gastroenterology. 2007;132:1618–20.

Geider S, Baronnet A, Cerini C, et al. Pancreatic lithostathine as a calcite habit modifier. J Biol Chem. 1996;271:26302–6.

Gerasimenko JV, Lur G, Sherwood MW, et al. Pancreatic protease activation by alcohol metabolite depends on Ca^{2+} release via acid store IP3 receptors. Proc Natl Acad Sci U S A. 2009;106(26):10758–63. doi:10.1073/pnas.0904818106.

Goto M, Nakano I, Kimura T, Miyahara T, Kinjo M, Nawata H. New chronic pancreatitis model with diabetes induced by cerulein plus stress in rats. Dig Dis Sci. 1995;40(11):2356–63.

Gouyon B, Lévy P, Ruszniewski P, Zins M, Hammel P, Vilgrain V, Sauvanet A, Belghiti J, Bernades P. Predictive factors in the outcome of pseudocysts complicating alcoholic chronic pancreatitis. Gut. 1997;41:821–5.

Graversen C, Olesen SS, Olesen AE, Steimle K, Farina D, Wilder-Smith OHG, Bouwense SAW, van Goor H, Drewes AM. The analgesic effect of pregabalin in patients with chronic pain is reflected by changes in pharmaco-EEG spectral indices. Br J Clin Pharmacol. 2012;73:363–72.

Gress T, Muller-Pillasch F, Elsasser HP, et al. Enhancement of transforming growth factor beta 1 expression in the rat pancreas during regeneration from caerulein-induced pancreatitis. Eur J Clin Investig. 1994;24(10):679–85.

Grippo PJ, Venkatasubramanian PN, Knop RH, et al. Visualization of mouse pancreas architecture using MR microscopy. Am J Pathol. 2011;179(2):610–8. doi:10.1016/j.ajpath.2011.04.007.

Gross J, Carlson RI, Brauer AW, et al. Isolation, characterization, and distribution of an unusual pancreatic human secretory protein. J Clin Invest. 1985;76:2115–26.

Gukovskaya AS, Mareninova OA, Odinokova IV, et al. Cell death in pancreatitis: effects of alcohol. J Gastroenterol Hepatol. 2006;21(Suppl 3):S10–3. doi:10.1111/j.1440-1746.2006.04571.x.

Gukovsky I, Lugea A, Shahsahebi M, et al. A rat model reproducing key pathological responses of alcoholic chronic pancreatitis. Am J Physiol Gastrointest Liver Physiol. 2008;294(1):G68–79. doi:10.1152/ajpgi.00006.2007.

Gupte AR, Forsmark CE. Chronic pancreatitis. Curr Opin Gastroenterol. 2014;30(5):500–5. doi:10.1097/MOG.0000000000000094.

Halangk W, Lerch MM, Brandt-Nedelev B, et al. Role of cathepsin B in intracellular trypsinogen activation and the onset of acute pancreatitis. J Clin Invest. 2000;106(6):773–81. doi:10.1172/JCI9411.

Harada H, Ueda O, Kochi F, Kobayashi T, Komazawa M. Comparative studies on viscosity and concentration of protein and hexosamine in pure pancreatic juice. Gastroenterol Jpn. 1981;16(6):623–6.

Harding HP, Zeng H, Zhang Y, et al. Diabetes mellitus and exocrine pancreatic dysfunction in perk-/- mice reveals a role for translational control in secretory cell survival. Mol Cell. 2001;7(6):1153–63.

Haroutounian S, Nikolajsen L, Bendtsen TF, Finnerup NB, Kristensen AD, Hasselstrom JB, Jensen TS. Primary afferent input critical for maintaining spontaneous pain in peripheral neuropathy. Pain. 2014;155:1272–9.

Hartel M, di Mola FF, Selvaggi F, et al. Vanilloids in pancreatic cancer: potential for chemotherapy and pain management. Gut. 2006;55:519–28.

Hayakawa T, Harada H, Noda A, et al. Lactoferrin in pure pancreatic juice in chronic pancreatitis. Am J Gastroenterol. 1983;78(4):222.

Hayakawa T, Kondo T, Shibata T, et al. Trypsin(ogen) content of pancreatic calculi in chronic calcified pancreatitis in man. Dig Dis Sci. 1994;39:1345–50.

Heinricher MM, Tavares I, Leith JL, Lumb BM. Descending control of nociception: specificity, recruitment and plasticity. Brain Res Rev. 2009;60:214–25.

Hillebrandt S, Wasmuth HE, Weiskirchen R, et al. Complement factor 5 is a quantitative trait gene that modifies liver fibrogenesis in mice and humans. Nat Genet. 2005;37(8):835–43. doi:10.1038/ng1599.

Hingorani SR, Wang L, Multani AS, et al. Trp53R172H and KrasG12D cooperate to promote chromosomal instability and widely metastatic pancreatic ductal adenocarcinoma in mice. Cancer Cell. 2005;7(5):469–83. doi:10.1016/j.ccr.2005.04.023.

Hoogerwerf WA, Gondesen K, Xiao S-Y, Winston JH, Willis WD, Pasricha PJ. The role of mast cells in the pathogenesis of pain in chronic pancreatitis. BMC Gastroenterol. 2005;5:8.

Huang W, Booth DM, Cane MC, et al. Fatty acid ethyl ester synthase inhibition ameliorates ethanol-induced Ca^{2+}-dependent mitochondrial dysfunction and acute pancreatitis. Gut. 2014;63(8):1313–24. doi:10.1136/gutjnl-2012-304058.

Hughes MS, Shenoy M, Liu L, Colak T, Mehta K, Pasricha PJ. Brain-derived neurotrophic factor is upregulated in rats with chronic pancreatitis and mediates pain behavior. Pancreas. 2011;40:551–6.

Iimuro Y, Frankenberg MV, Arteel GE, Bradford BU, Wall CA, Thurman RG. Female rats exhibit greater susceptibility to early alcohol-induced liver injury than males. Am J Phys. 1997;272(5 Pt 1):G1186–94.

Irving HM, Samokhvalov AV, Rehm J. Alcohol as a risk factor for pancreatitis. A systematic review and meta-analysis. JOP. 2009;10(4):387–92.

Isaksson G, Lundquist I, Ihse I. Effects on the exocrine and endocrine pancreas of duct occlusion with two different tissue glues in the rat. Eur Surg Res. 1983;15(3):136–44.

Jensen AR, Matzen P, Malchow-Møller A, Christoffersen I. Pattern of pain, duct morphology, and pancreatic function in chronic pancreatitis. A comparative study. Scand J Gastroenterol. 1984;19:334–8.

Jin CX, Naruse S, Kitagawa M, et al. Pancreatic stone protein of pancreatic calculi in chronic calcified pancreatitis in man. JOP. 2002;3:54–61.

Juel J, Olesen SS, Olesen AE, Poulsen JL, Dahan A, Wilder-Smith O, Madzak A, Frøkjær JB, Drewes AM. Study protocol for a randomised, double-blinded, placebo-controlled, clinical trial of S-ketamine for pain treatment in patients with chronic pancreatitis (RESET trial). BMJ Open. 2015;5:e007087.

Kahl S, Zimmermann S, Genz I, Schmidt U, Pross M, Schulz HU, Malfertheiner P. Biliary strictures are not the cause of pain in patients with chronic pancreatitis. Pancreas. 2004;28:387–90.

Kalvaria I, Bornman PC, Marks IN, Girdwood AH, Bank L, Kottler RE. The spectrum and natural history of common bile duct stenosis in chronic alcohol-induced pancreatitis. Ann Surg. 1989;210:608–13.

Kanno H, Nose M, Itoh J, Taniguchi Y, Kyogoku M. Spontaneous development of pancreatitis in the MRL/Mp strain of mice in autoimmune mechanism. Clin Exp Immunol. 1992;89(1):68–73.

Kara ME. The anatomical study on the rat pancreas and its ducts with emphasis on the surgical approach. Ann Anat. 2005;187(2):105–12. doi:10.1016/j.aanat.2004.10.004.

Keith RG, Keshavjee SH, Kerenyi NR. Neuropathology of chronic pancreatitis in humans. Can J surgery. 1985;28:207–11.

Keller J, Aghdassi AA, Lerch MM, Mayerle JV, Layer P. Tests of pancreatic exocrine function—clinical significance in pancreatic and non-pancreatic disorders. Best Pract Res Clin Gastroenterol. 2009;23(3):425–39. doi:10.1016/j.bpg.2009.02.013.

Kimura Y, Torimura T, Ueno T, Inuzuka S, Tanikawa K. Transforming growth factor beta 1, extracellular matrix, and inflammatory cells in wound repair using a closed duodenal loop pancreatitis model rat. Immunohistochemical study. Scand J Gastroenterol. 1995;30(7):707–14.

Kishi S, Takeyama Y, Ueda T, et al. Pancreatic duct obstruction itself induces expression of alpha smooth muscle actin in pancreatic stellate cells. J Surg Res. 2003;114(1):6–14.

Klöppel G. Chronic pancreatitis, pseudotumors and other tumor-like lesions. Mod Pathol. 2007;20(Suppl 1):S113–31. doi:10.1038/modpathol.3800690.

Klöppel G. Histopathologie der chronischen Pankreatitis. In: Beger HG, Büchler MW, Dralle H, Lerch MM, Malfertheiner P, Mössner J, Riemann JF, editors. Erkrankungen des Pankreas. Berlin: Springer; 2013. p. 86–91.

Kloppel G, Detlefsen S, Feyerabend B. Fibrosis of the pancreas: the initial tissue damage and the resulting pattern. Virchows Arch. 2004;445(1):1–8. doi:10.1007/s00428-004-1021-5.

Kohl J. Anaphylatoxins and infectious and non-infectious inflammatory diseases. Mol Immunol. 2001;38(2–3):175–87.

Kono H, Nakagami M, Rusyn I, et al. Development of an animal model of chronic alcohol-induced pancreatitis in the rat. Am J Physiol Gastrointest Liver Physiol. 2001;280(6):G1178–86.

Lampel M, Kern HF. Acute interstitial pancreatitis in the rat induced by excessive doses of a pancreatic secretagogue. Virchows Arch A Pathol Anat Histol. 1977;373(2):97–117.

Lankisch PG, Löhr-Happe A, Otto J, Creutzfeldt W. Natural course in chronic pancreatitis. Pain, exocrine and endocrine pancreatic insufficiency and prognosis of the disease. Digestion. 1993;54:148–55.

Lankisch PG, Breuer N, Bruns A, Weber-Dany B, Lowenfels AB, Maisonneuve P. Natural history of acute pancreatitis: a long-term population-based study. Am J Gastroenterol. 2009;104(11):2797–2805.; , quiz 2806. doi:10.1038/ajg.2009.405.

Latremoliere A, Woolf CJ. Central sensitization: a generator of pain hypersensitivity by central neural plasticity. J Pain. 2009;10:895–926.

Laugier R. Dynamic endoscopic manometry of the response to secretin in patients with chronic pancreatitis. Endoscopy. 1994;26:222–7.

Layer PH. Motor cycles and other cycles in chronic pancreatitis. Gastroenterology. 1995;109:316–9.

Lelic D, Olesen SS, Hansen TM, Valeriani M, Drewes AM. Functional reorganization of brain networks in patients with painful chronic pancreatitis. Eur J Pain. 2014; doi:10.1002/j.1532-2149.2013.00442.x.

Lerch MM, Gorelick FS. Models of acute and chronic pancreatitis. Gastroenterology. 2013;144(6):1180–93. doi:10.1053/j.gastro.2012.12.043.

Levy P, Dominguez-Munoz E, Imrie C, Lohr M, Maisonneuve P. Epidemiology of chronic pancreatitis: burden of the disease and consequences. United European Gastroenterol J. 2014;2(5):345–54. doi:10.1177/2050640614548208.

Li J, Guo M, Hu B, Liu R, Wang R, Tang C. Does chronic ethanol intake cause chronic pancreatitis?: evidence and mechanism. Pancreas. 2008;37(2):189–95. doi:10.1097/MPA.0b013e31816459b7.

Lieb JG II, Forsmark CE, Lieb JG, Forsmark CE. Review article: pain and chronic pancreatitis. Aliment Pharmacol Ther. 2009;29:706–19.

Lieber CS, DeCarli LM. Liquid diet technique of ethanol administration: 1989 update. Alcohol Alcohol. 1989;24(3):197–211.

Lieber CS, Jones DP, Decarli LM. Effects of prolonged ethanol intake: production of fatty liver despite adequate diets. J Clin Invest. 1965;44:1009–21. doi:10.1172/JCI105200.

Liu L, Shenoy M, Pasricha PJ. Substance P and calcitonin gene related peptide mediate pain in chronic pancreatitis and their expression is driven by nerve growth factor. JOP. 2011;12:389–94.

Lohse J, Kraemer R. Calcium binding to the"stone protein" isolated from pancreatic stones of patients with chronic calcified pancreatitis. Hoppe Seylers Z Physiol Chem. 1984;365:549–54.

Lohse J, Vérnie HJ, Sarles H. Studies on pancreatic stones. I. In vitro dissolution. Digestion. 1981;21:125–32.

Lugea A, Gukovsky I, Gukovskaya AS, Pandol SJ. Nonoxidative ethanol metabolites alter extracellular matrix protein content in rat pancreas. Gastroenterology. 2003;125(6):1845–59.

Lugea A, Gong J, Nguyen J, Nieto J, French SW, Pandol SJ. Cholinergic mediation of alcohol-induced experimental pancreatitis. Alcohol Clin Exp Res. 2010;34(10):1768–81. doi:10.1111/j.1530-0277.2010.01264.x.

Malfertheiner P, Büchler M, Stanescu A, Ditschuneit H. Pancreatic morphology and function in relationship to pain in chronic pancreatitis. Int J Pancreatol. 1987;2:59–66.

Manes G, Büchler M, Pieramico O, Di Sebastiano P, Malfertheiner P. Is increased pancreatic pressure related to pain in chronic pancreatitis? Int J Pancreatol. 1994;15:113–7.

Mariani A, Bernard JP, Provansal-Cheylan M, et al. Differences of pancreatic stone morphology and content in patients with pancreatic lithiasis. Dig Dis Sci. 1991;36:1509–16.

Marrache F, Tu SP, Bhagat G, et al. Overexpression of interleukin-1betainthemurinepancreasresultsinchronic pancreatitis. Gastroenterology. 2008;135(4):1277–87. doi:10.1053/j.gastro.2008.06.078.

McIlwrath SL, Westlund KN. Pharmacological attenuation of chronic alcoholic pancreatitis induced hypersensitivity in rats. World J Gastroenterol. 2015;21(3):836–53. doi:10.3748/wjg.v21.i3.836.

Meier T, Wasner G, Faust M, Kuntzer T, Ochsner F, Hueppe M, Bogousslavsky J, Baron R. Efficacy of lidocaine patch 5% in the treatment of focal peripheral neuropathic pain syndromes: a randomized, double- blind, placebo-controlled study. Pain. 2003;106: 151–8.

Menke A, Yamaguchi H, Gress TM, Adler G. Extracellular matrix is reduced by inhibition of transforming growth factor beta1 in pancreatitis in the rat. Gastroenterology. 1997;113(1):295–303.

Miyahara T, Kawabuchi M, Goto M, Nakano I, Nada O, Nawata H. Morphological study of pancreatic endocrine in an experimental chronic pancreatitis with diabetes induced by stress and cerulein. Ultrastruct Pathol. 1999;23(3):171–80.

Miyauchi M, Suda K, Kuwayama C, Abe H, Kakinuma C. Role of fibrosis-related genes and pancreatic duct obstruction in rat pancreatitis models: implications for chronic pancreatitis. Histol Histopathol. 2007;22(10):1119–27.

Moran RA, James T, Pasricha PJ. Pancreatic pain. Curr Opin Gastroenterol. 2015;31:407–15.

Mori M, Fu X, Chen L, Zhang G, Higuchi K. Hereditary pancreatitis model WBN/Kob rat strain has a unique haplotype in the Pdwk1 region on chromosome 7. Exp Anim. 2009;58(4):409–13.

Mullady DK, Yadav D, Amann ST, et al. Type of pain, pain-associated complications, quality of life, disability and resource utilisation in chronic pancreatitis: a prospective cohort study. Gut. 2011;60: 77–84.

Multigner L, Daudon M, Montalto G, et al. Radiolucent pancreatic stones. New Engl J Med. 1986;314:248.

Muniraj T, Aslanian HR, Farrell J, Jamidar PA. Chronic pancreatitis, a comprehensive review and update. Part I: epidemiology, etiology, risk factors, genetics, pathophysiology, and clinical features. Dis Mon. 2014;60(12):530–50. doi:10.1016/j.disamonth.2014.11.002.

Nagai H, Ohtsubo K. Pancreatic lithiasis in the aged. Its clinicopathology and pathogenesis. Gastroenterology. 1984;86:331–8.

Nakamura M, Oka M, Iizuka N, et al. Osteopontin expression in chronic pancreatitis. Pancreas. 2002;25: 182–7.

Nakayama S, Nishio A, Yamashina M, et al. Acquired immunity plays an important role in the development of murine experimental pancreatitis induced by alcohol and lipopolysaccharide. Pancreas. 2014;43(1):28–36. doi:10.1097/MPA.0b013e3182a7c76b.

Neuschwander-Tetri BA, Bridle KR, Wells LD, Marcu M, Ramm GA. Repetitive acute pancreatic injury in the mouse induces procollagen alpha1(I) expression colocalized to pancreatic stellate cells. Lab Investig. 2000a;80(2):143–50.

Neuschwander-Tetri BA, Burton FR, Presti ME, et al. Repetitive self-limited acute pancreatitis induces pancreatic fibrogenesis in the mouse. Dig Dis Sci. 2000b;45(4):665–74.

Noda A, Hayakawa T, Kondo T, et al. Pancreatic stones dissolution with dimethadione (DMO). I. In vitro dissolution. Jpn J Gastroenterol. 1984;81:101–7.

Noda A, Ibuki E, Murayama H, Hase S. Bromhexine hydrochloride eliminates protein plugs and relieves attacks of pancreatitis. Pancreas. 1997;15:209–11.

Novis BH, Bornman PC, Girdwood AW, Marks IN. Endoscopic manometry of the pancreatic duct and sphincter zone in patients with chronic pancreatitis. Dig Dis Sci. 1985;30:225–8.

Ohashi K, Kim JH, Hara H, Aso R, Akimoto T, Nakama K. WBN/Kob rats. A new spontaneously occurring model of chronic pancreatitis. Int J Pancreatol. 1990;6(4):231–47.

Ohashi S, Nishio A, Nakamura H, et al. Overexpression of redox-active protein thioredoxin-1 prevents development of chronic pancreatitis in mice. Antioxid Redox Signal. 2006;8(9–10):1835–45. doi:10.1089/ars.2006.8.1835.

Okazaki K, Yamamoto Y, Ito K. Endoscopic measurement of papillary sphincter zone and pancreatic main ductal pressure in patients with chronic pancreatitis. Gastroenterology. 1986;91:409–18.

Olesen SS, Brock C, Krarup AL, Funch-Jensen P, Arendt-Nielsen L, Wilder-Smith OH, Drewes AM. Descending inhibitory pain modulation is impaired in patients with chronic pancreatitis. Clin Gastroenterol Hepatol. 2010a;8:724–30.

Olesen SS, Frøkjær JB, Lelic D, Valeriani M, Drewes AM. Pain-associated adaptive cortical reorganisation in chronic pancreatitis. Pancreatology. 2010b;10:742–51.

Olesen SS, Hansen TM, Graversen C, Steimle K, Wilder-Smith OHG, Drewes AM. Slowed EEG rhythmicity in patients with chronic pancreatitis: evidence of abnormal cerebral pain processing? Eur J Gastroenterol Hepatol. 2011;23:418–24.

Olesen SS, Graversen C, Bouwense SA, van Goor H, Wilder-Smith OH, Drewes AM. Quantitative sensory testing predicts pregabalin efficacy in painful chronic pancreatitis. PLoS One. 2013a;8:e57963.

Olesen SS, Hansen TM, Graversen C, Valeriani M, Drewes AM. Cerebral excitability is abnormal in patients with painful chronic pancreatitis. Eur J Pain. 2013b;17:46–54.

Pandol SJ, Lugea A, Mareninova OA, et al. Investigating the pathobiology of alcoholic pancreatitis. Alcohol Clin Exp Res. 2011;35(5):830–7. doi:10.1111/j.1530-0277.2010.01408.x.

Patel AG, Toyama MT, Alvarez C, Nguyen TN, Reber PU, Ashley SW, Reber HA. Pancreatic interstitial pH in human and feline chronic pancreatitis. Gastroenterology. 1995;109:1639–45.

Perides G, Tao X, West N, Sharma A, Steer ML. A mouse model of ethanol dependent pancreatic fibrosis. Gut. 2005;54(10):1461–7. doi:10.1136/gut.2004.062919.

Perkins PS, Rutherford RE, Pandol SJ. Effect of chronic ethanol feeding on digestive enzyme synthesis and mRNA content in rat pancreas. Pancreas. 1995;10(1):14–21.

Pfutzer RH, Tadic SD, Li HS, et al. Pancreatic cholesterol esterase, ES-10, and fatty acid ethyl ester synthase III gene expression are increased in the pancreas and liver but not in the brain or heart with long-term ethanol feeding in rats. Pancreas. 2002;25(1):101–6.

Pitchumoni CS. Special problems of tropical pancreatitis. Clin Gastroenterol. 1984;13(3):941–59.

Pitchumoni CS, Viswanathan KV, Gee Varghese PJ, et al. Ultrastructure and elemental composition of human pancreatic calculi. Pancreas. 1987;2:152–8.

Piubello W, Vantini I, Scuro LA, Novelli P, Benini L, Brocco G, Cavallini G. Gastric secretion, gastroduodenal histological changes, and serum gastrin in chronic alcoholic pancreatitis. Am J Gastroenterol. 1982;77:105–10.

Prinz RA, Aranha GV, Greenlee HB. Combined pancreatic duct and upper gastrointestinal and biliary tract drainage in chronic pancreatitis. Arch Surg. 1985;120:361–6.

Puig-Divi V, Molero X, Salas A, Guarner F, Guarner L, Malagelada JR. Induction of chronic pancreatic disease by trinitrobenzene sulfonic acid infusion into rat pancreatic ducts. Pancreas. 1996;13(4):417–24.

Puig-Divi V, Molero X, Vaquero E, Salas A, Guarner F, Malagelada J. Ethanol feeding aggravates morphological and biochemical parameters in experimental chronic pancreatitis. Digestion. 1999;60(2):166–74.

Renner IG, Rinderknecht H, Valenzuela JE, et al. Studies of pure pancreatic secretion in chronic alcoholic subjects without pancreatic insufficiency. Scand J Gastroenterol. 1980;15:241–4.

Renou C, Grandval P, Ville E, Laugier R. Endoscopic treatment of the main pancreatic duct: correlations among morphology, manometry, and clinical follow-up. Int J Pancreatol. 2000;27:143–9.

Rolny P, Arlebäck A, Järnerot G, Andersson T. Endoscopic manometry of the sphincter of Oddi and pancreatic duct in chronic pancreatitis. Scand J Gastroenterol. 1986;21:415–20.

Sarles H, Bernard JP. Lithostathine and pancreatic lithogenesis. Gastroenterol Int Ed Int. 1991;4:130–4.

Sarles H, Lebreuil G, Tasso F, et al. A comparison of alcoholic pancreatitis in rat and man. Gut. 1971;12(5):377–88.

Sarnthein J, Stern J, Aufenberg C, Rousson V, Jeanmonod D. Increased EEG power and slowed dominant frequency in patients with neurogenic pain. Brain. 2006;129:55–64.

Sato T, Miyashita E, Yamauchi H, Matsuno S. The role of surgical treatment for chronic pancreatitis. Ann Surg. 1986;203:266–71.

Saunders JH, Cargill JM, Wormsley KG. Gastric secretion of acid in patients with pancreatic disease. Digestion. 1978;17:365–9.

Schneider L, Pietschmann M, Hartwig W, et al. Alcohol pretreatment increases hepatic and pulmonary injury in experimental pancreatitis. Pancreatology. 2009;9(3):258–66. doi:10.1159/000181176.

Schulze S, Thorsgaard Pedersen N, Jørgensen MJ, Møllmann KM, Rune SJ. Association between duodenal bulb ulceration and reduced exocrine pancreatic function. Gut. 1983;24:781–3.

Schütte K, Waldthaler A, Malfertheiner P. Klinik der chronischen Pankreatitis. In: Beger HG, Büchler MW, Dralle H, Lerch MM, Malfertheiner P, Mössner J, Riemann JF, editors. Erkrankungen des Pankreas. Berlin: Springer; 2013. p. 92–4.

Schwaiger T, van den Brandt C, Fitzner B, et al. Autoimmune pancreatitis in MRL/Mp mice is a T cell-mediated disease responsive to cyclosporine A and rapamycin treatment. Gut. 2014;63(3):494–505. doi:10.1136/gutjnl-2012-303635.

Schwartz ES, La JH, Scheff NN, Davis BM, Albers KM, Gebhart GF. TRPV1 and TRPA1 antagonists prevent the transition of acute to chronic inflammation and pain in chronic pancreatitis. J Neurosci. 2013;33:5603–11.

Scoggins CR, Meszoely IM, Wada M, Means AL, Yang L, Leach SD. p53-dependent acinar cell apoptosis triggers epithelial proliferation in duct-ligated murine pancreas. Am J Physiol Gastrointest Liver Physiol. 2000;279(4):G827–36.

Seleznik GM, Reding T, Romrig F, et al. Lymphotoxin beta receptor signaling promotes development of autoimmune pancreatitis. Gastroenterology. 2012;143(5):1361–74. doi:10.1053/j.gastro.2012.07.112.

Sendler M, Dummer A, Weiss FU, et al. Tumour necrosis factor alpha secretion induces protease activation and acinar cell necrosis in acute experimental pancreatitis in mice. Gut. 2013;62(3):430–9. doi:10.1136/gutjnl-2011-300771.

Sendler M, Beyer G, Mahajan UM, et al. Complement component 5 mediates development of fibrosis, via activation of stellate cells, in 2 mouse models of chronic pancreatitis. Gastroenterology. 2015;149(3):765–76. e10. doi:10.1053/j.gastro.2015.05.012.

Sharer N, Schwarz M, Malone G, et al. Mutations of the cystic fibrosis gene in patients with chronic pancreatitis. N Engl J Med. 1998;339(10):645–52. doi:10.1056/NEJM199809033391001.

Snouwaert JN, Brigman KK, Latour AM, et al. An animal model for cystic fibrosis made by gene targeting. Science. 1992;257(5073):1083–8.

Steele CW, Karim SA, Foth M, et al. CXCR2 inhibition suppresses acute and chronic pancreatic inflammation. J Pathol. 2015;237(1):85–97. doi:10.1002/path.4555.

Steinberg AD, Roths JB, Murphy ED, Steinberg RT, Raveche ES. Effects of thymectomy or androgen administration upon the autoimmune disease of MRL/Mp-lpr/lpr mice. J Immunol. 1980;125(2):871–3.

Stewart TA. The human reg gene encodes pancreatic stone protein. Biochem J. 1989;260:622–3.

Tanaka T, Ichiba Y, Fujii Y, Itoh H, Kodama O, Dohi K. New canine model of chronic pancreatitis due to chronic ischemia with incomplete pancreatic duct obstruction. Digestion. 1988;41(3):149–55.

Tanaka T, Miura Y, Matsugu Y, Ichiba Y, Ito H, Dohi K. Pancreatic duct obstruction is an aggravating factor in the canine model of chronic alcoholic pancreatitis. Gastroenterology. 1998;115(5):1248–53.

Tatsumi Y, Lichtenberger LM. Molecular association of trinitrobenzenesulfonic acid and surface phospholipids in the development of colitis in rats. Gastroenterology. 1996;110(3):780–9.

Toma H, Winston J, Micci MA, Shenoy M, Pasricha PJ. Nerve growth factor expression is up-regulated in the rat model of L-arginine-induced acute pancreatitis. Gastroenterology. 2000;119:1373–81.

Treuting PM, Dintzis SM, Liggitt D, Charles W. Pancreas. In: Treuting PM, Dintzis SM, Montine KS, editors. Comparative anatomy and histology: a mouse and human atlas. New York: Elsevier; 2012. p. 203–9.

Tsujimoto T, Tsuruzono T, Hoppo K, Matsumura Y, Yamao J, Fukui H. Effect of bromhexine hydrochloride therapy for alcoholic chronic pancreatitis. Alcohol Clin Exp Res. 2005;29(suppl 12):272S–6S.

Tsukamoto H, Towner SJ, Yu GS, French SW. Potentiation of ethanol-induced pancreatic injury by dietary fat. Induction of chronic pancreatitis by alcohol in rats. Am J Pathol. 1988;131(2):246–57.

Tuteja AK, Biskupiak J, Stoddard GJ, Lipman AG. Opioid-induced bowel disorders and narcotic bowel syndrome in patients with chronic non-cancer pain. Neurogastroenterol Motil. 2010;22:424–30, e96.

Tuveson DA, Hingorani SR. Ductal pancreatic cancer in humans and mice. Cold Spring Harb Symp Quant Biol. 2005;70:65–72. doi:10.1101/sqb.2005.70.040.

Tympner F. Selectively aspirated pure pancreatic secretion. Viscosity, trypsin activity, protein concentration and lactoferrin content of pancreatic juice in chronic pancreatitis. Hepatogastroenterology. 1981;28:169–72.

Ugljesić M, Bulajić M, Milosavljević T, Stimec B. Endoscopic manometry of the sphincter of Oddi and pancreatic duct in patients with chronic pancreatitis. Int J Pancreatol. 1996;19:191–5.

Ulmasov B, Oshima K, Rodriguez MG, Cox RD, Neuschwander-Tetri BA. Differences in the degree of cerulein-induced chronic pancreatitis in C57BL/6 mouse substrains lead to new insights in identification of potential risk factors in the development of chronic pancreatitis. Am J Pathol. 2013;183(3):692–708. doi:10.1016/j.ajpath.2013.05.020.

Unal E, Atalay S, Tolan HK, et al. Biliopancreatic duct injection of ethanol as an experimental model of acute and chronic pancreatitis in rats. Int J Clin Exp Med. 2015;8(1):304–10.

Van Laethem JL, Robberecht P, Resibois A, Deviere J. Transforming growth factor beta promotes development of fibrosis after repeated courses of acute pancreatitis in mice. Gastroenterology. 1996;110(2):576–82.

Vaquero E, Molero X, Tian X, Salas A, Malagelada JR. Myofibroblast proliferation, fibrosis, and defective pancreatic repair induced by cyclosporin in rats. Gut. 1999;45(2):269–77.

Vaso A, Adahan HM, Gjika A, Zahaj S, Zhurda T, Vyshka G, Devor M. Peripheral nervous system origin of phantom limb pain. Pain. 2014;155:1384–91.

Vera-Portocarrero LP, Xie JY, Yie JX, Kowal J, Ossipov MH, King T, Porreca F. Descending facilitation from the rostral ventromedial medulla maintains visceral pain in rats with experimental pancreatitis. Gastroenterology. 2006;130:2155–64.

Vestergaard H, Kruse A, Rokkjaer M, Frobert O, Thommesen P, Funch-Jensen P. Endoscopic manometry of the sphincter of Oddi and the pancreatic and biliary ducts in patients with chronic pancreatitis. Scand J Gastroenterol. 1994;29:188–92.

Vijungco JD, Prinz RA. Management of biliary and duodenal complications of chronic pancreatitis. World J Surg. 2003;27:1258–70.

Wang RN, Kloppel G, Bouwens L. Duct- to islet-cell differentiation and islet growth in the pancreas of duct-ligated adult rats. Diabetologia. 1995;38(12):1405–11.

Wang Y, Wrennall JA, Cai Z, Li H, Sheppard DN. Understanding how cystic fibrosis mutations disrupt CFTR function: from single molecules to animal models. Int J Biochem Cell Biol. 2014;52:47–57. doi:10.1016/j.biocel.2014.04.001.

Warshaw AL, Banks PA, Fernández-Del Castillo C. AGA technical review: treatment of pain in chronic pancreatitis. Gastroenterology. 1998;115:765–76.

Watanabe S, Abe K, Anbo Y, Katoh H. Changes in the mouse exocrine pancreas after pancreatic duct ligation: a qualitative and quantitative histological study. Arch Histol Cytol. 1995;58(3):365–74.

Watkins-Chow DE, Pavan WJ. Genomic copy number and expression variation within the C57BL/6J inbred mouse strain. Genome Res. 2008;18(1):60–6. doi:10.1101/gr.6927808.

Weiss FU, Simon P, Bogdanova N, et al. Complete cystic fibrosis transmembrane conductance regulator gene sequencing in patients with idiopathic chronic pancreatitis and controls. Gut. 2005;54(10):1456–60. doi:10.1136/gut.2005.064808.

Weiss FU, Schurmann C, Guenther A, et al. Fucosyltransferase 2 (FUT2) non-secretor status and blood group B are associated with elevated serum lipase activity in asymptomatic subjects, and an increased risk for chronic pancreatitis: a genetic association study. Gut. 2015;64(4):646–56. doi:10.1136/gutjnl-2014-306930.

Whitcomb DC. Genetics of alcoholic and nonalcoholic pancreatitis. Curr Opin Gastroenterol. 2012;28(5):501–6. doi:10.1097/MOG.0b013e328356e7f3.

Whitcomb DC, Gorry MC, Preston RA, et al. Hereditary pancreatitis is caused by a mutation in the cationic trypsinogen gene. Nat Genet. 1996;14(2):141–5. doi:10.1038/ng1096-141.

Whitcomb DC, LaRusch J, Krasinskas AM, et al. Common genetic variants in the CLDN2 and PRSS1-PRSS2 loci alter risk for alcohol-related and sporadic pancreatitis. Nat Genet. 2012;44(12):1349–54. doi:10.1038/ng.2466.

White TT, Bourde J. A new observation on human intraductal pancreatic pressure. Surg Gynecol Obstet. 1970;130:275–8.

Wilcox CM, Yadav D, Ye T, et al. Chronic pancreatitis pain pattern and severity are independent of abdominal imaging findings. Clin Gastroenterol Hepatol. 2015;13:552–60,quiz e28–9.

Willert RP, Woolf CJ, Hobson AR, Delaney C, Thompson DG, Aziz Q. The development and maintenance of human visceral pain hypersensitivity is dependent on the *N*-methyl-D-aspartate receptor. Gastroenterology. 2004;126:683–92.

Wolf MJ, Seleznik GM, Zeller N, Heikenwalder M. The unexpected role of lymphotoxin beta receptor signaling in carcinogenesis: from lymphoid tissue formation to liver and prostate cancer development. Oncogene. 2010;29(36):5006–18. doi:10.1038/onc.2010.260.

Wong GY, Gavva NR. Therapeutic potential of vanilloid receptor TRPV1 agonists and antagonists as analgesics: recent advances and setbacks. Brain Res Rev. 2009;60:267–77.

Woodruff TM, Nandakumar KS, Tedesco F. Inhibiting the C5-C5areceptoraxis. Mol Immunol. 2011;48(14):1631–42. doi:10.1016/j.molimm.2011.04.014.

Woolf CJ. Central sensitization: implications for the diagnosis and treatment of pain. Pain. 2011;152:S2–15.

Woolf CJ, Salter MW. Neuronal plasticity: increasing the gain in pain. Science. 2000;288:1765–9.

Woolf CJ, Safieh-Garabedian B, Ma QP, Crilly P, Winter J. Nerve growth factor contributes to the generation of inflammatory sensory hypersensitivity. Neuroscience. 1994;62:327–31.

Xu G-Y, Winston JH, Shenoy M, Yin H, Pendyala S, Pasricha PJ. Transient receptor potential vanilloid 1 mediates hyperalgesia and is up-regulated in rats with chronic pancreatitis. Gastroenterology. 2007;133:1282–92.

Yadav D, Lowenfels AB. The epidemiology of pancreatitis and pancreatic cancer. Gastroenterology. 2013;144(6):1252–61. doi:10.1053/j.gastro.2013.01.068.

Yadav D, Timmons L, Benson JT, Dierkhising RA, Chari ST. Incidence, prevalence, and survival of chronic pancreatitis: a population-based study. Am J Gastroenterol. 2011;106(12):2192–9. doi:10.1038/ajg.2011.328.

Yadav D, O'Connell M, Papachristou GI. Natural history following the first attack of acute pancreatitis. Am J Gastroenterol. 2012;107(7):1096–103. doi:10.1038/ajg.2012.126.

Yamamoto M, Otani M, Otsuki M. A new model of chronic pancreatitis in rats. Am J Physiol Gastrointest Liver Physiol. 2006;291(4):G700–8. doi:10.1152/ajpgi.00502.2005.

Yarnitsky D, Granot M, Nahman-Averbuch H, Khamaisi M, Granovsky Y. Conditioned pain modulation predicts duloxetine efficacy in painful diabetic neuropathy. Pain. 2012;153:1193–8.

Zambreanu L, Wise RG, Brooks JCW, Iannetti GD, Tracey I. A role for the brainstem in central sensitisation in humans. Evidence from functional magnetic resonance imaging. Pain. 2005;114:397–407.

Zhao HF, Ito T, Gibo J, et al. Anti-monocyte chemoattractant protein 1 gene therapy attenuates experimental chronic pancreatitis induced by dibutyltin dichloride in rats. Gut. 2005;54(12):1759–67. doi:10.1136/gut.2004.049403.

Zhu Y, Colak T, Shenoy M, Liu L, Pai R, Li C, Mehta K, Pasricha PJ. Nerve growth factor modulates TRPV1 expression and function and mediates pain in chronic pancreatitis. Gastroenterology. 2011;141:370–7.

Pathogenetics of Chronic Pancreatitis

6

Zhuan Liao, Zhao-Shen Li, David N. Cooper, Claude Férec, and Jian-Min Chen

Abbreviations

CEL	Carboxyl ester lipase
CFTR	Cystic fibrosis transmembrane conductance regulator
CLDN2	Claudin-2
CPA1	Carboxypeptidase A1
CTRC	Chymotrypsin C
ERS	Endoplasmic reticulum stress
FUT2	Fucosyltransferase 2
GWAS	Genome-wide association study
ICP	Idiopathic chronic pancreatitis
MODY	Maturity-onset diabetes of the young
NACP	Nonalcoholic chronic pancreatitis
NAHR	Non-allelic homologous recombination
NMD	Nonsense-mediated mRNA decay
OR	Odds ratio
PCR	Polymerase chain reaction
RAP	Recurrent acute pancreatitis
RT-PCR	Reverse transcription polymerase chain reaction
SNP	Single nucleotide polymorphism
VNTR	Variable number tandem repeat

Chronic pancreatitis is a condition that is associated with the progressive inflammation of the pancreas which over time gives rise to irreversible morphological changes accompanied by impairment of both exocrine and endocrine functions (Majumder and Chari 2016). Over the last 20 years, molecular genetics has played an increasingly important role in elucidating the

Z. Liao • Z.-S. Li
Department of Gastroenterology, Changhai Hospital, the Second Military Medical University, Shanghai, China

Shanghai Institute of Pancreatic Diseases, Shanghai, China

D.N. Cooper
Institute of Medical Genetics, School of Medicine, Cardiff University, Cardiff, UK

C. Férec
Institut National de la Santé et de la Recherche Médicale (INSERM), Brest U1078, France

Faculté de Médecine et des Sciences de la Santé, Université de Bretagne Occidentale (UBO), Brest, France

Etablissement Français du Sang (EFS)—Bretagne, Brest, France

Laboratoire de Génétique Moléculaire et d'Histocompatibilité, Centre Hospitalier Universitaire (CHU) Brest, Hôpital Morvan, Brest, France

J.-M. Chen, M.D., Ph.D. (✉)
Institut National de la Santé et de la Recherche Médicale (INSERM), Brest U1078, France

Faculté de Médecine et des Sciences de la Santé, Université de Bretagne Occidentale (UBO), Brest, France

Etablissement Français du Sang (EFS)—Bretagne, Brest, France
e-mail: Jian-Min.Chen@univ-brest.fr

Z.-S. Li et al. (eds.), *Chronic Pancreatitis*, DOI 10.1007/978-981-10-4515-8_6

aetiology of chronic pancreatitis. The dawn of the new era in the genetic analysis of autosomal dominant hereditary pancreatitis (OMIM #167800) was heralded by the mapping of a disease locus to the long arm of chromosome 7 (Le Bodic et al. 1996; Pandya et al. 1996; Whitcomb et al. 1996b) and the subsequent identification of a gain-of-function missense mutation (i.e., p.Arg122His) in the cationic trypsinogen gene (*PRSS1*; OMIM #276000) (Whitcomb et al. 1996a). Thereafter, a steady stream of chronic pancreatitis susceptibility (or protective) variants in different genes has been reported. The analysis of variants in four specific genes, all highly expressed in human pancreatic acinar cells [*PRSS1*, *PRSS2* (encoding anionic trypsinogen; OMIM #601564), *SPINK1* (encoding pancreatic secretory trypsin inhibitor; OMIM #167790) and *CTRC* (encoding chymotrypsin C, which specifically degrades all human trypsinogen/trypsin isoforms (OMIM #601405) (Szmola and Sahin-Tóth 2007))] has firmly established the importance of a homeostatic balance between the activation and inactivation of trypsinogen within the pancreas, thereby defining a trypsin-dependent pathway in the pathogenesis of chronic pancreatitis. Whereas gain-of-function missense mutations and copy number variants in *PRSS1* (Le Maréchal et al. 2006; Whitcomb et al. 1996a) and loss-of-function variants in *SPINK1* (Witt et al. 2000) and *CTRC* (Masson et al. 2008b; Rosendahl et al. 2008) predispose to chronic pancreatitis, loss-of-function variants in *PRSS1* (Boulling et al. 2015; Chen et al. 2003; Derikx et al. 2015; Whitcomb et al. 2012) and *PRSS2* (Witt et al. 2006) protect against the disease.

In past years, we have comprehensively reviewed the genetics and pathogenesis of chronic pancreatitis (Chen and Férec 2009, 2012). Herein we summarize the main developments of the last 5 years, focusing on (i) the conservative assessment of the major genetic causes of idiopathic chronic pancreatitis (ICP), (ii) the emerging pathway of misfolding-induced endoplasmic reticulum stress (ERS) in the aetiology of chronic pancreatitis, (iii) new findings from the first genome-wide association study (GWAS) performed on chronic pancreatitis, (iv) the association of rare functional *CPA1* variants with chronic pancreatitis, (v) the involvement of *CEL–HYB* alleles in chronic pancreatitis, and (vi) some other recent developments. The interested reader is invited to consult several other recent review articles that provide slightly different perspectives (Aghdassi et al. 2015; Masamune 2014; Mounzer and Whitcomb 2013; Paliwal et al. 2014; Ravi Kanth and Nageshwar Reddy 2014).

1 A Conservative Assessment of the Major Genetic Causes of ICP

ICP may be defined as chronic pancreatitis in the absence of any obvious precipitating factors (e.g., alcohol abuse) and a family history of the disease (Chen and Férec 2009). We have recently attempted to make a conservative assessment of the major genetic causes of ICP in a group of 253 young French patients. To this end, we analysed for the first time not only micro-lesions (comprising coding sequence variants and variants at intron/exon boundaries) but also gross genomic rearrangements in the four firmly established chronic pancreatitis genes [namely *PRSS1*, *SPINK1*, *CTRC* and *CFTR* (cystic fibrosis transmembrane conductance regulator; OMIM #602421)]. We classified the sequence variants/genotypes into three categories (viz. causative, contributory or neutral) taking into consideration the following four parameters: (i) their allele frequencies in both patient and normal control populations, (ii) their presumed or experimentally confirmed functional effects, (iii) the relative importance of their associated genes in the pathogenesis of chronic pancreatitis, and (iv) gene-gene interactions wherever applicable. Adoption of this strategy allowed us to assess the pathogenic relevance of specific variants/genotypes to their respective carriers to an unprecedented degree (Masson et al. 2013). The genetic cause of ICP could be unequivocally assigned in 23.7% of individuals in the study group. A strong genetic susceptibility factor was also identified in an additional 24.5% of cases. Taken together, up to 48.2% of the studied ICP patients were found to display evidence of a genetic basis for their disease phenotype (Masson et al. 2013).

2 The Emerging Pathway of Misfolding-Induced ERS in the Aetiology of Chronic Pancreatitis

In eukaryotic cells, the endoplasmic reticulum is essential for the folding and trafficking of secretory proteins. Environmental insults or increased protein synthesis often lead to protein misfolding in the organelle, the accumulation of misfolded or unfolded proteins—known as ERS—and the activation of the adaptive unfolded protein response to restore homeostasis. However, misfolded proteins that result from heritable mutations may cause persistent ERS leading to genetic disease (Oakes and Papa 2015; Wang and Kaufman 2016).

That a subset of chronic pancreatitis-associated variants might exert their effect through misfolding-induced ERS was first suggested in 2009. Unlike some *in vitro* expressed PRSS1 mutants including p.Ala16Val, p. Asn29Ile, p.Asn29Thr and p.Arg122His which were secreted normally, the p.Arg116Cys mutant exhibited significant protein misfolding both in the test tube and in living cells; further, in cells expressing the p.Arg116Cys mutant, the ERS markers immunoglobulin-binding protein (BiP) and the spliced form of the X-box binding protein-1 (XBP1s) were both elevated (Kereszturi et al. 2009a). Additional chronic pancreatitis-associated rare variants in the *PRSS1* and *CTRC* genes were recently found to exert their effects in a way consistent with the misfolding-induced ERS mechanism (Beer et al. 2013; Schnúr et al. 2014). Furthermore, defective *CPA1* variants (see Sect. 4) were often characterized by significantly decreased secretion, intracellular retention and degradation, implying involvement of misfolding-induced ERS; expression of the p.Asn256Lys variant, which was found in 7 chronic pancreatitis patients but not in controls, resulted in ERS in AR42J rat acinar cells (Witt et al. 2013).

3 The First GWAS Study of Chronic Pancreatitis

The year 2012 witnessed the publication of the first GWAS study of chronic pancreatitis (Whitcomb et al. 2012).

3.1 Identification of a Protective Single Nucleotide Polymorphism in the *PRSS1-PRSS2* Locus

In the GWAS study, the minor T allele of a common single nucleotide polymorphism (SNP), rs10273639:C/T, located 408 base-pairs upstream of the translational initiation codon of the *PRSS1* gene, was found to be significantly overrepresented in the control group as compared with the patient group (Whitcomb et al. 2012). This finding has been supported by several follow-up studies (Avanthi et al. 2015; Derikx et al. 2015; Giri et al. 2016; Masamune et al. 2015; Paliwal et al. 2016). Consistent with conferring a protective role against chronic pancreatitis, the minor T allele was associated with lower expression of *PRSS1* mRNA in human pancreatic tissue as compared with the major C allele (Whitcomb et al. 2012). However, as with many GWAS findings [for a review, see (Zhang et al. 2014)], whether the rs10273639 T allele is the causal variant or not remains unknown.

In general, proximal promoter regions of tissue-specific genes are enriched for regulatory elements (Forrest et al. 2014). We wondered whether rs10273639 was in linkage disequilibrium with another polymorphism within the proximal promoter of *PRSS1*. We therefore resequenced the promoter region of *PRSS1* in 287 French individuals of European ancestry and found that rs4726576:C/A, which is located 204 bp upstream of the translational initiation codon of *PRSS1*, is in perfect linkage disequilibrium ($r^2 = 1$) with rs10273639:C/T. Employing promoter reporter gene assays in both rat pancreatic acinar AR42J cell and mouse parenchymal pancreatic tissue models, we provided evidence to support the view that it is the minor A allele of rs4726576 which underlies the aforementioned protective effect (Boulling et al. 2015).

The identification of a polymorphism other than that identified in the original studies as being the causal variant may have diagnostic implications since the two variants of interest may not always be in perfect linkage disequilibrium. Indeed, when we calculated linkage disequilibrium between rs4726576 and rs10273639 from the 1000 Genomes Project Phase 3 data, we found that the degree of linkage disequilibrium varies significantly between five meta-populations: r^2 values in South Asian, European, Asian, American, and African were 1.000, 0.996, 0.994, 0.977, and 0.797, respectively (Boulling et al. 2015). The problem appeared to be most serious in the African meta-population: whereas the TC diplotype (i.e., rs10273639T in *cis* with rs4726576C) carriers, who accounted for 5.5% of subjects, should be regarded as carrying a risk allele, they would have been ascertained as carrying a protective allele if the minor T allele of rs10273639 were thought to be causal (Nemeth and Sahin-Tóth 2014).

More recently, we extended our resequencing of the *PRSS1* promoter region (Boulling et al. 2015) to 626 French Caucasians (242 ICP patients and 384 controls). We discovered three additional variants (c.-184G>A, c.-173C>T and c.-147C>T), each being found only once in either a patient or a control. We analysed these three variants, together with a known *PRSS1* promoter variant (c.-30_-28delTCC) long considered to be causative for chronic pancreatitis (Férec et al. 1999), by luciferase promoter reporter assay in AR42J cells treated with dexamethasone. This analysis revealed that c.-30_-28delTCC resulted in reduced rather than increased *PRSS1* gene expression, suggesting that it is not a chronic pancreatitis risk factor as originally claimed. Moreover, we provided evidence that c.-147C>T probably confers protection against chronic pancreatitis by reducing the affinity of an ATF4 transcription factor binding site (Boulling et al. 2016). That loss of function regulatory variants in the promoter region of the *PRSS1* gene protect against chronic pancreatitis (Boulling et al. 2015, 2016; Whitcomb et al. 2012) complement previous observations that gains of trypsinogen copy number cause or predispose to the disease (Le Maréchal et al. 2006; Masson et al. 2008a).

3.2 Identification of a Risk SNP in the *CLDN2* Locus

The GWAS study also identified a SNP in the X-linked and pancreas-expressed *CLDN2* (claudin-2; OMIM #300520) locus that appeared to be significantly associated with chronic pancreatitis (Whitcomb et al. 2012). Supporting data were obtained from multiple replication studies (Avanthi et al. 2015; Derikx et al. 2015; Giri et al. 2016; Masamune et al. 2015; Paliwal et al. 2016). The *CLDN2* risk allele was reported to be associated with the atypical localization of CLDN2 in pancreatic acinar cells, but whether this allele is the causal variant underlying the chronic pancreatitis or simply a linkage disequilibrium marker remains to be clarified.

4 Rare Functional *CPA1* Variants and Chronic Pancreatitis

Procarboxypeptidase A1 is the precursor and inactive form of the digestive enzyme carboxypeptidase A1 (CPA1; OMIM #114850). Procarboxypeptidase A1, a component of the pancreatic zymogen activation cascade (Chen and Férec 2009), is the sec most abundantly synthesized protein after trypsinogens in the pancreatic juice (Scheele et al. 1981). Earlier findings from the study of the *PRSS1*, *PRSS2*, *SPINK1* and *CTRC* genes prompted Witt and colleagues to analyse the *CPA1* as a candidate gene for chronic pancreatitis (Witt et al. 2013). They found an overrepresentation of functionally defective *CPA1* variants (defined as having enzyme activity <20% of the wild-type) in German patients with nonalcoholic chronic pancreatitis (NACP; including idiopathic and familial subtypes) as compared with controls (3.1%

(29/944) vs. 0.1% (5/3938); odds ratio (OR) = 24.9, $P = 1.5 \times 10^{-16}$). The association was strongest for the German patients aged ≤10 years, where the detection frequency was nearly 10% (22/228) and the corresponding OR was as high as 84.0 (Witt et al. 2013). Functionally impaired *CPA1* variants were also found to be significantly overrepresented in NACP patients in a European replication study, albeit with an approximately seven-fold lower OR and a much higher *P* value (Witt et al. 2013). Replications in two small Asian cohorts provided further supporting data (Witt et al. 2013). However, given the remarkable differences in the occurrence and distribution of rare functional *CPA1* variants between the different populations and the small sizes of the two Asian cohorts so far analysed, further independent replication in larger studies is required (MacArthur et al. 2014).

The two other human pancreatic carboxypeptidase genes, *CPA2* and *CPB1*, were recently analysed in 477 Japanese patients with chronic pancreatitis (234 alcoholic, 243 nonalcoholic) and in 497 German patients with nonalcoholic chronic pancreatitis by targeted next-generation sequencing and/or Sanger sequencing. Secretion and the enzymatic activity of *CPA2* and *CPB1* variants were both determined after transfection into HEK 293T cells. None of the *CPA2* or *CPB1* variants, including those resulting in a marked loss of function, were found to be overrepresented in patients with chronic pancreatitis (Nakano et al. 2015).

5 *CEL-HYB* Alleles and Chronic Pancreatitis

5.1 *CEL-HYB* Allele Discovery

CEL encodes carboxyl ester lipase (OMIM #114840), a digestive enzyme synthesized and secreted in abundance by the pancreatic acinar cells (Holmes and Cox 2011). The *CEL* gene is highly polymorphic by virtue of a 33-bp variable number tandem repeat (VNTR) in its eleventh and last exon; the repeat number varies from 9 to 23 in the normal population, the most common allele containing 16 repeats (Lindquist et al. 2002). Single nucleotide deletions occurring within this VNTR region have been reported to cause autosomal dominant maturity-onset diabetes of the young (MODY) (Raeder et al. 2006).

MODY is characterized by endocrine and exocrine dysfunctions of the pancreas. Therefore, Fjeld and colleagues analysed *CEL* as a candidate gene for chronic pancreatitis (Fjeld et al. 2015). They found that a hybrid allele (*CEL-HYB*), involving the *CEL* gene and its tandemly linked pseudogene *CELP*, was significantly overrepresented in chronic pancreatitis cases as compared with controls, firstly in a discovery cohort of patients with familial chronic pancreatitis and then in three replication cohorts of patients with ICP. This hybrid allele resulted from non-allelic homologous recombination (NAHR) occurring between *CEL* intron 10 and *CELP* intron 10′. The consequent replacement of the eleventh and last exon of *CEL* by *CELP* exon 11′ was predicted to yield a premature stop codon within the third "pseudo" 33-bp VNTR (Fig. 6.1a). The truncated CPA1 enzyme is more stable than its wild-type counterpart and induced autophagy in cellular models (Fjeld et al. 2015). Autophagy is a homeostatic process or regulated destructive mechanism of the cell that disassembles unnecessary or dysfunctional components (Klionsky 2008). It is widely implicated in many pathophysiological processes such as cancer, metabolic and neurodegenerative disorders, and cardiovascular and pulmonary diseases (Choi et al. 2013). Findings from experimental models and genetically altered mice demonstrated that this principal cellular degradative pathway was also impaired in pancreatitis (Gukovskaya and Gukovsky 2012).

5.2 The *CEL-HYB* Allele Probably Represents an Ethnicity-Specific Risk Factor

The patients analysed in the Fjeld study were solely of European ancestry (Fjeld et al. 2015).

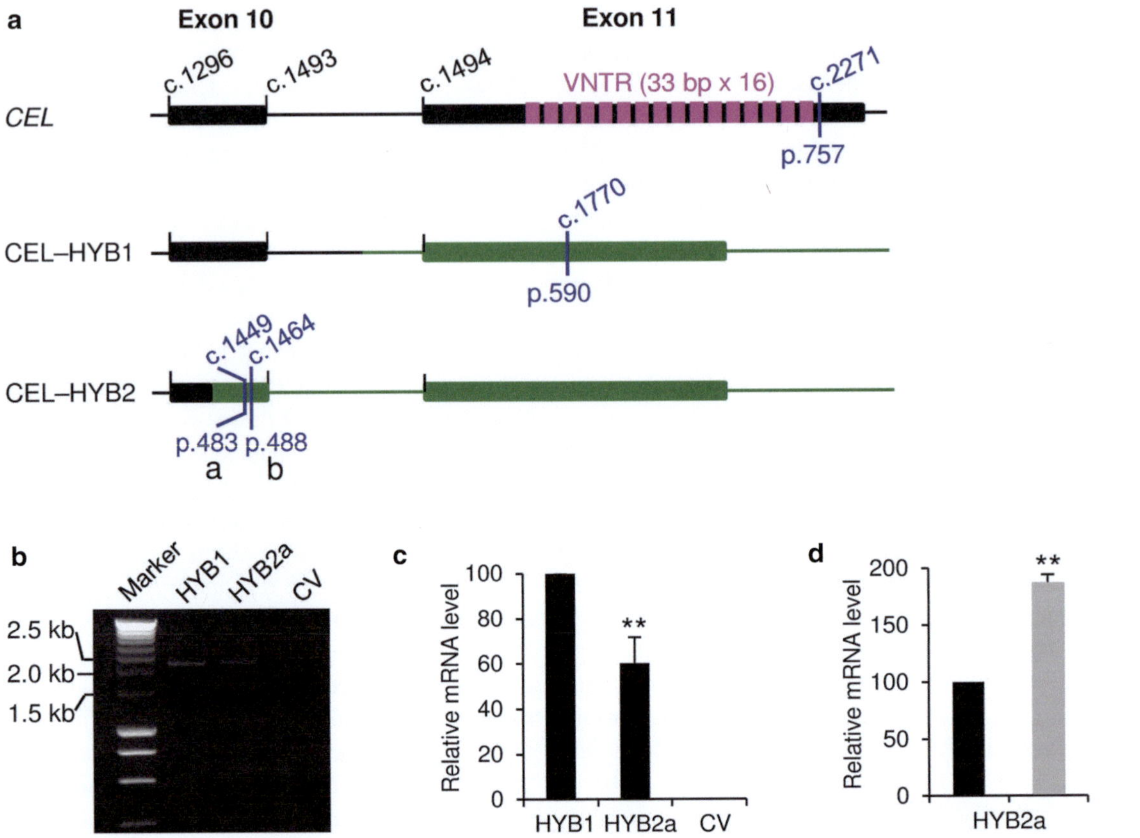

Fig. 6.1 (**a**) Key differences between *CEL-HYB1* [originally termed *CEL-HYB* (Fjeld et al. 2015)], *CEL-HYB2* and the wild-type *CEL* gene in terms of the defining exon 10, intron 10 and exon 11 sequences. The gene structure of *CEL* (*in black*) and that of the replacement *CELP* sequences (*in green*) within *CEL-HYB1* and *CEL-HYB2* were described in accordance with GenBank accession number AF072711.1. In *CEL*, the VNTRs within exon 11 are indicated in *purple*; nucleotide positions of the exon 10 boundaries and the beginning of exon 11 are numbered by reference to the A of the translational initiation codon ATG as c.1; the translational termination codon is denoted by a *vertical blue bar*, with the last coding nucleotide and the amino acid position of the translational termination codon being numbered above and below the bar. In *CEL-HYB1*, *CEL-HYB2a* and *CEL-HYB2b*, the presumed premature stop codons are indicated in a similar manner. (**b**) A representative gel showing the RT-PCR analyses of HEK293T cells transfected with expression constructs carrying the full-length *CEL-HYB1* and *CEL-HYB2a* genomic sequences. Sanger sequencing of the approximately 2.2-kb *CEL-HYB1* and *CEL-HYB2a* products revealed that all introns were spliced correctly. *CV* control vector. (**c**) Relative mRNA expression levels of *CEL-HYB2a* versus *CEL-HYB1 in vitro* as determined by quantitative RT-PCR analyses. *CV* control vector. (**d**) Relative mRNA expression levels of *CEL-HYB2a* in transfected cells with (*grey*) and without (*black*) cycloheximide treatment as determined by quantitative RT-PCR analyses. $^{**}P < 0.01$. Reprinted from Gastroenterology, Vol 150, Zou WB, Boulling A, Masamune A, Issarapu P, Masson E, Wu H, Sun XT, Hu LH, Zhou DZ, He L, Fichou Y, Nakano E, Hamada S, Kakuta Y, Kume K, Isayama H, Paliwal S, Mani KR, Bhaskar S, Cooper DN, Férec C, Shimosegawa T, Chandak GR, Chen JM, Li ZS, Liao Z, No association between *CEL-HYB* hybrid allele and chronic pancreatitis in Asian populations, 1558–1560.e5, Copyright (2016), with permission from Elsevier

We therefore attempted to replicate the association between *CEL-HYB* and chronic pancreatitis in three Asian (Chinese, Japanese, and Indian) populations. Contrary to expectation, we failed to identify the aforementioned *CEL-HYB* allele in any of our three cohorts (Zou et al. 2016c).

Instead, we found an alternative *CEL-HYB* allele, which was not found to be associated with ICP in any of our cohorts. This alternative allele resulted from an NAHR event occurring within a 239-bp sequence tract affecting the intron 9/exon 10 boundary of *CEL* and the intron 9′/exon 10′ boundary of *CELP* (Fig. 6.1a). To distinguish the two *CEL-HYB* alleles, we termed them respectively *CEL-HYB1* and *CEL-HYB2*. *CEL-HYB2* was further divided into two subtypes by reference to three SNPs present within the substituting *CELP* sequence (Zou et al. 2016c).

The allele frequency of *CEL-HYB1* in healthy German and French populations is approximately 0.4% (Fjeld et al. 2015). *CEL-HYB1* thus falls into the category of rare variants in accordance with current terminology (Manolio et al. 2009; Tennessen et al. 2012). Given that most rare variants are population-specific (Tennessen et al. 2012), *CEL-HYB1* most likely represents an ethnicity-specific disease risk factor. This issue could be clarified by the analysis of *CEL-HYB1* in an independent cohort of European ancestry such as the North American Pancreatitis Study II cohort (LaRusch et al. 2015).

5.3 Molecular Mechanisms Underlying the Contrasting Phenotypes of *CEL-HYB1* and *CEL-HYB2*

The contrasting phenotypic consequences of *CEL-HYB1* and *CEL-HYB2* imply very different effects on gene expression and/or protein function. In this regard, we noted that whereas *CEL-HYB2* variants harbour a premature stop codon within the second last exon, *CEL-HYB1* variants harbour a premature stop codon within the last exon (Fig. 6.1a). We therefore surmised that *CEL-HYB2* mRNAs could be subject to significant degradation by nonsense-mediated mRNA decay (NMD); by contrast, this may not be the case for *CEL-HYB1* because mRNAs that harbour a stop codon in the final exon usually escape degradation by NMD (Karam et al. 2013). To test these postulates, we amplified the full-length genomic *CEL-HYB2a* and *CEL-HYB1* sequences by means of polymerase chain reaction (PCR) from their corresponding carriers and cloned the resulting PCR products into the pcDNA3.1/V5-His-TOPO vector. Reverse transcription polymerase chain reaction (RT-PCR) analyses of mRNAs from subsequently transfected HEK293T cells indicated lower *CEL–HYB2a* mRNA expression as compared to *CEL-HYB1* (Fig. 6.1b). Further quantitative RT-PCR analyses demonstrated that the mRNA expression of *CEL-HYB2a* accounted for only 60% of that of *CEL-HYB1* (Fig. 6.1c). Finally, we tested whether the mRNA expression level of *CEL-HYB2a* could be increased by treatment of the transfected cells with cycloheximide, a known NMD inhibitor (Pereverzev et al. 2015) and found this to be the case (Fig. 6.1d). Consequently, we concluded that mRNA expression from the *CEL-HYB2a* allele is significantly reduced by NMD. We believe that this conclusion should apply to *CEL-HYB2b* due to its high sequence similarity with *CEL-HYB2a* (refer to Fig. 6.1a).

Finally, it is important to mention that pancreatic exocrine function has been found to be normal in *Cel*-knockout mice (Vesterhus et al. 2010). This finding, taken together with the significant degradation of *CEL-HYB2a* mRNA by NMD, was held to account for the apparent lack of any association between *CEL-HYB2a* and chronic pancreatitis (Zou et al. 2016c).

5.4 Implications for Variant Discovery in Complex Regions of the Human Genome

Classical molecular genetic techniques including long-range PCR, cloning and Sanger DNA sequencing were employed to identify and characterize the *CEL-HYB1* allele. Indeed, it is unlikely that the *CEL-HYB1* allele would have been discovered by the current high-throughput methodologies such as GWAS of common variants and whole exome sequencing. This suggests that many of the disease-associated variants that occur in complex regions of the human genome will fail to be identified by currently used high-throughput screening techniques (Fjeld et al. 2015).

6 Some Other Recent Developments

6.1 A Comprehensive Functional Annotation of *SPINK1* Intronic Variants

In vitro functional analysis often represents the only practical means to ascertain the pathogenicity of patient-derived sequence variants, particularly when they are individually rare. Various examples have recently been provided in the context of *SPINK1* intronic variants.

A mini-gene splicing assay is currently the most frequently used method to evaluate the effect of intronic variants on splicing. The *SPINK1* c.101A > G (p.Asn34Ser) variant and the four intronic variants in linkage disequilibrium with it were previously subjected to such analysis (Kereszturi et al. 2009b). These variants were also analysed in the context of a full gene splicing assay wherein the full-length *SPINK1* genomic sequence (approximately 7 kb stretching from the translational initiation codon to the stop codon of the gene) was cloned into the pcDNA3.1/V5-His-TOPO vector (Boulling et al. 2012). This latter expression system is strongly representative of the *in vivo* situation, as indicated by the observed splicing patterns of the wild-type sequence and two *SPINK1* splice site variants, c.87 + 1G>A and c.194 + 2T>C (Zou et al. 2016a). Employing this assay system, we confirmed previous conclusions with respect to two known pathogenic variants and five presumed non-pathogenic variants, establishing that seven previously reported variants of unknown clinical significance were not of pathological significance (Zou et al. 2016a). We also excluded all ten newly found intronic variants from a pilot resequencing study of the *SPINK1* gene from further consideration of their pathological relevance (Zou et al. 2016b).

6.2 An Explanation for Why No Chronic Pancreatitis-Predisposing Variants in the *PRSS2* Gene Have Ever Been Described

Anionic trypsinogen (encoded by *PRSS2*) is the second major and functional trypsinogen isoform in the human pancreatic juice after cationic trypsinogen (encoded by *PRSS1*); the two trypsinogen isoforms share 89% similarity at the amino acid sequence level (Chen et al. 2013b). It has been something of a puzzle that no variants in the *PRSS2* gene have ever been reported to predispose to chronic pancreatitis (Chen et al. 1999; Idris et al. 2005; Whitcomb et al. 1996b; Witt et al. 2006). Recently, a plausible explanation was put forward to account for this (Jancso and Sahin-Tóth 2016). Having compared CTRC-related biochemical properties of anionic and cationic trypsinogens, these authors concluded that anionic trypsinogen is controlled by CTRC in such a manner that individual natural *PRSS2* mutations could not render the mutant anionic trypsin stable enough to promote intra-pancreatic activation.

6.3 A Novel Disease-Causing Gene Conversion Mutation in the *PRSS1* Gene

Gene conversion, one of the two mechanisms of homologous recombination, involves the unidirectional transfer of genetic material from a 'donor' sequence to a highly homologous 'acceptor' (Chen et al. 2007). The *PRSS1* gene and four of its five paralogs are tandemly linked on chromosome 7q35 (see below for *PRSS3* translocated to chromosome 9). These clustered paralogs share approximately 91% nucleotide sequence similarity, providing the molecular basis for gene conversion occurring between them (Chen et al. 2013a). Several chronic pancreatitis-causing mutations in the *PRSS1* gene have been previously considered to result from gene conversion (Chen et al. 2000; Chen and Férec 2000a, b; Teich et al. 2005). Recently, a new gene conversion affecting the *PRSS1* gene was found in two unrelated patients with chronic pancreatitis. This event resulted in the replacement of 24–71 nucleotides in exon 3 of the *PRSS1* gene by the corresponding sequence of *PRSS3P2*, one of the pseudo-trypsinogen genes. The mutant *PRSS1* allele was predicted to encode a protein with three missense mutations including the disease-causing p.Arg122His (Rygiel et al. 2015).

6.4 A Chronic-Pancreatitis-Associated *CTRC* Variant Resembling One of the Evolutionary Signatures of Human Mesotrypsinogen in Terms of Biochemical Properties

Mesotrypsinogen (encoded by *PRSS3*) is the third and last functional trypsinogen isoform (Chen et al. 2013b). *PRSS1* and *PRSS2* are both located on chromosome 7q35 whereas *PRSS3* was translocated to chromosome 9p13 some 15–20 million years ago (Rowen et al. 2005). This translocation liberated *PRSS3* from its shared functional or regulatory constraints exerted at the original locus, reflected by the dramatic differences between mesotrypsinogen and the cationic and anionic trypsinogens in terms of their expression levels in the pancreas and their biochemical properties (Nyaruhucha et al. 1997; Rinderknecht et al. 1984; Szmola et al. 2003). Remarkably, virtually all the unique properties of mesotrypsin may be attributed to an ancestral mutation that replaced a glycine residue at position 198 with an arginine (i.e., the amino acid position 198 is arginine in mesotrypsinogen but glycine in both cationic and anionic trypsinogens); the mutation of Arg198 in mesotrypsin back to Gly converted mesotrypsin to a normal trypsin (Szmola et al. 2003). Therefore, p.Gly198Arg represents part of the evolutionary signature of mesotrypsinogen.

A *CTRC* variant, p.Gly214Arg, was identified in a subject with chronic pancreatitis in Slovakia (Szabó et al. 2015a). Biochemical characterization demonstrated that the mutant CTRC had increased activity on a small chromogenic peptide substrate but was markedly defective in cleaving bovine β-casein or the natural CTRC substrates human cationic trypsinogen and procarboxypeptidase A1. Consequently, the *CTRC* p.Gly214Arg mutation was considered to be analogous to the evolutionary p.Gly198Arg mutation in human mesotrypsin, which rendered this trypsin isoform resistant to proteinaceous inhibitors and conferred its ability to cleave these inhibitors (Szabó et al. 2015a). This finding nicely illustrates "how the same natural mutation in homologous pancreatic serine proteases can evolve a new physiological role or lead to pathology, determined by the biological context of protease function" (Szabó et al. 2015a).

6.5 The Common *CTRC* Synonymous Variant (c.180C>T) Increases Risk of Chronic Pancreatitis But Not Recurrent Acute Pancreatitis

Based on a review of clinical studies, Yadav and colleagues concluded that approximately 1/3 of patients with acute pancreatitis will develop recurrent acute pancreatitis (RAP) and approximately 1/3 of RAP patients will develop chronic pancreatitis (Yadav 2011; Yadav et al. 2012; Yadav and Lowenfels 2013). Patients with hereditary pancreatitis and those with a predisposing environmental factor such as alcohol abuse and smoking have the highest progression rate.

LaRush and co-workers evaluated the occurrence of *CTRC* variants in a total of 694 patients with chronic pancreatitis, 448 patients with RAP, and 1017 controls from the North American

Pancreatitis Study II cohort (LaRusch et al. 2015). They detected rare *CTRC* variants such as p. Ala73Thr and p.Arg254Trp in the chronic pancreatitis and/or RAP patients but the low detection rate and small sample sizes prevented them from obtaining a significant association. However, they found that the common synonymous variant, c.180C>T, was significantly associated with chronic pancreatitis but not RAP (LaRusch et al. 2015). The c.180C>T variant had been previously reported to be overrepresented in a small cohort (N = 42) of French patients with familial chronic pancreatitis (Masson et al. 2008b) and Indian patients with tropical chronic pancreatitis (Derikx et al. 2009; Paliwal et al. 2013).

The important message emanating from the finding of an association of the *CTRC* c.180C>T variant with chronic pancreatitis but not RAP is that loss of CTRC function accelerates progression from RAP to chronic pancreatitis (LaRusch et al. 2015). The c.180C>T variant was also found to be significantly associated with *CFTR* or *SPINK1* variants, alcohol and smoking, suggesting the involvement of complex genetic-genetic and genetic-environmental interactions in driving the rapid disease progression (LaRusch et al. 2015). These findings notwithstanding, whether the *CTRC* c.180C>T variant is itself functional or whether it instead represents a linkage disequilibrium marker, remains to be clarified.

6.6 Biological Mechanism Underlying *CFTR* Variants That Increase the Risk of Pancreatitis But Not Cystic Fibrosis

In the human exocrine pancreas, CFTR is predominantly expressed in the apical plasma membrane of the ductal and centroacinar cells, wherein its major function is thought to prevent the formation of protein plugs that predispose to pancreatic injury via dilution and alkalinisation of the protein-rich acinar secretions (Chen and Férec 2009). A diverse range of *CFTR* variants have been associated with idiopathic and alcoholic chronic pancreatitis, but the underlying biological mechanisms are unclear in most cases. The risk of pancreatitis in patients with cystic fibrosis appears to be determined by the type of *CFTR* mutation; somewhat paradoxically, it is the mild genotypes that confer an increased risk of pancreatitis as compared with the moderate-severe genotypes (Ooi et al. 2011). A recent study has shed light on this paradox. LaRusch and colleagues identified several *CFTR* variants in patients with chronic pancreatitis (and often sinus infections) and male infertility, but not other symptoms of cystic fibrosis (LaRusch et al. 2014). These mutant CFTR channels were shown to secrete chloride, which is important in the sweat glands, lung and intestine, but not bicarbonate, which is important in the pancreas, sinuses and male reproductive tract (LaRusch et al. 2014). In other words, these *CFTR* variants cause a selective bicarbonate defect in channel function, affecting organs that utilize CFTR for bicarbonate secretion but sparing organs that utilize CFTR for chloride secretion. Presumably, some *CFTR* variants may affect both channel functions but their respective effects may differ between variants.

6.7 ABO Blood Type B and Fucosyltransferase 2 Non-secretor Status as Genetic Risk Factors for Chronic Pancreatitis

Elevated serum lipase activity, at least three times the upper limit of normal, is a diagnostic marker of acute pancreatitis. Weiss and coworkers recently performed a two-step analysis to investigate whether high serum lipase activity confers an increased risk of chronic pancreatitis (Weiss et al. 2015). First, they found a significant association between higher serum lipase activity and three SNPs as well as the fucosyltransferase 2 (FUT2) non-secretor status (homozygosity for the *FUT2* p.Trp134Ter mutation) and the ABO blood type B by performing a GWAS on 3966 German volunteers from the population-based Study-of-Health-in-Pomerania with replication in 1444 blood donors. Then, they analysed FUT2 non-secretor status and ABO blood type B in more than 1000 patients with chronic pancreatitis, demonstrating a significant association for both factors (Weiss et al. 2015). These findings remain to be replicated using larger sample sizes and taking into considerations environmental factors (Kirsten et al. 2016; Weiss et al. 2016).

Conclusions

As opined by Molven and colleagues, the description of the *CEL* genetic variants associated with pancreatic disease suggests that there may be multiple pathways that lead to the development of chronic pancreatitis (Molven et al. 2016). In support of this idea, these authors cited the recent description of a mutation in the *PNLIP* gene (encoding pancreatic lipase) in two brothers with probable chronic pancreatitis (Behar et al. 2014; Szabó et al. 2015b). Because *CEL* and *PNLIP* have no apparent role in trypsinogen activation, risk variants found in these genes should predispose to chronic pancreatitis through a trypsin-independent pathway. It is clear that in the 20th anniversary year of the 1996 landmark discovery of the *PRSS1* gain-of-function missense mutation causing hereditary pancreatitis (Whitcomb et al. 1996a), our understanding of the pathogenetics of chronic pancreatitis is still very far from complete.

Acknowledgments The work was supported by the Conseil Régional de Bretagne, the Association des Pancréatites Chroniques Héréditaires, the Association de Transfusion Sanguine et de Biogénétique Gaetan Saleun, and the Institut National de la Santé et de la Recherche Médicale (INSERM), France; and the National Natural Science Foundation of China (81470884 and 81422010 to ZL), the Shuguang Program of Shanghai Education Development Foundation and Shanghai Municipal Education Commission (15SG33 to ZL) and the Chang Jiang Scholars Program of Ministry of Education (Q2015190 to ZL), China.

References

Aghdassi AA, Weiss FU, Mayerle J, Lerch MM, Simon P. Genetic susceptibility factors for alcohol-induced chronic pancreatitis. Pancreatology. 2015;15:S23–31.

Avanthi SU, Ravi Kanth VV, Agarwal J, Lakhtakia S, Gangineni K, Rao GV, Reddy DN, Talukdar R. Association of claudin2 and *PRSS1-PRSS2* polymorphisms with idiopathic recurrent acute and chronic pancreatitis: a case-control study from India. J Gastroenterol Hepatol. 2015;30:1796–801.

Beer S, Zhou J, Szabo A, Keiles S, Chandak GR, Witt H, Sahin-Tóth M. Comprehensive functional analysis of chymotrypsin C (*CTRC*) variants reveals distinct loss-of-function mechanisms associated with pancreatitis risk. Gut. 2013;62:1616–24.

Behar DM, Basel-Vanagaite L, Glaser F, Kaplan M, Tzur S, Magal N, Eidlitz-Markus T, Haimi-Cohen Y, Sarig G, Bormans C, Shohat M, Zeharia A. Identification of a novel mutation in the *PNLIP* gene in two brothers with congenital pancreatic lipase deficiency. J Lipid Res. 2014;55:307–12.

Boulling A, Chen JM, Callebaut I, Férec C. Is the *SPINK1* p.Asn34Ser missense mutation *per se* the true culprit within its associated haplotype? Webmed Central Gene. 2012;3:WMC003084.

Boulling A, Sato M, Masson E, Genin E, Chen JM, Férec C. Identification of a functional *PRSS1* promoter variant in linkage disequilibrium with the chronic pancreatitis-protecting rs10273639. Gut. 2015;64:1837–8.

Boulling A, Abrantes A, Masson E, Cooper DN, Robaszkiewicz M, Chen JM, Férec C. Discovery and functional annotation of *PRSS1* promoter variants in chronic pancreatitis. Hum Mutat. 2016;37:1149–52.

Chen JM, Férec C. Gene conversion-like missense mutations in the human cationic trypsinogen gene and insights into the molecular evolution of the human trypsinogen family. Mol Genet Metab. 2000a;71:463–9.

Chen JM, Férec C. Origin and implication of the hereditary pancreatitis-associated N21I mutation in the cationic trypsinogen gene. Hum Genet. 2000b;106:125–6.

Chen JM, Férec C. Chronic pancreatitis: genetics and pathogenesis. Annu Rev Genomics Hum Genet. 2009;10:63–87.

Chen JM, Férec C. Genetics and pathogenesis of chronic pancreatitis: the 2012 update. Clin Res Hepatol Gastroenterol. 2012;36:334–40.

Chen JM, Audrézet MP, Mercier B, Quéré I, Férec C. Exclusion of anionic trypsinogen and mesotrypsinogen involvement in hereditary pancreatitis without cationic trypsinogen gene mutations. Scand J Gastroenterol. 1999;34:831–2.

Chen JM, Raguénès O, Férec C, Deprez PH, Verellen-Dumoulin C. A CGC>CAT gene conversion-like event resulting in the R122H mutation in the cationic trypsinogen gene and its implication in the genotyping of pancreatitis. J Med Genet. 2000;37:E36.

Chen JM, Le Maréchal C, Lucas D, Raguénès O, Férec C. "Loss of function" mutations in the cationic trypsinogen gene (*PRSS1*) may act as a protective factor against pancreatitis. Mol Genet Metab. 2003;79:67–70.

Chen JM, Cooper DN, Chuzhanova N, Férec C, Patrinos GP. Gene conversion: mechanisms, evolution and human disease. Nat Rev Genet. 2007;8:762–75.

Chen JM, Cooper DN, Férec C. Trypsinogen genes: insights into molecular evolution from the study of pathogenic mutations. In: eLS. Chichester: Wiley. 2013a. http://www.els.net. doi: 10.1002/9780470015902.a0006140.pub3.

Chen JM, Radisky ES, Férec C. Human trypsins. In: Rawlings ND, Salvesen GS, editors. Handbook of proteolytic enzymes. Oxford: Academic; 2013b. p. 2600–9.

Choi AM, Ryter SW, Levine B. Autophagy in human health and disease. N Engl J Med. 2013;368:651–62.

Derikx MH, Szmola R, te Morsche RH, Sunderasan S, Chacko A, Drenth JP. Tropical calcific pancreatitis and its association with *CTRC* and *SPINK1* (p.N34S) variants. Eur J Gastroenterol Hepatol. 2009;21:889–94.

Derikx MH, Kovacs P, Scholz M, Masson E, Chen JM, Ruffert C, Lichtner P, Te Morsche RH, Cavestro GM, Férec C, Drenth JP, Witt H, Rosendahl J. Polymorphisms at *PRSS1-PRSS2* and *CLDN2-MORC4* loci associate with alcoholic and non-alcoholic chronic pancreatitis in a European replication study. Gut. 2015;64:1426–33.

Férec C, Raguénès O, Salomon R, Roche C, Bernard JP, Guillot M, Quéré I, Faure C, Mercier B, Audrézet MP, Guillausseau PJ, Dupont C, Munnich A, Bignon JD, Le Bodic L. Mutations in the cationic trypsinogen gene and evidence for genetic heterogeneity in hereditary pancreatitis. J Med Genet. 1999;36:228–32.

Fjeld K, Weiss FU, Lasher D, Rosendahl J, Chen JM, Johansson BB, Kirsten H, Ruffert C, Masson E, Steine SJ, Bugert P, Cnop M, Grutzmann R, Mayerle J, Mossner J, Ringdal M, Schulz HU, Sendler M, Simon P, Sztromwasser P, Torsvik J, Scholz M, Tjora E, Férec C, Witt H, Lerch MM, Njolstad PR, Johansson S, Molven A. A recombined allele of the lipase gene *CEL* and its pseudogene *CELP* confers susceptibility to chronic pancreatitis. Nat Genet. 2015;47:518–22.

Forrest AR, Kawaji H, Rehli M, Baillie JK, de Hoon MJ, Haberle V, Lassmann T, Kulakovskiy IV, Lizio M, Itoh M, Andersson R, Mungall CJ, Meehan TF, Schmeier S, Bertin N, Jorgensen M, Dimont E, Arner E, Schmidl C, Schaefer U, Medvedeva YA, Plessy C, Vitezic M, Severin J, Semple C, Ishizu Y, Young RS, Francescatto M, Alam I, Albanese D, Altschuler GM, Arakawa T, Archer JA, Arner P, Babina M, Rennie S, Balwierz PJ, Beckhouse AG, Pradhan-Bhatt S, Blake JA, Blumenthal A, Bodega B, Bonetti A, Briggs J, Brombacher F, Burroughs AM, Califano A, Cannistraci CV, Carbajo D, Chen Y, Chierici M, Ciani Y, Clevers HC, Dalla E, Davis CA, Detmar M, Diehl AD, Dohi T, Drablos F, Edge AS, Edinger M, Ekwall K, Endoh M, Enomoto H, Fagiolini M, Fairbairn L, Fang H, Farach-Carson MC, Faulkner GJ, Favorov AV, Fisher ME, Frith MC, Fujita R, Fukuda S, Furlanello C, Furino M, Furusawa J, Geijtenbeek TB, Gibson AP, Gingeras T, Goldowitz D, Gough J, Guhl S, Guler R, Gustincich S, Ha TJ, Hamaguchi M, Hara M, Harbers M, Harshbarger J, Hasegawa A, Hasegawa Y, Hashimoto T, Herlyn M, Hitchens KJ, Ho Sui SJ, Hofmann OM, Hoof I, Hori F, Huminiecki L, Iida K, Ikawa T, Jankovic BR, Jia H, Joshi A, Jurman G, Kaczkowski B, Kai C, Kaida K, Kaiho A, Kajiyama K, Kanamori-Katayama M, Kasianov AS, Kasukawa T, Katayama S, Kato S, Kawaguchi S, Kawamoto H, Kawamura YI, Kawashima T, Kempfle JS, Kenna TJ, Kere J, Khachigian LM, Kitamura T, Klinken SP, Knox AJ, Kojima M, Kojima S, Kondo N, Koseki H, Koyasu S, Krampitz S, Kubosaki A, Kwon AT, Laros JF, Lee W, Lennartsson A, Li K, Lilje B, Lipovich L, Mackay-Sim A, Manabe R, Mar JC, Marchand B, Mathelier A, Mejhert N, Meynert A, Mizuno Y, de Lima Morais DA, Morikawa H, Morimoto M, Moro K, Motakis E, Motohashi H, Mummery CL, Murata M, Nagao-Sato S, Nakachi Y, Nakahara F, Nakamura T, Nakamura Y, Nakazato K, van Nimwegen E, Ninomiya N, Nishiyori H, Noma S, Noazaki T, Ogishima S, Ohkura N, Ohimiya H, Ohno H, Ohshima M, Okada-Hatakeyama M, Okazaki Y, Orlando V, Ovchinnikov DA, Pain A, Passier R, Patrikakis M, Persson H, Piazza S, Prendergast JG, Rackham OJ, Ramilowski JA, Rashid M, Ravasi T, Rizzu P, Roncador M, Roy S, Rye MB, Saijyo E, Sajantila A, Saka A, Sakaguchi S, Sakai M, Sato H, Savvi S, Saxena A, Schneider C, Schultes EA, Schulze-Tanzil GG, Schwegmann A, Sengstag T, Sheng G, Shimoji H, Shimoni Y, Shin JW, Simon C, Sugiyama D, Sugiyama T, Suzuki M, Suzuki N, Swoboda RK, t Hoen PA, Tagami M, Takahashi N, Takai J, Tanaka H, Tatsukawa H, Tatum Z, Thompson M, Toyodo H, Toyoda T, Valen E, van de Wetering M, van den Berg LM, Verado R, Vijayan D, Vorontsov IE, Wasserman WW, Watanabe S, Wells CA, Winteringham LN, Wolvetang E, Wood EJ, Yamaguchi Y, Yamamoto M, Yoneda M, Yonekura Y, Yoshida S, Zabierowski SE, Zhang PG, Zhao X, Zucchelli S, Summers KM, Suzuki H, Daub CO, Kawai J, Heutink P, Hide W, Freeman TC, Lenhard B, Bajic VB, Taylor MS, Makeev VJ, Sandelin A, Hume DA, Carninci P, Hayashizaki Y. A promoter-level mammalian expression atlas. Nature. 2014;507:462–70.

Giri AK, Midha S, Banerjee P, Agrawal A, Mehdi SJ, Dhingra R, Kaur I, Ramesh Kumar G, Lakhotia R, Ghosh S, Das K, Mohindra S, Rana S, Bhasin DK, Garg PK, Bharadwaj D. Common variants in *CLDN2* and *MORC4* genes confer disease susceptibility in patients with chronic pancreatitis. PLoS One. 2016;11:e0147345.

Gukovskaya AS, Gukovsky I. Autophagy and pancreatitis. Am J Physiol Gastrointest Liver Physiol. 2012;303:G993–G1003.

Holmes RS, Cox LA. Comparative structures and evolution of vertebrate carboxyl ester lipase (*CEL*) genes and proteins with a major role in reverse cholesterol transport. Cholesterol. 2011;2011:781643.

Idris MM, Bhaskar S, Reddy DN, Mani KR, Rao GV, Singh L, Chandak GR. Mutations in anionic trypsinogen gene are not associated with tropical calcific pancreatitis. Gut. 2005;54:728–9.

Jancso Z, Sahin-Tóth M. Tighter control by chymotrypsin C (CTRC) explains lack of association between human anionic trypsinogen and hereditary pancreatitis. J Biol Chem. 2016;291:12897–905.

Karam R, Wengrod J, Gardner LB, Wilkinson MF. Regulation of nonsense-mediated mRNA decay: implications for physiology and disease. Biochim Biophys Acta. 2013;1829:624–33.

Kereszturi E, Szmola R, Kukor Z, Simon P, Weiss FU, Lerch MM, Sahin-Tóth M. Hereditary pancreatitis caused by mutation-induced misfolding of human cationic trypsinogen: a novel disease mechanism. Hum Mutat. 2009a;30:575–82.

Kereszturi E, Kiraly O, Sahin-Tóth M. Minigene analysis of intronic variants in common *SPINK1* haplotypes associated with chronic pancreatitis. Gut. 2009b;58:545–9.

Kirsten H, Scholz M, Kovacs P, Grallert H, Peters A, Strauch K, Frank J, Rietschel M, Nothen MM, Witt H, Rosendahl J. Genetic variants of lipase activity in chronic pancreatitis. Gut. 2016;65:184–5.

Klionsky DJ. Autophagy revisited: a conversation with Christian de Duve. Autophagy. 2008;4:740–3.

LaRusch J, Jung J, General IJ, Lewis MD, Park HW, Brand RE, Gelrud A, Anderson MA, Banks PA, Conwell D, Lawrence C, Romagnuolo J, Baillie J, Alkaade S, Cote G, Gardner TB, Amann ST, Slivka A, Sandhu B, Aloe A, Kienholz ML, Yadav D, Barmada MM, Bahar I, Lee MG, Whitcomb DC. Mechanisms of *CFTR* functional variants that impair regulated bicarbonate permeation and increase risk for pancreatitis but not for cystic fibrosis. PLoS Genet. 2014;10:e1004376.

LaRusch J, Lozano-Leon A, Stello K, Moore A, Muddana V, O'Connell M, Diergaarde B, Yadav D, Whitcomb DC. The common chymotrypsinogen C (*CTRC*) variant G60G (C.180T) increases risk of chronic pancreatitis but not recurrent acute pancreatitis in a North American population. Clin Transl Gastroenterol. 2015;6:e68.

Le Bodic L, Bignon JD, Raguénès O, Mercier B, Georgelin T, Schnee M, Soulard F, Gagne K, Bonneville F, Muller JY, Bachner L, Férec C. The hereditary pancreatitis gene maps to long arm of chromosome 7. Hum Mol Genet. 1996;5:549–54.

Le Maréchal C, Masson E, Chen JM, Morel F, Ruszniewski P, Levy P, Férec C. Hereditary pancreatitis caused by triplication of the trypsinogen locus. Nat Genet. 2006;38:1372–4.

Lindquist S, Blackberg L, Hernell O. Human bile salt-stimulated lipase has a high frequency of size variation due to a hypervariable region in exon 11. Eur J Biochem. 2002;269:759–67.

MacArthur DG, Manolio TA, Dimmock DP, Rehm HL, Shendure J, Abecasis GR, Adams DR, Altman RB, Antonarakis SE, Ashley EA, Barrett JC, Biesecker LG, Conrad DF, Cooper GM, Cox NJ, Daly MJ, Gerstein MB, Goldstein DB, Hirschhorn JN, Leal SM, Pennacchio LA, Stamatoyannopoulos JA, Sunyaev SR, Valle D, Voight BF, Winckler W, Gunter C. Guidelines for investigating causality of sequence variants in human disease. Nature. 2014;508:469–76.

Majumder S, Chari ST. Chronic pancreatitis. Lancet. 2016;387:1957–66.

Manolio TA, Collins FS, Cox NJ, Goldstein DB, Hindorff LA, Hunter DJ, McCarthy MI, Ramos EM, Cardon LR, Chakravarti A, Cho JH, Guttmacher AE, Kong A, Kruglyak L, Mardis E, Rotimi CN, Slatkin M, Valle D, Whittemore AS, Boehnke M, Clark AG, Eichler EE, Gibson G, Haines JL, Mackay TF, McCarroll SA, Visscher PM. Finding the missing heritability of complex diseases. Nature. 2009;461:747–53.

Masamune A. Genetics of pancreatitis: the 2014 update. Tohoku J Exp Med. 2014;232:69–77.

Masamune A, Nakano E, Hamada S, Kakuta Y, Kume K, Shimosegawa T. Common variants at *PRSS1-PRSS2* and *CLDN2-MORC4* loci associate with chronic pancreatitis in Japan. Gut. 2015;64:1345–6.

Masson E, Le Maréchal C, Chandak GR, Lamoril J, Bezieau S, Mahurkar S, Bhaskar S, Reddy DN, Chen JM, Férec C. Trypsinogen copy number mutations in patients with idiopathic chronic pancreatitis. Clin Gastroenterol Hepatol. 2008a;6:82–8.

Masson E, Chen JM, Scotet V, Le Maréchal C, Férec C. Association of rare chymotrypsinogen C (*CTRC*) gene variations in patients with idiopathic chronic pancreatitis. Hum Genet. 2008b;123:83–91.

Masson E, Chen JM, Audrezet MP, Cooper DN, Férec C. A conservative assessment of the major genetic causes of idiopathic chronic pancreatitis: data from a comprehensive analysis of *PRSS1*, *SPINK1*, *CTRC* and *CFTR* genes in 253 young French patients. PLoS One. 2013;8:e73522.

Molven A, Fjeld K, Lowe ME. Lipase genetic variants in chronic pancreatitis: when the end is wrong, all's not well. Gastroenterology. 2016;150:1515–8.

Mounzer R, Whitcomb DC. Genetics of acute and chronic pancreatitis. Curr Opin Gastroenterol. 2013;29:544–51.

Nakano E, Geisz A, Masamune A, Niihori T, Hamada S, Kume K, Kakuta Y, Aoki Y, Matsubara Y, Ebert K, Ludwig M, Braun M, Groneberg DA, Shimosegawa T, Sahin-Tóth M, Witt H. Variants in pancreatic carboxypeptidase genes *CPA2* and *CPB1* are not associated with chronic pancreatitis. Am J Physiol Gastrointest Liver Physiol. 2015;309:G688–94.

Nemeth BC, Sahin-Tóth M. Human cationic trypsinogen (*PRSS1*) variants and chronic pancreatitis. Am J Physiol Gastrointest Liver Physiol. 2014;306:G466–73.

Nyaruhucha CN, Kito M, Fukuoka SI. Identification and expression of the cDNA-encoding human mesotrypsin

(ogen), an isoform of trypsin with inhibitor resistance. J Biol Chem. 1997;272:10573–8.
Oakes SA, Papa FR. The role of endoplasmic reticulum stress in human pathology. Annu Rev Pathol. 2015;10:173–94.
Ooi CY, Dorfman R, Cipolli M, Gonska T, Castellani C, Keenan K, Freedman SD, Zielenski J, Berthiaume Y, Corey M, Schibli S, Tullis E, Durie PR. Type of *CFTR* mutation determines risk of pancreatitis in patients with cystic fibrosis. Gastroenterology. 2011;140:153–61.
Paliwal S, Bhaskar S, Mani KR, Reddy DN, Rao GV, Singh SP, Thomas V, Chandak GR. Comprehensive screening of chymotrypsin C (*CTRC*) gene in tropical calcific pancreatitis identifies novel variants. Gut. 2013;62:1602–6.
Paliwal S, Bhaskar S, Chandak GR. Genetic and phenotypic heterogeneity in tropical calcific pancreatitis. World J Gastroenterol. 2014;20:17314–23.
Paliwal S, Bhaskar S, Nageshwar Reddy D, Rao GV, Thomas V, Singh SP, Chandak GR. Association analysis of *PRSS1-PRSS2* and *CLDN2-MORC4* variants in nonalcoholic chronic pancreatitis using tropical calcific pancreatitis as model. Pancreas. 2016;45:1153–7.
Pandya A, Blanton SH, Landa B, Javaheri R, Melvin E, Nance WE, Markello T. Linkage studies in a large kindred with hereditary pancreatitis confirms mapping of the gene to a 16-cM region on 7q. Genomics. 1996;38:227–30.
Pereverzev AP, Gurskaya NG, Ermakova GV, Kudryavtseva EI, Markina NM, Kotlobay AA, Lukyanov SA, Zaraisky AG, Lukyanov KA. Method for quantitative analysis of nonsense-mediated mRNA decay at the single cell level. Sci Rep. 2015;5:7729.
Raeder H, Johansson S, Holm PI, Haldorsen IS, Mas E, Sbarra V, Nermoen I, Eide SA, Grevle L, Bjorkhaug L, Sagen JV, Aksnes L, Sovik O, Lombardo D, Molven A, Njolstad PR. Mutations in the *CEL* VNTR cause a syndrome of diabetes and pancreatic exocrine dysfunction. Nat Genet. 2006;38:54–62.
Ravi Kanth V, Nageshwar Reddy D. Genetics of acute and chronic pancreatitis: an update. World J Gastrointest Pathophysiol. 2014;5:427–37.
Rinderknecht H, Renner IG, Abramson SB, Carmack C. Mesotrypsin: a new inhibitor-resistant protease from a zymogen in human pancreatic tissue and fluid. Gastroenterology. 1984;86:681–92.
Rosendahl J, Witt H, Szmola R, Bhatia E, Ozsvari B, Landt O, Schulz HU, Gress TM, Pfutzer R, Lohr M, Kovacs P, Bluher M, Stumvoll M, Choudhuri G, Hegyi P, te Morsche RH, Drenth JP, Truninger K, Macek M Jr, Puhl G, Witt U, Schmidt H, Buning C, Ockenga J, Kage A, Groneberg DA, Nickel R, Berg T, Wiedenmann B, Bodeker H, Keim V, Mossner J, Teich N, Sahin-Tóth M. Chymotrypsin C (CTRC) variants that diminish activity or secretion are associated with chronic pancreatitis. Nat Genet. 2008;40:78–82.
Rowen L, Williams E, Glusman G, Linardopoulou E, Friedman C, Ahearn ME, Seto J, Boysen C, Qin S, Wang K, Kaur A, Bloom S, Hood L, Trask BJ. Interchromosomal segmental duplications explain the unusual structure of *PRSS3*, the gene for an inhibitor-resistant trypsinogen. Mol Biol Evol. 2005;22:1712–20.
Rygiel AM, Beer S, Simon P, Wertheim-Tysarowska K, Oracz G, Kucharzik T, Tysarowski A, Niepokoj K, Kierkus J, Jurek M, Gawlinski P, Poznanski J, Bal J, Lerch MM, Sahin-Tóth M, Weiss FU. Gene conversion between cationic trypsinogen (*PRSS1*) and the pseudogene trypsinogen 6 (*PRSS3P2*) in patients with chronic pancreatitis. Hum Mutat. 2015;36:350–6.
Scheele G, Bartelt D, Bieger W. Characterization of human exocrine pancreatic proteins by two-dimensional isoelectric focusing/sodium dodecyl sulfate gel electrophoresis. Gastroenterology. 1981;80:461–73.
Schnúr A, Beer S, Witt H, Hegyi P, Sahin-Tóth M. Functional effects of 13 rare *PRSS1* variants presumed to cause chronic pancreatitis. Gut. 2014;63:337–43.
Szabó A, Ludwig M, Hegyi E, Szépeová R, Witt H, Sahin-Tóth M. Mesotrypsin signature mutation in a chymotrypsin C (*CTRC*) variant associated with chronic pancreatitis. J Biol Chem. 2015a;290:17282–92.
Szabó A, Xiao X, Haughney M, Spector A, Sahin-Tóth M, Lowe ME. A novel mutation in *PNLIP* causes pancreatic triglyceride lipase deficiency through protein misfolding. Biochim Biophys Acta. 2015b;1852:1372–9.
Szmola R, Sahin-Tóth M. Chymotrypsin C (caldecrin) promotes degradation of human cationic trypsin: identity with Rinderknecht's enzyme Y. Proc Natl Acad Sci U S A. 2007;104:11227–32.
Szmola R, Kukor Z, Sahin-Tóth M. Human mesotrypsin is a unique digestive protease specialized for the degradation of trypsin inhibitors. J Biol Chem. 2003;278:48580–9.
Teich N, Nemoda Z, Kohler H, Heinritz W, Mossner J, Keim V, Sahin-Tóth M. Gene conversion between functional trypsinogen genes *PRSS1* and *PRSS2* associated with chronic pancreatitis in a six-year-old girl. Hum Mutat. 2005;25:343–7.
Tennessen JA, Bigham AW, O'Connor TD, Fu W, Kenny EE, Gravel S, McGee S, Do R, Liu X, Jun G, Kang HM, Jordan D, Leal SM, Gabriel S, Rieder MJ, Abecasis G, Altshuler D, Nickerson DA, Boerwinkle E, Sunyaev S, Bustamante CD, Bamshad MJ, Akey JM. Evolution and functional impact of rare coding variation from deep sequencing of human exomes. Science. 2012;337:64–9.
Vesterhus M, Raeder H, Kurpad AJ, Kawamori D, Molven A, Kulkarni RN, Kahn CR, Njolstad PR. Pancreatic function in carboxyl-ester lipase knockout mice. Pancreatology. 2010;10:467–76.
Wang M, Kaufman RJ. Protein misfolding in the endoplasmic reticulum as a conduit to human disease. Nature. 2016;529:326–35.
Weiss FU, Schurmann C, Guenther A, Ernst F, Teumer A, Mayerle J, Simon P, Volzke H, Radke D, Greinacher A, Kuehn JP, Zenker M, Volker U, Homuth G, Lerch

MM. Fucosyltransferase 2 (FUT2) non-secretor status and blood group B are associated with elevated serum lipase activity in asymptomatic subjects, and an increased risk for chronic pancreatitis: a genetic association study. Gut. 2015;64:646–56.

Weiss FU, Schurmann C, Teumer A, Mayerle J, Simon P, Volzke H, Greinacher A, Kuehn JP, Zenker M, Volker U, Homuth G, Lerch MM. ABO blood type B and fucosyltransferase 2 non-secretor status as genetic risk factors for chronic pancreatitis. Gut. 2016;65:353–4.

Whitcomb DC, Gorry MC, Preston RA, Furey W, Sossenheimer MJ, Ulrich CD, Martin SP, Gates LK Jr, Amann ST, Toskes PP, Liddle R, McGrath K, Uomo G, Post JC, Ehrlich GD. Hereditary pancreatitis is caused by a mutation in the cationic trypsinogen gene. Nat Genet. 1996a;14:141–5.

Whitcomb DC, Preston RA, Aston CE, Sossenheimer MJ, Barua PS, Zhang Y, Wong-Chong A, White GJ, Wood PG, Gates LK Jr, Ulrich C, Martin SP, Post JC, Ehrlich GD. A gene for hereditary pancreatitis maps to chromosome 7q35. Gastroenterology. 1996b;110:1975–80.

Whitcomb DC, LaRusch J, Krasinskas AM, Klei L, Smith JP, Brand RE, Neoptolemos JP, Lerch MM, Tector M, Sandhu BS, Guda NM, Orlichenko L, Alkaade S, Amann ST, Anderson MA, Baillie J, Banks PA, Conwell D, Cote GA, Cotton PB, DiSario J, Farrer LA, Forsmark CE, Johnstone M, Gardner TB, Gelrud A, Greenhalf W, Haines JL, Hartman DJ, Hawes RA, Lawrence C, Lewis M, Mayerle J, Mayeux R, Melhem NM, Money ME, Muniraj T, Papachristou GI, Pericak-Vance MA, Romagnuolo J, Schellenberg GD, Sherman S, Simon P, Singh VP, Slivka A, Stolz D, Sutton R, Weiss FU, Wilcox CM, Zarnescu NO, Wisniewski SR, O'Connell MR, Kienholz ML, Roeder K, Barmada MM, Yadav D, Devlin B. Common genetic variants in the *CLDN2* and *PRSS1-PRSS2* loci alter risk for alcohol-related and sporadic pancreatitis. Nat Genet. 2012;44:1349–54.

Witt H, Luck W, Hennies HC, Classen M, Kage A, Lass U, Landt O, Becker M. Mutations in the gene encoding the serine protease inhibitor, Kazal type 1 are associated with chronic pancreatitis. Nat Genet. 2000;25:213–6.

Witt H, Sahin-Tóth M, Landt O, Chen JM, Kahne T, Drenth JP, Kukor Z, Szepessy E, Halangk W, Dahm S, Rohde K, Schulz HU, Le Marechal C, Akar N, Ammann RW, Truninger K, Bargetzi M, Bhatia E, Castellani C, Cavestro GM, Cerny M, Destro-Bisol G, Spedini G, Eiberg H, Jansen JB, Koudova M, Rausova E, Macek M Jr, Malats N, Real FX, Menzel HJ, Moral P, Galavotti R, Pignatti PF, Rickards O, Spicak J, Zarnescu NO, Bock W, Gress TM, Friess H, Ockenga J, Schmidt H, Pfutzer R, Lohr M, Simon P, Weiss FU, Lerch MM, Teich N, Keim V, Berg T, Wiedenmann B, Luck W, Groneberg DA, Becker M, Keil T, Kage A, Bernardova J, Braun M, Guldner C, Halangk J, Rosendahl J, Witt U, Treiber M, Nickel R, Férec C. A degradation-sensitive anionic trypsinogen (PRSS2) variant protects against chronic pancreatitis. Nat Genet. 2006;38:668–73.

Witt H, Beer S, Rosendahl J, Chen JM, Chandak GR, Masamune A, Bence M, Szmola R, Oracz G, Macek M Jr, Bhatia E, Steigenberger S, Lasher D, Buhler F, Delaporte C, Tebbing J, Ludwig M, Pilsak C, Saum K, Bugert P, Masson E, Paliwal S, Bhaskar S, Sobczynska-Tomaszewska A, Bak D, Balascak I, Choudhuri G, Nageshwar Reddy D, Rao GV, Thomas V, Kume K, Nakano E, Kakuta Y, Shimosegawa T, Durko L, Szabo A, Schnur A, Hegyi P, Rakonczay Z Jr, Pfutzer R, Schneider A, Groneberg DA, Braun M, Schmidt H, Witt U, Friess H, Algul H, Landt O, Schuelke M, Kruger R, Wiedenmann B, Schmidt F, Zimmer KP, Kovacs P, Stumvoll M, Bluher M, Muller T, Janecke A, Teich N, Grutzmann R, Schulz HU, Mossner J, Keim V, Lohr M, Férec C, Sahin-Tóth M. Variants in *CPA1* are strongly associated with early onset chronic pancreatitis. Nat Genet. 2013;45:1216–20.

Yadav D. Recent advances in the epidemiology of alcoholic pancreatitis. Curr Gastroenterol Rep. 2011;13:157–65.

Yadav D, Lowenfels AB. The epidemiology of pancreatitis and pancreatic cancer. Gastroenterology. 2013;144:1252–61.

Yadav D, O'Connell M, Papachristou GI. Natural history following the first attack of acute pancreatitis. Am J Gastroenterol. 2012;107:1096–103.

Zhang X, Bailey SD, Lupien M. Laying a solid foundation for Manhattan—'setting the functional basis for the post-GWAS era'. Trends Genet. 2014;30:140–9.

Zou WB, Boulling A, Masson E, Cooper DN, Liao Z, Li ZS, Férec C, Chen JM. Clarifying the clinical relevance of *SPINK1* intronic variants in chronic pancreatitis. Gut. 2016a;65:884–6.

Zou WB, Masson E, Boulling A, Cooper DN, Li ZS, Liao Z, Férec C, Chen JM. Digging deeper into the intronic sequences of the *SPINK1* gene. Gut. 2016b;65:1055–6.

Zou WB, Boulling A, Masamune A, Issarapu P, Masson E, Wu H, Sun XT, Hu LH, Zhou DZ, He L, Fichou Y, Nakano E, Hamada S, Kakuta Y, Kume K, Isayama H, Paliwal S, Mani KR, Bhaskar S, Cooper DN, Férec C, Shimosegawa T, Chandak GR, Chen JM, Li ZS, Liao Z. No association between *CEL-HYB* hybrid allele and chronic pancreatitis in Asian populations. Gastroenterology. 2016c;150:1558–60. e5

Diagnosis of Chronic Pancreatitis

7

Xin-Ying Tang, An-Jing Zhao, Jin Yu, Jin-Huan Lin, Wen-Bin Zou, Zhuan Liao, Zhao-Shen Li, Song Su, Mao-Jin Xu, Jutta Keller, Peter Layer, Yun Bian, Jian-Ping Lu, Li Wang, Liang-Hao Hu, Lei Xin, Jian-Wei Zhu, Fei Jiang, and Zhen-Dong Jin

1 Diagnosis of Chronic Pancreatitis

Xin-Ying Tang, An-Jing Zhao, Jin Yu, Jin-Huan Lin, Wen-Bin Zou, Zhuan Liao, and Zhao-Shen Li

1.1 Diagnostic Criteria of Chronic Pancreatitis

It is difficult to some extent to make the definitive diagnosis of chronic pancreatitis, especially if the disease is not recognized by the physicians treating the patients. Basing on the presence of several different diagnostic characters of the CP, the Zürich workshop on alcoholic

Xin-Ying Tang, An-Jing Zhao, and Jin Yu contributed equally to this work.

X.-Y. Tang, M.D. • A.-J. Zhao, M.D. • J.-H. Lin, M.D.
W.-B. Zou, M.D. • Z. Liao, M.D. (✉)
Z.-S. Li, M.D. (✉) • L.-H. Hu, M.D. • L. Xin, M.D.
Department of Gastroenterology, Changhai Hospital, The Second Military Medical University, Shanghai, China

Shanghai Institute of Pancreatic Diseases, Shanghai, China
e-mail: liaozhuan@smmu.edu.cn; zhaoshenli@hotmail.com

J. Yu, M.D.
Department of Gastroenterology, Changhai Hospital, The Second Military Medical University, Shanghai, China

Shanghai Institute of Pancreatic Diseases, Shanghai, China

Tibet Military General Hospital, Tibet, China

S. Su, M.D.
Department of Gastroenterology, The 307 Hospital of Academy of Military Medical Science, Beijing 100171, China

Department of Internal Medicine, Changhai Hospital, Second Military Medical University, Shanghai 200433, China

M.-J. Xu, M.D. (✉)
Department of Internal Medicine, Changhai Hospital, Second Military Medical University, Shanghai 200433, China
e-mail: xumaojinch@126.com

J. Keller, M.D. (✉) • P. Layer
Department of Internal Medicine, Israelitic Hospital, Orchideenstieg 14, 22297 Hamburg, Germany
e-mail: j.keller@ik-h.de

Y. Bian, M.D., Ph.D.
Department of Radiology, Changhai Hospital, The Second Military Medical University, Shanghai 200433, China

Department of Radiology, The 411st Hospital of Chinese PLA, Shanghai 200081, China

J.-P. Lu, M.D. • L. Wang, M.D. (✉)
Department of Radiology, Changhai Hospital, The Second Military Medical University, Shanghai 200433, China
e-mail: wangli_changhai@163.com

J.-W. Zhu, M.D. • F. Jiang, M.D. • Z.-D. Jin, M.D. (✉)
Department of Gastroenterology, Changhai Hospital, The Second Military Medical University, Shanghai, China
e-mail: zhendjin@126.com

Z.-S. Li et al. (eds.), *Chronic Pancreatitis*, DOI 10.1007/978-981-10-4515-8_7

chronic pancreatitis proposed a classification in which CP was divided into 'probable' and 'definite' (Ammann 1997). There is a similar grading recommended by the Japan Pancreas Society (Homma et al. 1997). In 2007, Schneider and his colleagues established a new MANNHEIM classification system referring to the understandings of the Zürich workshop, but they decided to include smaller amounts of alcohol intake as risk factors for the development of CP than before, as well as a subgroup of 'borderline' CP into the classification system. The M-ANNHEIM diagnostic criteriaof CP are listed in (Schneider et al. 2007).

1.2 The Cambridge Classification

The Cambridge classification established distinct criteria in which it described equivocal, mild, moderate, and severe changes by imaging with ERCP (Sarner and Cotton 1984a, b; Axon et al. 1984). The Cambridge classification also categorized pancreatic imaging findings on CT and abdominal US just like the grading of ERCP changes (Sarner and Cotton 1984a, b; Axon et al. 1984). However, the grading according to CT and US had difficulty in distinguishing between mild and moderate changes. Since the early 1980s, EUS has been widely used in the diagnosis of CP and pancreatic cancer. Thus, it has detected several characteristic findings which were described in details (Wiersema et al. 1993; Catalano et al. 1998; Sahai et al. 1998; Kahl and Malfertheiner 2005; Nattermann et al. 1993). According to the Cambridge classification, the suggestions for using various imaging means to grade morphological changes are summarized.

1.3 M-ANNHEIM Score and M-ANNHEIM Severity Index

M-ANNHEIM classification system also provides a scoring system to determine the severity of the chronic pancreatitis.

There is a diagnostic challenge existing in the judgement of PEI. On account of the administration of different stimulants of the gland and the measurement of different parameters, it's difficult to compare (Etemad and Whitcomb 2001). In this system, pancreatic insufficiency was divided as mild, moderate and severe pancreatic insufficiency based on recommendations of Lankisch and colleagues (1983).

Based on the presence or absence of clinical characters as described by the M-ANNHEIM scoring, the points are added together to yield an overall score of clinical severity, which allows the division of patients according to the M-ANNHEIM severity index. Gives a general review on the different steps and the corresponding tables necessary to classify patients according to the M-ANNHEIM classification system.

The M-ANNHEIM classification system provides us with the chance to categorize patients according to disease etiology (Table C2-2) and to compare clinical progresses of CP according to stages (Table C2-3) and severity of the disease. To be honest, the M-ANNHEIM classification gives a totally new approach to investigation and treatment of patients with CP. According to this context, the M-ANNHEIM classification offers a framework for combining and comparing interinstitutional data. The classification needs clinical information that can be acquired from the patients in a simple way. The proposed staging of the disease (Table C2-3) and the prioritization of clinical and therapeutic characters closely reflect the clinical presentation of the disease and clearly distinguish between different grades of disease severity. The MANNHEIM system expands the consensus of the Cambridge classification and incorporates imaging information obtained from EUS and MRI. Thus, different progresses of CP can be compared by the disease duration together with the stage and severity of the disease. The M-ANNHEIM system accelerates the progression of prospective studies of chronic diseases.

1.4 Symptoms and Signs

Chronic pancreatitis is thought to be the end result of a long-term inflammatory process that results in both morphological and structural changes (Gupta and Toskes 2005). This has been proposed as a two-step process in which functional and structural impairment of pancreatic secretion activates zymogens, thus resulting in local destruction of glandular tissue and eventually fibrosis (Gupta and Toskes 2005). This may also leads to marked pancreatic structural changes including the formation of pseudocysts and ductal strictures. Moreover, repeated cycles of increasing damage and inflammation ultimately contribute to both exocrine and endocrine insufficiency (Gupta and Toskes 2005; Singer et al. 1985; Steer et al. 1995).

1.5 Symptoms

1.5.1 Abdominal Pain

The most common symptom of CP is abdominal pain, found in 60~100% of the patients and most of the pain is located in the left and upper abdomen. The pain could radiates to the back, with different frequency and duration of episodes. During the remission, patients may feel continuously uncomfortable and even faint pain. Episodic pain is a definite symptom of CP and it is classically described as constant pain in the epigastric area with radiation to the back (Pitchumoni 1998). Painful episodes last roughly a week and are often accompanied by fatigue, nausea, vomiting, food avoidance, and weight loss (Braganza et al. 2011). It has been estimated that overall 5–10% of patients with CP, especially those with late-onset idiopathic diseases, do not suffer from abdominal pain (Pitchumoni 1998). In the beginning of the disease, the interval of abdominal pain is relatively long, then it becomes shorter as the pain occurs more frequent with longer duration each time, indicating exacerbation of the symptom. Pain patterns (Table 7.1) are originally scored into one of five patterns based on the American Gastrointestinal Association's technical review (Warshaw et al. 1998).

CP is mostly found in mid-aged men, induced by intemperate drinking and meal. Pain is typically worsened with food intake and may be ameliorated without some kinds of precipitating food. Pain can be alleviated when patients sit or bend their knees and the position is called "Pancreas Position", but exacerbating pain would occur when patients lie down. Doctors from Changhai Hospital reported 42 cases of CP children, with the average age of 11.7 years old. The figures also demonstrate that upper abdominal pain accounted for 78.5% (Wang et al. 2009a). The severity of the pain is mostly grouped into light and serious rather than using pain scores. The mechanism of abdominal pain has not been clear so far. It may result from increasing inner pressure of pancreatic ducts and pancreatic parenchyma caused by pancreatic duct obstruction, nerve stimulation by inflammatory products in the pancreatic tissue, nerve inflammatory cell infiltration around pancreas, increasing sensitivity of spinal cord and central nervous system with pain (Braganza et al. 2011; Navaneethan and Venkataraman 2010; Ceyhan et al. 2007; Vardanyan and Rilo 2010; Drenes et al. 2008).

Table 7.1 Pain patterns based on the American Gastrointestinal Association's technical review (Warshaw et al. 1998)

Pain patterns
Episodic mild to moderate pain
Constant mild to moderate pain
Typically pain free between episodes of severe pain
Constant mild pain with episodes of severe pain
Constant pain

1.5.2 Pancreatic Exocrine Insufficiency

More than 90% of pancreatic exocrine function loss will cause significant exocrine insufficiency (Affronti 2011). The main symptoms are anorexia, upper abdomen fullness and distension after meal, intolerant with greasy food, weight loss etc. Due to lipase and protease secretion decrease, food cannot be fully digested and absorbed leading to steatorrhea (Dimagno and Dimagno 2011) patients' daily stool frequency varies from 3 to 30, with the excreta presenting light color, large quantity, foam and cacosmia. Microscopic examination can find lipid droplets and muscle fibers. Due to poor fat absorption, the patients may appear fat-soluble vitamin deficiency symptoms, such as night blindness, rough

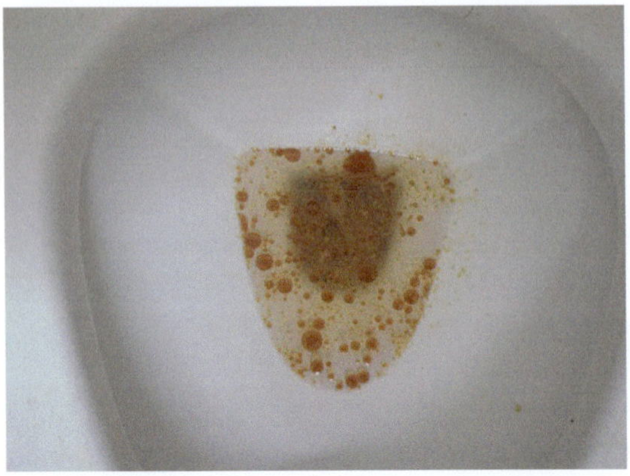

Fig. 7.1 Typical steatorrhea

skin, bleeding tendency etc (Pezzilli 2009). Typical steatorrhea is showed in Fig. 7.1.

1.5.3 Pancreatic Endocrine Insufficiency

About 1/3 of patients have dominant diabetes, other 1/3 glucose metabolism disorder just showing glucose tolerance abnormal (Singer et al. 1985). Contrary to primary diabetes, diabetes resulting from CP rarely cause retinopathy, nephropathy, atherosclerosis and ketoacidosis. This may be due to the locality, non-uniformity, and slow progression of pancreatic parenchymal damage caused by CP.

1.6 Signs

Simple CP patients without any positive signs have the same acute onset clinical manifestations as that of acute pancreatitis. Patients have acute pain and take the pancreas position to alleviate the pain and abdomen tenderness. A smooth and soft mass can be palpable when pancreatic pseudocyst form.

Patients of CP can also have ascites sometimes, such ascites resulting from the pancreatic pseudocyst or stenosis, expanded ducts of pancreatic leakage into the abdominal cavity. Ascites is intractable, containing non-bloody fluids with protein higher than 25 g/L, less inflammatory cells, and significantly higher concentration of amylase than that in serum.

A small number of patients may present with jaundice, and yellow skin and sclera can be found in physical examination. consistent jaundice may result from pancreatic pseudocyst that compresses common bile duct or chronic Inflammation Invasion of pancreatic head and lower common bile duct stenosis. In addition, enlarged pancreatic pseudocysts could compress the stomach, duodenum and portal vein, leading to upper gastrointestinal obstruction and portal hypertension (pancreatic/regional/left portal hypertension).

1.7 Laboratory Tests

Tests for chronic pancreatitis are aimed to assist in differential and etiological diagnosis, as well as to characterize CP-induced endocrine or exocrine insufficiency. Currently, there are no specific serological markers for diagnosis of CP (Steer et al. 1995).

1.7.1 Routine Tests

White blood cell counts and electrolytes are generally normal in routine laboratory tests. CP with alcoholic liver often has abnormal liver function. Five to ten percent of CP due to pancreatic edema or fibrosis caused by increased pressure of common bile duct and pancreatic duct can result in higher levels of bilirubin and alkaline phosphatase.

Exocrine insufficiency caused by poor absorption can present a large number of fecal fat that can be diagnosed by Sudan fecal stain. Endocrine insufficiency should be checked by the fasting blood glucose, glucose tolerance test, glycosylated hemoglobin, insulin and C peptide. Blood glucose monitoring is necessary if "brittle diabetes" is considered.

Serum amylase and lipase may be normal or slightly high, especially in acute onset. Amylase in chest ascites is often significantly increased. When combined with pseudocyst, amylase can also elevate. As fibrosis in the glands progresses, the synthetic trypsin is greatly reduced, without abnormality of amylase levels.

There are mainly two isozymes, namely, Pam (derived from the pancreas) and Sam (derived from the salivary glands and other tissues); other isozymes are phenotype of the two or post-translational modifications. Serum total amylase levels are affected by Sam and Pam amylase, respectively. The tests of these two isozymes can improve diagnostic value.

Studies have shown that 74–100% of Pam levels are reduced in CP with severe pancreatic exocrine insufficiency, while mild or moderate pancreatic exocrine insufficiency only reduces Pam levels by 12–42%. However, serum Pam in hyperamylasemia caused by pancreatic pseudocyst and acute attack of CP is almost in the normal range despite exocrine insufficiency.

1.7.2 Tumor Markers

Tumor markers are commonly used in the differential diagnosis of CP and pancreatic cancer. For pancreatic cancer, carbohydrate antigen 19-9 (CA19-9) is most widely used and considered as the most sensitive and valuable tumor markers. Compared pancreatic cancer, CA19-9 can increase to varying degrees in a small number of CP, but only with mild elevation. Pancreatic cancer is highly suggestive if CA19-9 continues to increase to more than twice as the initial level.

1.7.3 Differential Diagnosis

External factors of CP include alcohol, smoking and certain drugs. Intrinsic factors can be identified by laboratory tests, including genetic factors, hypercalcemia, hyperparathyroidism, hyperlipidemia, lipoprotein lipase deficiency and chronic renal failure, etc. Cystic fibrosis mainly involves the gastrointestinal tract and respiratory system, and when it involves pancreas, chronic pancreatitis is highly suspected. Sweat with increased sodium chloride content is characterized by this disease. Sweat chlorine has important diagnostic significance when it is more than 60 mmol/L in children (adult higher than 70 mmol/L), combined with sodium higher than 80 mmol/L and exclude adrenal insufficiency.

Autoimmune pancreatitis (AIP) is a special type of CP with high rate of clinical misdiagnosis so that differential diagnosis from CP and focal AIP is needed. AIP with abnormal serum autoimmune indicators of IgG4 is considered in the pathogenesis of AIP is of great significance. Serum IgG4 level is to identify AIP from common CP and it is a specific serum marker. Also, IgG4 levels can also reflect the reduction of hormone therapy Effect (Tetsuo et al. 2002; Okazaki et al. 2006; Chari et al. 2006; Morselli-Labate and Pezzilli 2009). Anti-nuclear antibody (ANA) and other autoimmune antibodies also have some diagnostic value. Studies have shown that the combination of IgG and IgG4 as a test index can significantly increase sensitivity, without the specificity significantly affected (Song et al. 2010). The study also showed that additional testing of ANA and RF does not increase diagnostic efficacy (Frulloni et al. 2009). It is worth noting that some patients with biliary and pancreatic tumors can also show positive IgG4. The incidence of AIP is low, so IgG4 positive predictive rate is low, and it could not be used to diagnose AIP alone. In addition to IgG4, several studies have attempted to filt new potentially identifiable serological markers, including AIP1-7, serum leptin, and adiponectin, which need further confirmation.

2 Endocrine Function Tests of Chronic Pancreatitis

Song Su, and Mao-Jin Xu

According to American Pancreatic Association Practice Guidelines, endocrine function tests in the diagnosis of chronic pancreatitis (CP) is of limited values. In patients with CP, diabetes mellitus is one of the most common metabolic diseases caused by pancreatic endocrine dysfunction. Diabetes mellitus together with mild pancreas imaging morphology or recurrent pseudocyst/pancreatitis can only give probable evidence instead of definitive evidence (Conwell et al. 2014; Sze et al. 2014). The relationship between CP and diabetes mellitus is complicated. For the sake of obesity or metabolic syndrome, some patients with earlier stages of CP develop type 2 diabetes mellitus (T2DM) . Patients with type 1 diabetes mellitus (T1DM) for a long time can also have CP, but the mechanism of this phenomenon is scarcely known (Chen et al. 2011; Cui and Andersen 2011). Considering the high prevalence and incidence of endocrine dysfunction, physicians should pay great attention to diabetes mellitus secondary to CP and detect it as an essential component of the complete diagnosis of CP.

2.1 Classification and Menace of Diabetes Mellitus Secondary to CP

Diabetes mellitus is an unfortunate but common complication of CP and can be observed in up to 26–80% of CP patients and 5–10% of all patients with diabetes mellitus in western populations (Cui and Andersen 2011; Delhaye et al. 2014; Rickels et al. 2013). Furthermore, CP patients with early onset of calcific disease, prior partial or total pancreatectomy, ongoing alcohol consumption and long-term duration of CP can be at a higher risk of diabetes mellitus (Rickels et al. 2013; Ito et al. 2007). According to the classification of American Diabetes Association, these diabetes mellitus secondary to CP refer to specific types of diabetes mellitus rather than type 1 or 2, classified as pancreatogenic diabetes mellitus (type 3c diabetes mellitus (T3cDM)). Patients with abnormal pancreatic imaging, pancreatic endocrine insufficiency and absence of diabetes-associated antibodies should be recognized as T3cDM (Delhaye et al. 2014; American Diabetes Association 2014).

T3cDM is typically characterized by "brittleness" in glycemic control due to loss of the glucagon response to hypoglycemia, inconsistent eating patterns associated with pain and/or nausea, and carbohydrate malabsorption. These features can also result in more frequent treatment-induced hypoglycemia (Cui and Andersen 2011; Rickels et al. 2013; Andersen 2012; Ewald and Bretzel 2013). In addition, in patients with T3cDM, complications such as micro- or macro-angiopathy, nephropathy, retinopathy and neuropathy are as common as those of T1DM (Delhaye et al. 2014). Moreover, the presence of T3cDM serves as an additional risk factor for developing pancreatic cancer, although CP is a risk factor for pancreatic cancer (Andersen et al. 2013; Gupte and Forsmark 2014).

2.2 Evaluation of CP Patients for Presence or Increased Risk of T3cDM

Currently, investigations for pancreatic endocrine dysfunction mainly consist of fasting serum glucose, oral glucose tolerance test, serum glycosylated hemoglobin (HbA1c), and serum C-peptide (Sze et al. 2014). Pancreas Fest 2012 recommends that fasting serum glucose and HbA1c tests should be repeated annually as initial evaluation. The diagnosis of increased risk or the presence of diabetes is as per endocrinology guidelines such as American Diabetes Association guidelines (Rickels et al. 2013; Andersen 2012). When impairment either in fasting glucose or in HbA1c is found, a standard 75g oral glucose tolerance test (OGTT) should be commenced to further clarify the diagnosis (Rickels et al. 2013). In line with the predominant insulin deficiency in T3cDM patients, hyperglycemia mainly manifests in the postprandial stage in these patients, whereas fasting hyperglycemia develops later. Thus, based on results of fasting glucose or HbA1c levels, T3cDM may easily be overlooked. In contrast, OGTT provides a more accurate diagnosis. A recent study demonstrated that when β-cells was reduced by 64%, diabetes could be diagnosed based on OGTT 2-h glucose levels. Whereas, a mean β-cells loss of 89–93% were needed when the HbA1c and fasting glucose were adopted as diagnostic criteria, respectively (Meier et al. 2012).

2.3 Differentiation Diagnosis of T3cDM from T1DM or T2DM

When it comes to the differentiation between T3cDM and T1DM or T2DM, several additional laboratory tests are needed. The presence of islet autoimmune markers (e.g., against glutamine acid decarboxylase, insulin, or islet cell antigen) is associated with T1DM. And the finding of evidence of insulin resistance (e.g. increased insulin secretion measured by C-peptide levels or acanthosis nigricans) is usually consistent with T2DM. These results can be used to distinguish T3cDM from T1DM or T2DM (Sze et al. 2014; Ewald and Bretzel 2013). However, if ambiguity remains, an absence of pancreatic polypeptide (PP) response to mixed-nutrient ingestion can be adopted as a specific indicator of T3cDM. The consensus statement from Pancreas Fest 2012 also recommend that the mixed-nutrient ingestion using a 12 ounces of Boost® or equivalent can be standardized and administered with prescribed pancreatic enzymes (Rickels et al. 2013). The non-diabetic subjects are characterized by four to sixfold increase of PP levels, whereas, CP patients demonstrate less than a double of basal values which is also reduced in CP patients (Cui and Andersen 2011). These features can distinguish T3cDM from T1DM in which PP levels can increase normally (Larsen et al. 1988; Rabiee et al. 2011), and from T2DM in which both basal and stimulated values of PP are elevated (Rickels et al. 2013; Glaser et al. 1988). But some authors argue that the sensitivity is low by measuring pancreatic polypeptide level to diagnose CP (Meier and Giese 2015; Eddes et al. 2001).

2.4 Assessment of Pancreatic Endocrine Reserve in CP Patients

In addition, when patients with CP are evaluated and followed up for total pancreatectomy with islet auto-transplantation (TPIAT), pancreatic endocrine reserve, and importantly functional β-cell mass should be assessed (Rickels et al. 2013). Serum C-peptide levels observed during either OGTT or mixed-nutrient meal testing can be used to estimate function β-cell mass. Despite the insulin or C-peptide response to glucose-potentiated arginine testing may be more accurate to measure β-cell secretory capacity, such testing is not widely accept (Rickels et al. 2013; Teuscher et al. 1998).

2.5 Other Pancreatic Endocrine Function Tests

Other pancreatic endocrine function test include glucagon, glucagon-like peptide-1 (GLP-1) and glucose-dependent insulinotropic polypeptide (GIP) (Cui and Andersen 2011).

Diminished pancreatic exocrine function has been reported to correlate with impairment of pancreatic β-cell function (Larsen et al. 1987). Although it is likely that reduction in β-cell mass results in the defect in insulin secretion, exocrine pancreatic insufficiency may also play a role in developing impaired insulin secretion by affecting the insulinotropic hormones GIP and GLP-1 (Meier and Giese 2015; Meier and Nauck 2010). The secretion of GIP and GLP-1 from enteroendocrine cells is associated with absorption of nutrients, so malabsorption in the proximal gut due to exocrine pancreatic insufficiency may impair GIP and GLP-1 secretion and thereby diminish postprandial insulin release (Knop et al. 2007; Ebert and Creutzfeldt 1980).

Glucagon secretion can also be impaired in CP patients (Meier and Giese 2015). A study on patients with advanced CP demonstrated that the glucagon counter-regulatory response to hypoglycemia is significantly reduced (Linde et al. 1977). When patients with CP associated T3cDM were treated with insulin or insulinotropic agents, an increased risk for large swings in blood glucose and frequent hypoglycemic episodes should be taken into account (Meier and Giese 2015). Therefore, early evaluation of glucagon level should also be performed in CP patients.

3 Pathophysiology and Diagnosis of Pancreatic Exocrine Insufficiency in Chronic Pancreatitis

Jutta Keller, and Peter Layer

3.1 Introduction

Pancreatic exocrine insufficiency is defined as partial or complete loss of digestive enzyme and bicarbonate secretion. While several pathomechanisms may impair intraluminal availability of pancreatic secretions, progressive destruction of functioning pancreatic tissue in chronic pancreatitis remains its most frequent cause. The pancreas has a large functional reserve, therefore, typical symptoms of pancreatic exocrine insufficiency such as steatorrhoea, weight loss and abdominal complaints caused by maldigestion usually become apparent in advanced stages, only. However, also patients with mild to moderate pancreatic exocrine insufficiency have an increased risk of nutritional deficiencies. This is one of the reasons why experts agree that pancreatic exocrine insufficiency should be searched for actively in patients with chronic pancreatitis and usually requires treatment (HaPanEU 2016). However, both, diagnosis and treatment of pancreatic exocrine insufficiency are demanding: available tests have either limited availability due to invasiveness and/or high costs or have limited sensitivity and specificity. Furthermore, galenic preparation of pancreatic enzyme supplements that ensures availability of enzymes in the small intestinal lumen together with meal components is challenging. This chapter focuses on pathophysiology and diagnosis of pancreatic exocrine insufficiency in chronic pancreatitis.

3.2 Pathophysiology

In chronic pancreatitis pancreatic exocrine insufficiency develops as a consequence of progressive inflammatory destruction of pancreatic tissue leading to reduced synthesis and secretion of bicarbonate and particularly pancreatic enzymes during meals. It is reported that in patients with chronic pancreatitis, pancreatic exocrine function is reduced by around 50–80% compared with healthy controls. On the other hand, 80–90% of chronic pancreatitis patients show some degree of pancreatic exocrine insufficiency (Keller and Layer 2005). In the majority of patients, that is in about 65–75%, morphologic alterations and functional impairment develop in parallel. Still, in rare cases, histologically proven chronic pancreatitis with pancreatic exocrine insufficiency can be present without visible morphologic alterations, even when using endoscopic ultrasound (Chowdhury et al. 2005; Conwell et al. 2007).

Due to the large reserve capacity of the pancreas, clinically overt malabsorption rarely occurs before pancreatic function is impaired more than 90% (DiMagno et al. 1973). Once this stage has been reached, marked reduction of enzyme output to less than 5% of normal has been shown to be associated with an about 40% malabsorption rate from a readily digestible low-calorie meal (Layer et al. 1997).

In alcoholic chronic pancreatitis, development of steatorrhea as a sign of overt malabsorption usually takes 10–20 years after diagnosis (Layer et al. 1994). Still, a minority of chronic pancreatitis patients—about 10%—may initially present with symptoms of maldigestion due to advanced pancreatic exocrine insufficiency (Layer et al. 1994). The risk of pancreatic exocrine insufficiency appears to be influenced by the aetiology of chronic pancreatitis. Different natural courses suggest that, compared with alcoholic and “late onset” idiopathic chronic pancreatitis, maldigestion may present later in “early onset” idiopathic chronic pancreatitis and hereditary disease, although hardly any study has directly compared the degree of exocrine insufficiency in patients with varying etiologies (Keller and Layer 2005; Layer et al. 1994; Hoffmeister et al. 2012). Smoking has an independent negative impact on pancreatic exocrine function (Luaces-Regueira et al. 2014; Rebours et al. 2012).

With regard to different macronutrients, lipid malabsorption with steatorrhea usually occurs earlier and is more severe than malabsorption of other nutrients. This is due to a combination of pathomechanisms that preferentially impair secretion and intraluminal availability of pancreatic lipase: lipase secretion decreases earlier compared with that of amylase and proteases as it is highly susceptible to pH and proteolytic destruction (Keller and Layer 2005; DiMagno et al. 1975). Moreover, in humans only gastric lipase can serve as an extrapancreatic source of lipolytic activity. Although it may be elevated, it does not compensate for pancreatic lipase deficiency (Carriere et al. 1993). In contrast, even after almost complete inactivation of pancreatic amylase activity, more than 80% of complex carbohydrates can be digested and absorbed (Layer et al. 1986), and the colonic flora can further metabolize malabsorbed carbohydrates leading to production of short chain fatty acids. These can be absorbed by the colon and thereby contribute to the overall caloric supply.

3.3 Clinical Symptoms of Pancreatic Exocrine Insufficiency

Typical symptoms of pancreatic exocrine insufficiency are steatorrhoea, abdominal discomfort, malnutrition, weight loss and symptoms of vitamin deficiency (Andersen 2007). Patients with steatorrhea typically report an increase in daily bowel movements, with fatty ("shiny"), bulky stools that are difficult to flush away ("sticky") (HaPanEU 2016). However, while it is important to evaluate the stool characteristics, they are neither sensitive nor specific for detection of steatorrhoea (Lankisch et al. 1996; Dumasy et al. 2004). Verification of steatorrhoea conventionally requires measurement of stool fat excretion exceeding 7 g fat per day during ingestion of a standard diet (DiMagno et al. 1973). Often steatorrhoea is accompanied by diarrhoea. This is partly caused by accelerated gastric emptying and intestinal transit in patients with exocrine insufficiency that can be reversed by enzyme supplementation (Layer et al. 1997; Keller and Layer 2015). It is self-evident that diagnosis of steatorrhea is not necessarily equivalent with diagnosis of chronic pancreatitis but may be due to a variety of other diseases including celiac disease and Crohn's disease.

Table 7.2 Clinical symptoms and signs of impaired absorption of lipid soluble vitamins in pancreatic exocrine insufficiency

Vitamin K deficiency—ecchymoses due to clotting
Vitamin E deficiency—ataxia, peripheral neuropathy
Vitamin A deficiency—impaired night vision, xerophthalmia
Vitamin D deficiency—contraction or muscle spasms, osteomalacia and osteoporosis

Potential clinical symptoms and signs of micronutrient deficiencies due to impaired absorption of lipid soluble vitamins are detailed in Table 7.2.

Further clinical consequences of pancreatic exocrine insufficiency can include hyperoxaluria, urinary oxalate stones, renal insufficiency, impairment of cognitive functioning and, thus, working ability (with resulting financial strain) and reduced overall quality of life (HaPanEU 2016).

Absorption of fat-soluble vitamins can be impaired even in patients with mild to moderate exocrine insufficiency (Haaber et al. 2000; Kalvaria et al. 1986; Mann et al. 2003a, b; Teichmann et al. 2007). Even after selective exclusion of patients with steatorrhea, exocrine insufficiency correlated with relelevant clinical consequences, i.e. osteoporotic fractures (Mann et al. 2008). Accordingly, not only severe pancreatic exocrine insufficiency but also mild to moderate forms appear to be of clinical relevance.

3.4 Pancreatic Function Tests

Although required for reliable diagnosis of pancreatic exocrine insufficiency, available pancreatic function tests are hampered by either limited availability due to invasiveness and/or high costs, or limited sensitivity and specificity. For clinical purposes, non-invasive tests are recommended (HaPanEU 2016; Hoffmeister et al. 2012) and, of these, stool tests are generally preferred. Invasive tests such as the secretin- or secretin-pancreozymin test are highly sensitive and specific and therefore generally accepted as reference method (Hoffmeister et al. 2012; Keller and Layer 2015). However, they are also compromised by high costs, complicated procedures and lack of standardization, Theoretically, they are still required for evaluation of new pancreatic function tests but they are hardly indicated in clinical situations.

3.5 Secretin Test

For this test, the patient needs to be intubated with a double-lumen nasoduodenal tube with one lumen placed in the gastric antrum and used for continuous aspiration of gastric secretions which are discarded, and the other located in the proximal duodenum for aspiration of duodenal juice. For reliable test results, pancreatin preparations, and nicotine and drugs with sedative or anticholinergic effects have to be discontinued at least 24 h in advance. Aspiration is performed for 30 min under basal conditions followed by a 60 min collection period with intravenous application of 1 U/kg secretin, followed by a second 60 min-stimulation period using a combination of secretin and cholecystokinin (CCK) or the CCK-analog cerulein (Keller and Layer 2015). However, the latter substances are currently not available in many countries so that secretin is used for stimulation, only. Following the test, secretion volume, bicarbonate concentration and activity of pancreatic enzymes (trypsin, chymotrypsin, lipase and amylase) need to be determined in duodenal juice samples.

Some specialized centers use endoscopy based modifications of the secretin test (Stevens et al. 2008; Stevens and Parsi 2011), e.g. by aspiration of duodenal juice through the suction channel of the endoscope at 15, 30, 45 and 60 min after secretin stimulation. A bicarbonate concentration >80 mmol/L in any of the samples is considered as normal. The endoscopic secretin test has demonstrated good sensitivity and specificity compared with conventional, tube based stimulation tests. Unfortunately, long operation time (1 h) binds considerable endoscopic resources. Reducing the length to 45 min with fluid collections at 30 and 45 min provides 94% accuracy compared with the 1 h test but further abbreviations appear to lead to inaccurate results, though it is feasible to inject secretin prior to endoscopy so that the duration of intubation can be limited (Stevens and Parsi 2011; Erchinger et al. 2013). CCK alone or CCK in combination with secretin has also been used in endoscopic function tests (Keller and Layer 2015; Stevens and Parsi 2011).

All tests using hormonal stimulation are contraindicated in patients with acute pancreatitis for the first 8–12 weeks after the acute episode.

3.6 Stool Tests

Fecal excretion of pancreatic enzymes correlates with duodenal enzyme secretion (Katschinski et al. 1997), and, compared with other enzymes, elastase-1 and chymotrypsin are very stable during intestinal transit. Therefore, these two enzymes appear suitable for stool testing.

The concentration of fecal elastase-1 in the stool sample is stable and cannot be influenced by pancreatin supplements, accordingly there is no need to discontinue pancreatic enzyme preparations, thus the measurement of fecal elastase-1 is the preferred and best available pancreatic function test. While the exact threshold depends on the method used for evaluation, normal stool concentration of elastase-1 usually exceeds 200 μg/g. Less than 100 μg/g stool are usually equivalent to severe pancreatic exocrine insufficiency. However, the diagnostic value is limited in early stages of chronic pancreatitis as the sensitivity is only 54–75% in mild to moderate pancreatic exocrine insufficiency (Hoffmeister et al. 2012). Moreover, specificity of fecal elastase-1 is rather low in the differential diagnosis of diarrhea, because stool dilution by increased stool-water content artificially decreases elastase-1 concentration (Keller et al. 2009).

The activity of chymotrypsin in stool can be tested photometrically, but sensitivity and specificity are even lower than that of fecal elastase-1 (Siegmund et al. 2004). Pancreatin supplementation needs to be discontinued at least 5 days as it is impossible to identify human and substituted porcine chymotrypsin, unless the chymotrypsin test is used to monitor a patient's compliance with enzyme supplementation in refractory cases. Three stool samples are needed for sensitivity improvement and this further explains why fecal elastase-1 measurements have mostly replaced chymotrypsin measurements nowadays.

3.7 Indirect Tests

While all tests described above are direct tests based on the measurement of secreted enzymes and bicarbonate, indirect pancreatic function tests described below investigate secondary effects which are due to the lack of enzymes (Chowdhury and Forsmark 2003). Among these, the fluorescein dilaurate (pancreolauryl test=PLT) and the NBT-PABA test (*N*-benzoyl-L-tyrosyl-*p*-aminobenzoic acid test) were frequently used but are no longer commercially available in many countries. Briefly, for these tests, the patient ingests a substrate that is metabolized by pancreatic enzymes. At least one of the metabolites is absorbed from the gut, conjugated, and excreted in urine, where it can be measured. Increased fecal excretion of the substrate and decreased urinary excretion of the degraded metabolite suggests pancreatic exocrine insufficiency (Keller and Layer 2015). To account for inter-individual variability of intestinal absorption and renal function, the fluorescein dilaurate test includes application of the absorbable metabolite (fluorescein) on a second day and the results of the test are expressed as the ratio of excreted fluorescein on the test and the control day in percent. A ratio of less than 20% is clearly abnormal (Keller and Layer 2015). A modified serum test simplifies the procedure but does not increase sensitivity and specificity (Siegmund et al. 2004).

3.8 ^{13}C-Breath Tests

Several breath tests using ^{13}C-labeled substrates for indirect measurement of pancreatic function have been developed during the recent years. As described above, lipase synthesis and secretion tend to be impaired earlier than those of other pancreatic enzymes in chronic pancreatitis. Therefore, tests using ^{13}C-labeled lipids are most promising and most frequently performed. The labeled lipids are ingested orally together with a test meal and need to be digested to monoglycerides and free fatty acids by pancreatic lipase prior to absorption. Hepatic metabolism of the absorbed lipids via β-oxidation eventually leads to production of $^{13}CO_2$ which enters the blood stream and is finally exhaled. Accordingly, intestinal lipolysis, the rate limiting step, is reflected by the ratio of breath $^{13}CO_2/^{12}CO_2$ over time (Vantrappen et al. 1989). Apart from diagnosing pancreatic exocrine insufficiency, breath tests using ^{13}C-labeled lipids can also be used to monitor the effect of enzyme replacement therapy (Dominguez-Munoz et al. 2007).

Available substrates for breath testing include 1,3 distearyl-2[^{13}C]-octanoate, uniformly labeled Hiolein® (mixture of long chain triglycerides) and cholesteryl-^{13}C-octanoate (Keller et al. 2009). The ^{13}C-mixed triglyceride breath test has several advantages over other lipid markers and is therefore most commonly used. Sensitivity and specificity of certain modifications of this non-invasive test reach 90% in comparison to the reference method (Iglesias-Garcia et al. 2003; Keller et al. 2011), and have been shown to also detect mild to moderate pancreatic exocrine insufficiency (Keller et al. 2011). For this modified version of the test subjects receive a standardized test meal, consisting of two slices of white bread, 20 g butter and 30 g chocolate cream. The chocolate cream is carefully mixed with 250 mg ^{13}C-mixed triglycerides. The meal is ingested within 10 min, together with 200 ml of water. In order to achieve a stable CO_2-production rate, it is important that subjects remain seated during the test. Breath samples are collected before ingestion of the test meal and every 30 min thereafter for 6 h (Keller et al. 2011). The breath $^{13}CO_2/^{12}CO_2$ isotope ratio can be determined by mass spectrometry or isotope-selective non-dispersive infrared spectrometry. A cumulative ^{13}C-exhalation below 26.8% of the dose administered is regarded as pathological (Keller et al. 2011).

A major disadvantage of this test version is the need for prolonged breath sampling. However, retrospective comparison of test results in a large group of patients has shown that an abbreviated version requiring breath sampling for 4 h still provides a high accuracy (Keller et al. 2014a).

Furthermore, the test has limitations in terms of specificity, i.e. false positive results have to be expected in non-pancreatic fat malabsorption (Keller et al. 2014b) and it is not yet available in several countries.

3.9 Fecal Fat Analysis

The reference method for diagnosis of steatorrhea is quantitative measurement of fecal fat excretion over 72 h during ingestion of a diet containing 100 g fat per day. Under these circumstances, a fecal fat excretion of more than 7 g/day fat is abnormal (Safdi et al. 2006). Often, fecal fat excretion seen in chronic pancreatitis is much higher (>20 g/day). Due to its numerous disadvantages including non-specificity for pancreatic disease, need for prolonged abstinence from pancreatic enzyme preparations and unpleasant sampling, storage and mixing of stool, it is no longer performed for clinical reasons in most centers (Keller and Layer 2015). Sudan staining of a random stool sample for fecal fat can be used alternatively but is relatively insensitive for fat malabsorption (Lieb and Draganov 2008).

3.10 Combined Morphological and Functional Investigations

Secretin-enhanced magnetic resonance cholangiopancreatography (S-MRCP) reveals ductal morphological alterations and simultaneously gives semi-quantitative information on functional changes by evaluation of the degree of duodenal filling (Balci et al. 2010). However, the number of appropriate studies is small and the sensitivity of this technique for pancreatic exocrine insufficiency appears to be limited (about 70%) (Schneider et al. 2006; Bilgin et al. 2008). Thus, normal duodenal filling does not rule out pancreatic exocrine insufficiency (Martinez et al. 2013). Endoscopic ultrasonography has recently also been combined with secretin-stimulation. Similar to S-MRCP, fluid filling in the descending part of duodenum was a predictor of pancreatic insufficiency (Engjom et al. 2015) but clinical usefulness of this method needs to be further evaluated.

3.11 Clinical Role of Pancreatic Function Tests

Since both morphological and functional impairment, can be the only sign of histologically proven chronic pancreatitis (Albashir et al. 2010), experts agree that a pancreatic function test can be required for the diagnosis of chronic pancreatitis (HaPanEU 2016). Proof of impaired exocrine function using function testing is particularly required for diagnosis in chronic pancreatitis patients with inconclusive morphological findings. Moreover, several diagnostic and classification systems take exocrine function into account (Layer et al. 1994; Ammann 1997; Buchler et al. 2009) but are usually only employed in clinical studies.

Function testing is also recommended in newly diagnosed chronic pancreatitis patients to screen for exocrine insufficiency (HaPanEU 2016), and national and international guidelines recommend repetitive testing at annual intervals in patients with previously normal results (HaPanEU 2016; Hoffmeister et al. 2012; Martinez et al. 2013), in order to detect maldigestion prior to the occurrence of overt clinical symptoms. Apart from this, function tests should be repeated when symptoms occur or deteriorate and can be attributable to pancreatic exocrine insufficiency (HaPanEU 2016). To evaluate the efficacy of enzyme replacement therapy, it is usually sufficient to verify clinical parameters such as the normalization of nutritional parameters and symptomatic improvement. However, when symptoms of exocrine insufficiency persist in spite of adequate pancreatic enzyme treatment indirect function tests that evaluate the effect of enzyme activity (^{13}C-mixed triglyceride breath test, acid steatocrit, quantitative fecal fat) are recommended in order to evaluate treatment efficacy (HaPanEU 2016).

From a practical point of view, verification of pancreatic exocrine insufficiency by a pathological pancreatic function test is a prerequisite for reimbursement of enzyme treatment in some countries.

4 Radiographic Examinations of Chronic Pancreatitis

Yun Bian, Jian-Ping Lu, and Li Wang

Diagnosing chronic pancreatitis (CP) in the advanced phase is easily. A standard abdominal radiograph (KUB) of pancreatic calcification can be confirmed. But diagnosing suspected and mild CP is difficult because State-of-the-art imagines cannot recognize these subtle ductal changes. Presently, the diagnosis of CP still relies mainly on the clinical and imagines. The clinical evaluation of CP typically includes radiography, computed tomography (CT), magnetic resonance (MR) imaging, and endoscopic retrograde cholangiopancreatography (ERCP) or endoscopic ultrasonography (EUS).

4.1 Transabdominal Ultrasound (TUS)

Transabdominal ultrasound (TUS) is generally used as the first imaging method for patients with suspected CP. The primary diagnostic findings of CP on abdominal US include pancreatic calcifications, a dilated pancreatic duct, gland atrophy or enlargement, irregular gland margins, pseudocysts, and changes in gland echotexture. The sensitivity reported for US in CP ranges from 49 to 96% (Rosch et al. 2000). The low sensitivity is partly a result of the difficulty of visualizing the pancreas from overlying bowel gas. One additional problem that can make the interpretation of abdominal ultrasonograpy challenging is the tremendous spectrum of changes that can occur in the pancreas as a consequence of aging. Changes in echotexture, pancreatic duct dilation, cystic cavities, and even ductal calcifications may develop with aging (Keller et al. 2014a). These findings mimic those in CP. It can be difficult or impossible in some patients to differentiate age-related changes from pathological CP. Nonetheless, TUS remains a very useful diagnostic test for CP and is often able to identify pancreatic cancer and biliary disease, as well as pseudocyst or biliary obstruction (Forsmark 2005). Abdominal ultrasonography is widely available, inexpensive, and risk-free.

4.2 Plain Abdominal Radiographs

A standard abdominal radiograph (KUB) may detect diffuse pancreatic calcification in very far-advanced CP. The finding of diffuse calcification is specific for CP but is quite insensitive (Fig. 7.2a, b). Although the sensitivity of this finding is limited (around 30–40%), a plain film of the abdomen should be the first diagnostic test used when attempting to evaluate chronic abdominal pain as a positive finding obviates the need for additional testing (Yamada 2008).

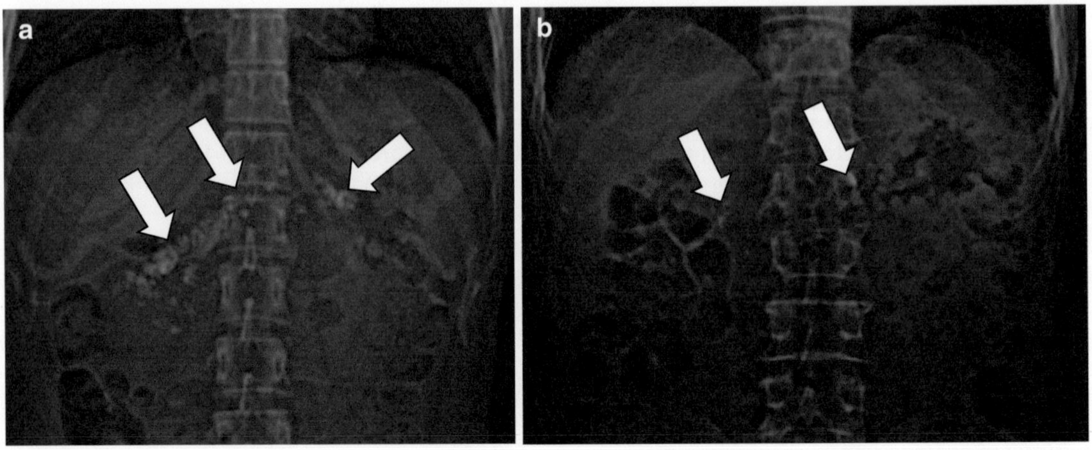

Fig. 7.2 Chronic pancreatitis on plain abdominal radiographs. (**a**, **b**) Of two alcoholic patients show multiple coarse calcifications in the topography of the pancreas (*arrows*)

4.3 Computed Tomography (CT)

In current practice, CT scan abdomen is often the initial investigation when CP is suspected. CT is the most sensitive and specific modality for depicting pancreatic calcifications, which may be tiny and punctate or larger and coarse (Muniraj et al. 2015). However, the early changes associated with chronic pancreatitis are more difficult to identify on CT. Characteristic findings on CT include dilatation of the pancreatic.

Optimal evaluation of the pancreas requires helical CT scanning using a pancreas-optimized protocol. This technology permits scanning of the complete pancreas during a single breath hold. Whenever possible, an oral contrast agent should be used to maximize pancreatic visualization and especially the duodenal wall, the papilla, and the duodenal pancreatic boundaries. Table 7.3 provides the typical imaging parameters that we employ.

4.4 CT Findings

4.4.1 Morphology

Inflammatory disease of pancreas characterized by irreversible damage to morphology and function. The size of the pancreatic gland, initially normal, becomes progressively smaller due to an increasing parenchymal atrophy characterized as uniform and diffuse (Fig. 7.3a, b). In extreme cases, the parenchyma may not be visible. Pancreas increased in size with inflammation, edema and cyst.

4.4.2 Pancreatic Duct

The spectrum of changes in the pancreatic duct are broad including dilatation, stricture, stenosis, intraductal calculi, occasionally side branch duct dilatation ("chain of lakes" or "string of pearls" appearance) (Fig. 7.4a–c). There may be stones inside the lumen of the main duct, sometimes the Santorini duct and the minor ducts. These stones arise from calcium deposits along the intraductal protein plugs.

4.4.3 Inflammatory Mass

Some patients with CP may have more than one mass-like lesion in the pancreas. The inflammatory mass may occur anywhere within the pancreas but is most common in the head of the gland. Due to fibrosis, the mass is hypo enhanced. The inflammatory mass may be associated with bile duct obstruction or duodenal obstruction, main pancreatic duct obstruction, or compression of the portal vein or superior mesenteric vein, thus mimicking most of the imaging features of pancreatic malignancy (Figs. 7.5a–c and 7.6a–c).

Table 7.3 Multidetector CT dedicated pancreatic protocol parameters

Parameter		Parameter	
Position	Supine position Head to food	FOV (mm × mm)	348,348
Scanning range	From thoracic cavity to pelvic cavity	Intravenous contrast agent	Iodine
Kvp	120	Trace point of contrast agent	Abdominal aorta superior the pancreas
mAs	150	Bolus tracking (Hu)	140
Collimation (mm)	128 × 0.625	Injection rate (mL/s)	3.0~4.0
Rotation time (s)	0.5	Arterial phase (s)	20~25
Section thickness (mm)	0.5	Pancreatic parenchymal phase(s)	60~70
Pitch factor (mm)	1.2	Portal venous phase (s)	110~130
Pitch (mm)	1.5	Window level (Hu)	350
Reconstructing space (mm)	1.0	Window width (Hu)	50

Note: *FOV* field of view

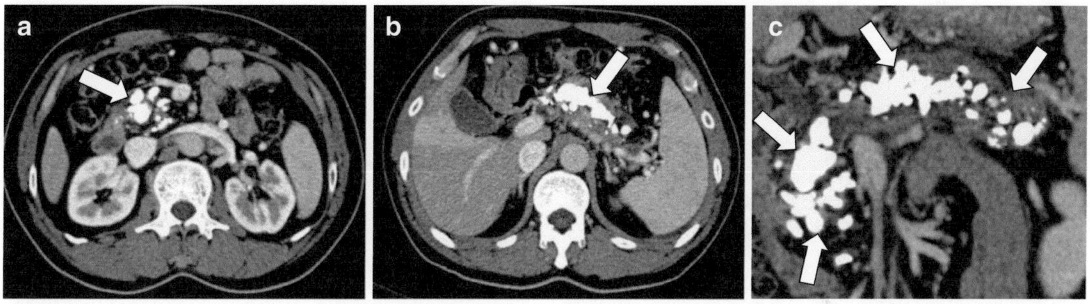

Fig. 7.3 Chronic pancreatitis on CT. CECT axial images (**a**, **b**) show a dilated pancreatic duct, multiple calcifications (*arrows*) throughout the pancreas, and parenchymal atrophy. Curved planar reconstruction image (**c**) show the multiple calcifications (*arrows*) throughout the pancreas (*arrows*), and parenchymal atrophy

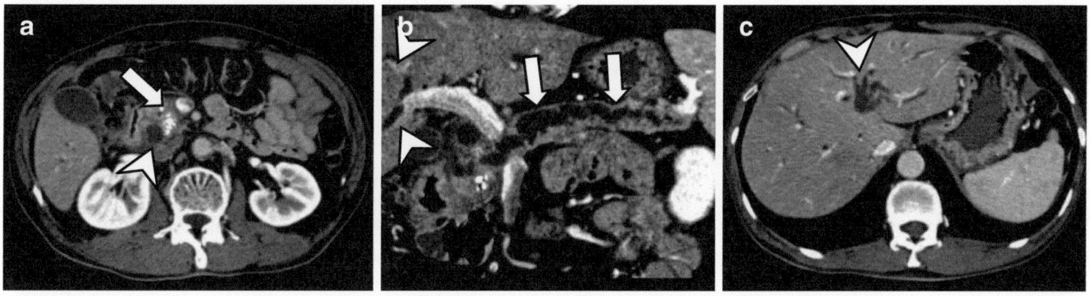

Fig. 7.4 Chronic pancreatitis on CT. CECT axial image (**a**) images show calcifications (*arrow*) and pseudocyst (*arrow head*) in the head of the pancreas, CECT axial (**b**) and coronal (**c**) images show irregular dilatation of the main pancreatic duct up to the level of the neck (*arrow*), as well as dilatation of the intra- and extrahepatic biliary system (*arrow heads*)

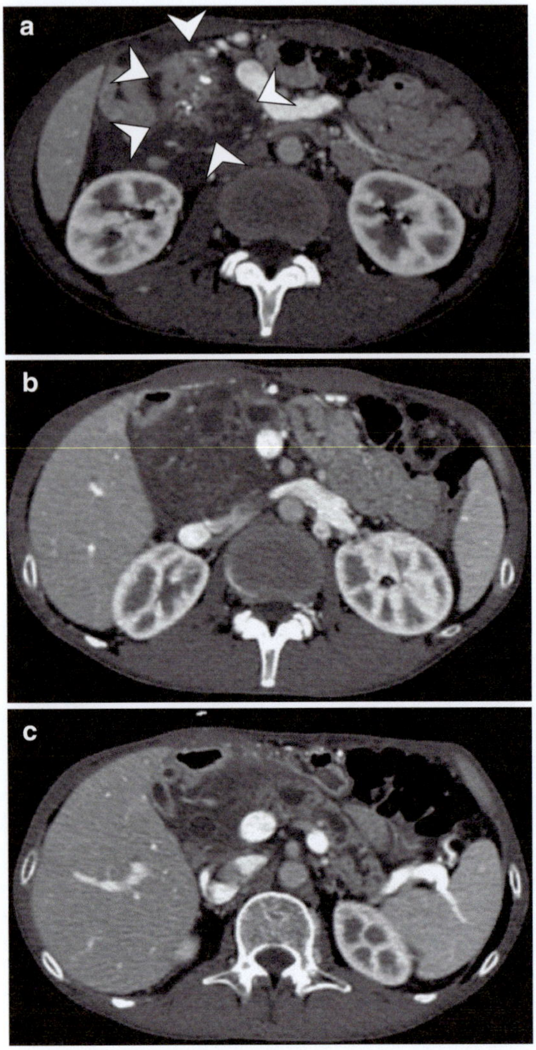

Fig. 7.5 Mass-forming pancreatitis on CT. CECT axial (**a**, **b**) images show the hypo enhanced and ill-defined mass (*arrow head*) in the head of the pancreas. Presence of calcification in the pancreatic head suggests underlying chronic pancreatitis in this patient. There are extreme fluid accumulation in the peripancreatic region. CECT axial (**c**) image shows the pancreas is reduced in size in the body-tail with the irregular dilatation of the main pancreatic duct

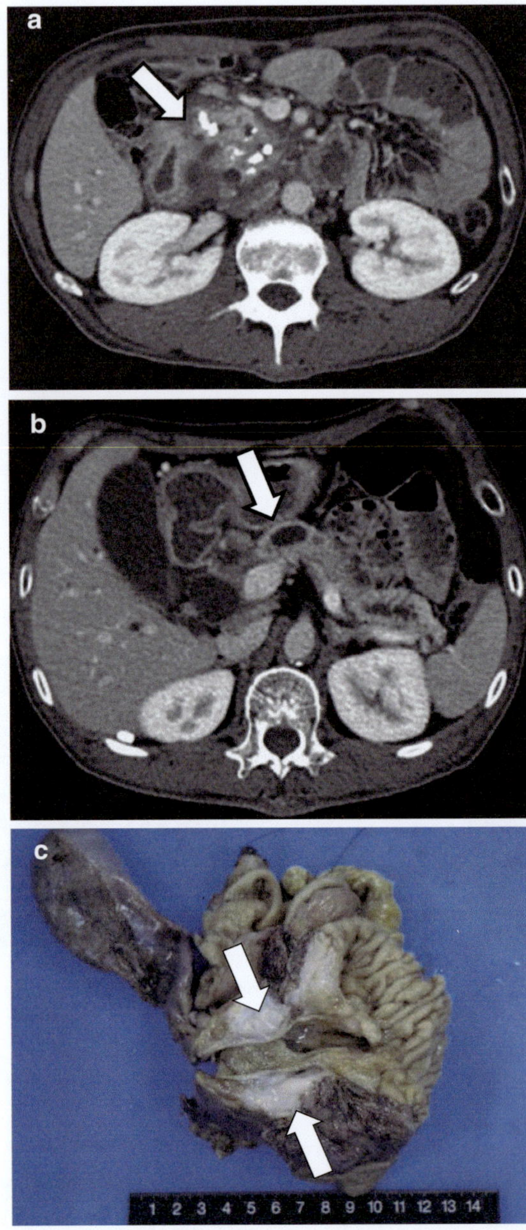

Fig. 7.6 Mass forming pancreatitis on CT. CECT axial (**a**) images show the hypo enhanced and ill-defined mass (*arrow head*) in the head of the pancreas. Presence of calcification and many retention cysts in the pancreatic head suggests mass forming pancreatitis in this patient. CECT axial (**b**) image shows parenchymal atrophy and the irregular dilatation of the pancreatic duct and its side branches. Photography of the gross specimen (**c**) reveals an ill-defined mass (*arrows*) in the pancreatic head

4.4.4 Pancreatic Pseudocysts

On CT, pseudocysts are round or oval in shape and have a relatively thin or thick capsule, which can calcify (Fig. 7.7a, b). The pseudocysts may locate anywhere. They contain fluid which is less than 15 Hounsfield units (HU); higher fluid attenuation values of 40–50 HU indicate intra cystic hemorrhage. Pseudocysts vary significantly in size and may communicate with the pancreatic duct.

4.4.5 Other Feathers

The other findings include (1) thickening of peripancreatic fascia (with acute attack), (2) the obstructive cholangiectasis (3) splenic vein thrombosis, splenomegaly, varices, and (4) may progress to thrombosis of portal vein (Fig. 7.8a, b).

4.5 Magnetic Resonance Imaging (MRI)

In recent years, MRI has been refined so as to become an ideal, noninvasive imaging technique. With appropriate contrast media, ultra-fast MRI can now provide simultaneous information on the morphology, ductal conditions (MRCP) and blood vessels in pancreatic lesions. MRCP is particularly good at imaging the pancreatic duct when it is dilated. Agreement is best when significant pancreatic ductal abnormalities are present, and when the pancreatic duct is dilated. With the advent of MRCP, the indications for invasive ERCP have to be redefined—usually being reserved for patients requiring additional interventional endoscopic therapy.

Our standard MR protocol for the evaluation to the pancreas includes T_1-weighted fat-suppressed 3D gradient echo, Tl-weighted in-phase, out-of phase, water and fat gradient echo, T_2-weighted single-shot echo-train spin-echo with/without fat suppression, and post-gadolinium imaging in the tri-phase (arterial phase, pancreatic parenchymal phase and portal venous phase). Table 7.4 provides the typical imaging parameters that we employ.

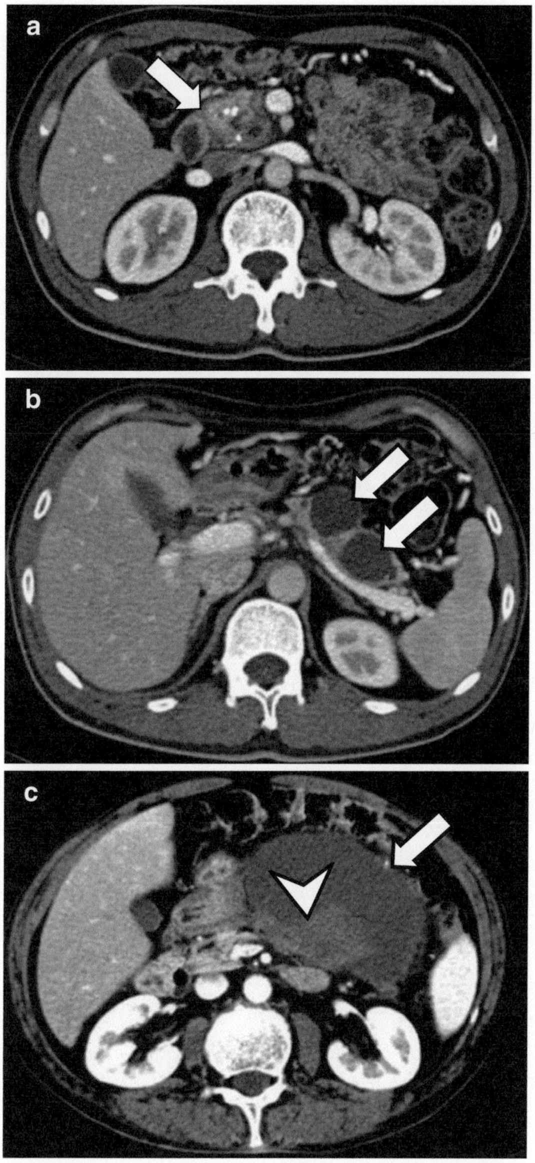

Fig. 7.7 Chronic pancreatitis and pancreatic pseudocyst on CT. A 38-year-old male with history of chronic pancreatitis and chronic upper back pain. CECT axial (**a**, **b**) images reveal multiple pancreatic calcifications in the head (*arrows*) and a bilobulated cystic lesion involving the body and tail of the pancreas (*arrow*). A 38-year-old male with history of chronic pancreatitis and chronic upper back pain. Contrast CT axial (**c**) images reveal parenchymal atrophy and a big round cystic lesion with hemorrhage (*arrow head*) involving the body and tail of the pancreas (*arrow*)

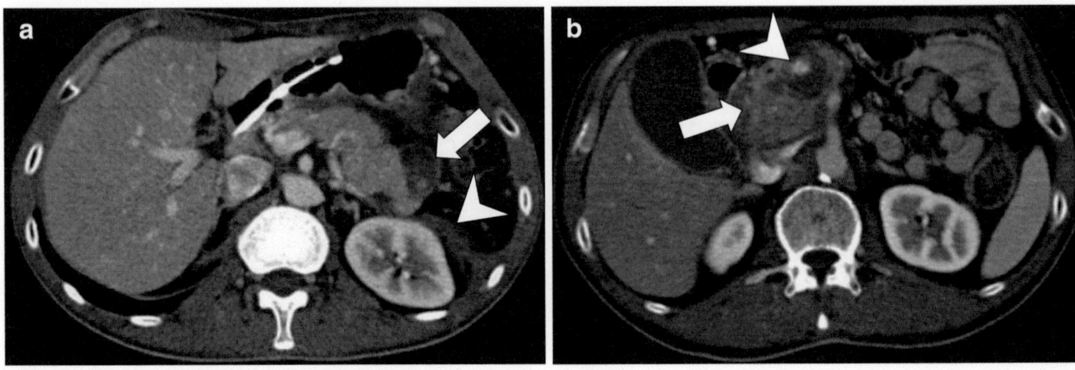

Fig. 7.8 Other findings of chronic pancreatitis on CT. CECT axial (**a**) image shows the pancreatic pseudocyst (*arrow*) and the peripancreatic fascia thickening (*arrow head*) in the tail of the pancreas. CECT axial (**b**) image shows the hypo enhanced mass (*arrow head*) in the head of the pancreas involves the superior mesenteric vein (*arrow*)

Table 7.4 3.0 T MR dedicated pancreatic protocol parameters

Parameter	T_1WI	T_2WI	T_2WI	MRCP	MRCP
Sequence	LAVA	FSE	SS-FES	–	–
Orientation	Axial	Axial	Axial	Axial	Axial
Space	3D	2D	2D	2D	3D
TR(ms)	4.25	2833	1530	7000	3333
TE(ms)	1.94	86.74	65	1271.81	387
Matrix	224×320	224 × 320	288 × 288	288 × 288	288 × 288
FOV(mm)	440×440	440 × 440	400 × 400	300 × 300	300 × 300
Section thickness (mm)	5	6	5	64	1.0
Intersectional gap	0	6	6	6	1.8
Flip angle	15°	–	–	–	
Fat suppression	Four phases	Yes	No	Yes	Yes
Respiratory	Breath hold	Triggering	Breath hold	Breath hold	Triggering
Tri-phase	15s, 20s, 40s	–	–	–	–
Contrast agent	Gd-DTPA, 0.1 ml/kg, an injection rate of 3.5 ml/s	–	–	–	–

Note: *T_1WI* T_1-weighted imaging, *T_2WI* T_2-weighted imaging, *MRCP* magnetic resonance cholangiopancreatography, *LAVA* liver acquisition with volume acceleration, *FSE* fast sequence echo, *SS-FSE* single shot fast sequence echo, *Four phases* water phase, fat phase, in phases, out phases, – no value, *TR* repetition time, *TE* echo time, *ms* millisecond, *mm* millimeter, *FOV* field of view, *2D* 2-dimensional

4.6 MR Findings

4.6.1 T_1 C+

Decreased T_1-weighted signal intensity of the gland owe to decreased protein content due to glandular atrophy and fibrosis (also contributing to T_1 hypo intensity). Furthermore, the fibrotic changes of the parenchyma result in attenuation of the vascular supply reflected by decreased enhancement on immediate post gadolinium images (Roth 2012) (Figs. 7.9a–d and 7.10a–c).

4.6.2 Fat-Suppressed T_2WI

Pseudocyst and necrotic areas show hyper intense. Gallstones and intraductal calculi show hypo intense or signal void.

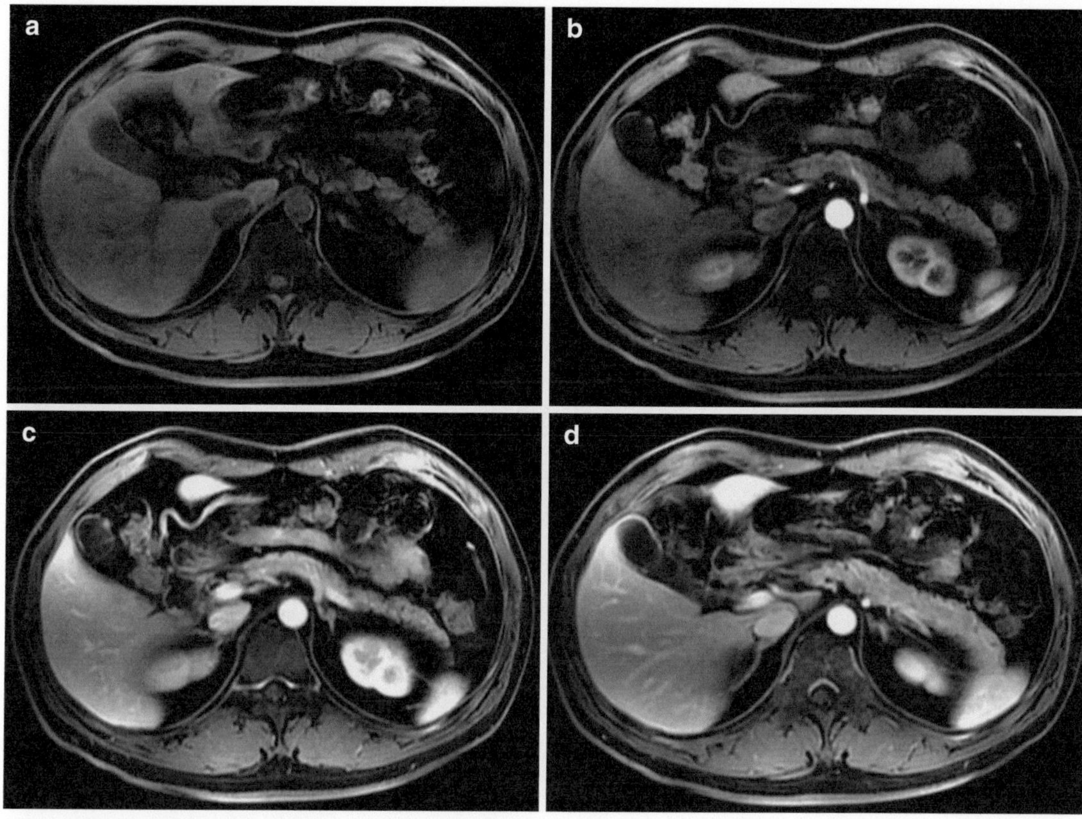

Fig. 7.9 Suspected chronic pancreatitis on MRI. A 46-year-old patient with isolated segmental finding. Axial T_1-weighted fat-saturated spoiled gradient echo image (**a**) demonstrate the normal size and signal of pancreas. Arterial phase (**b**), pancreatic parenchymal phase (**c**) and portal venous phase (**d**) show the delayed enhancement of pancreatic parenchyma

4.6.3 MRCP

In early stage CP, the ducts and more specifically the side branches are first involved. These changes correspond to the distribution of fibrosis that primarily involves the base of the side branch that will appear narrowed with a clubbed appearance. These changes are better detected by MRCP after secretin administration. In advanced stages of the disease, the diagnosis is easily established at MRCP by identifying structural changes involving both the MPD and the side branches, such as dilatation, narrowing or stricture formation, irregular contour, and filling defects (Fig. 7.10a, b). These changes are better detected by MRCP. The major limitation of MRCP concerns the detection of calcifications. Calcifications are seen as hypo intense filling defects surrounded by a bright fluid. When calcifications are grouped or scattered throughout the pancreas, the bright signal of the ducts is dramatically decreased, which may preclude their detection and makes unenhanced CT mandatory. Uniform dilatation of the main pancreatic duct and relative sparing or only mild dilatation of side branches are typical features of the obstructive type (secondary to a tumor) of CP in the advanced stage. In chronic calcifying pancreatitis, the side branches are also involved and MPD dilatation may be diffuse or focal as a consequence of the extent of surrounding fibrosis. The associated complications such as pseudocysts and bile duct strictures are also detected by MRCP (Fig. 7.11c).

4.6.4 Secretin-MRI and MRCP

Secretin administration stimulates fluid and bicarbonate secretion by the pancreas, thereby

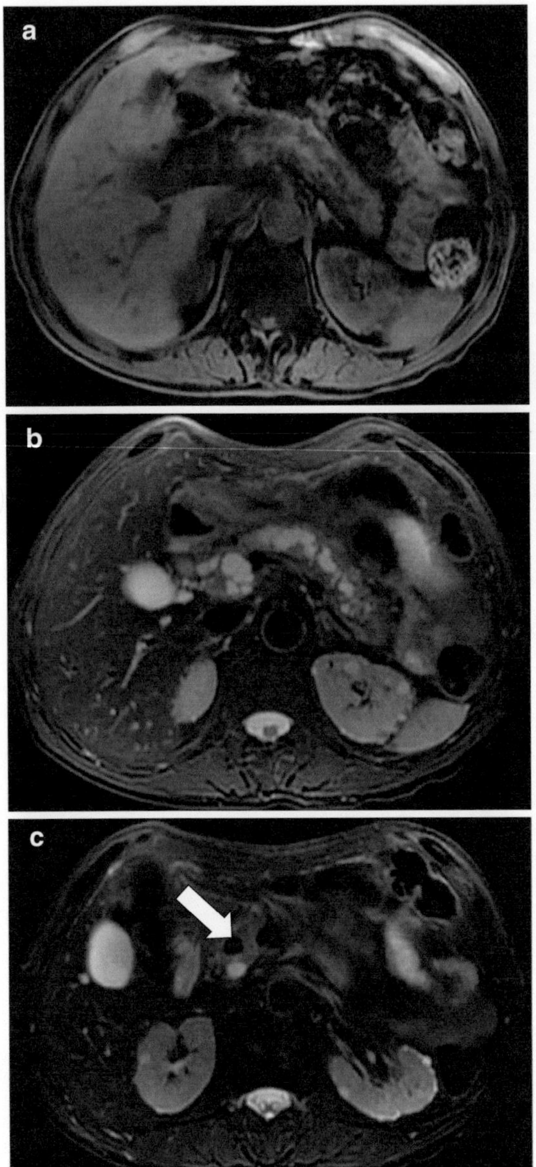

Fig. 7.10 Chronic pancreatitis on MRI. Axial T_1-weighted fat-saturated spoiled gradient echo image (**a**) and axial T_2-weighted fat-saturated spoiled gradient echo image (**b**, **c**) demonstrate atrophy of the pancreas with a dilated bead-like appearance of the main pancreatic duct, and filling defects in the head of the pancreas (*arrow*)

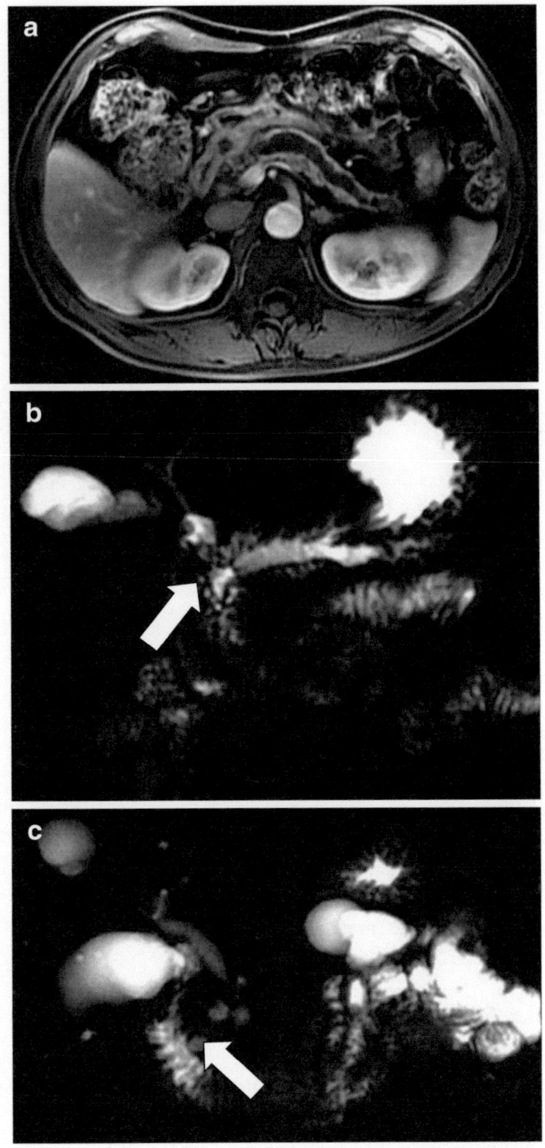

Fig. 7.11 Chronic pancreatitis on MRI. A 52-year-old male with history of recurrent severe epigastric pain. Axial T_1-weighted fat-saturated spoiled gradient echo image (**a**) and Coronal MRCP (**b**) demonstrate a dilatation of the main pancreatic duct, side-branch ectasia, and filling defects in the head of the pancreas (*arrow*). A 45-year-old male with chronic pancreatitis Coronal MRCP (**c**) shows severe strictures of the main duct with pseudocyst formation in the head (*arrow*)

improving pancreatic duct and side branch (Mensel et al. 2014a). For S-MRCP, 2-dimensional MR is repeated every 30 s for 10 min after intravenous administration of 0.2 μg/kg body weight of Human secretin. Pre- and post-secretin images are then compared for changes in main pancreatic ductal caliber (compliance), better visualization of ducts and side branches, sphincter of Oddi function, and the duodenal filling (Boninsegna

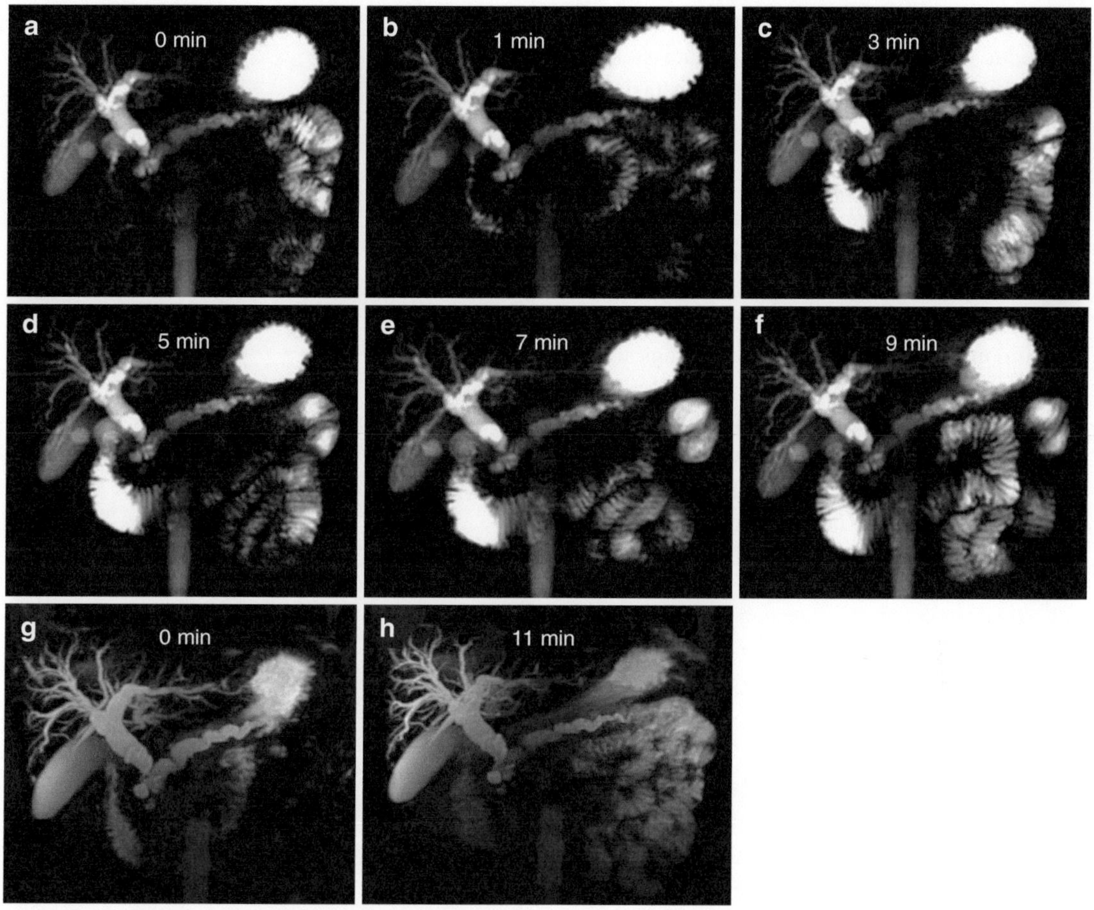

Fig. 7.12 Secretin-MRCP demonstrates the duodenal filling in a chronic pancreatitis. Before (**a**) and 1 (**b**), 3 (**c**), 5 (**d**), 7 (**e**), 9 min (**f**) after secretin administration on 2-dimensional MRCP. Before (**g**) and 9 min (**h**) after secretin administration on 3-dimensional MRCP. Progressive filling of duodenum with pancreatic juice, from the bulb to the genu inferius, is shown. The main pancreatic duct is better depicted after secretin administration

et al. 2015; Sandrasegaran et al. 2014; Mensel et al. 2014b; Ketwaroo et al. 2013) (Fig. 7.12a–h). Duodenal filling following S-MRCP is significantly reduced in CP patients with exocrine pancreatic insufficiency compared with healthy subjects (Bian et al. 2014). Pancreatic flow dynamics can be monitored after intravenous secretin administration, and measurement of the subsequent filling of the duodenum during MRCP can be used to evaluate the exocrine pancreatic function (Bian et al. 2013). Side-branch ectasia, mild ductal dilatation with loss of the normal gentle taper, and mural irregularities are the S-MRCP features of early-stage CP (Sherman et al. 2014). Secretin administration also increases the parenchymal signal intensity on T2WI. Decreased parenchymal signal is associated with loss of pancreatic acinar tissue (Lowenfels et al. 1993).

4.7 Differential Diagnosis

4.7.1 Pancreatic Ductal Adenocarcinoma (PDAC)

Patients with CP may also present with an apparent mass on cross-sectional imaging. Mass forming pancreatitis (MFP) need to be differentiated from PDAC. MFP and PC has similar findings: the hypo enhanced mass (arrow head) in the head of the pancreas, (2) the dilatation of the main pancreatic duct, (3) common bile duct stenosis Biochemical analysis has shown cholestasis and clinical jaundice.

Epidemiological studies have shown that the risk of development of PDAC is increased in patients with chronic pancreatitis (Lowenfels et al. 1993). In the subset of patients suffering from CP with IMH, PDAC was found in the pancreatic head in 3.5–6.8% (Lowenfels et al. 1993; Talamini et al. 1999). The follow findings which are suggestive of malignancy include (1) a focal low-density mass, (2) pancreatic duct dilation upstream from the mass, (3) atrophy of the pancreas upstream from the mass, (4) the lack of features of CP (especially calcification), (5) vascular compression or obstruction with the loss of the fat plane between blood vessels and the mass, and (6) metastatic disease (Fig. 7.13a–c).

However, some cases of CP and PDAC are impossible to differentiate without surgical excision and histology.

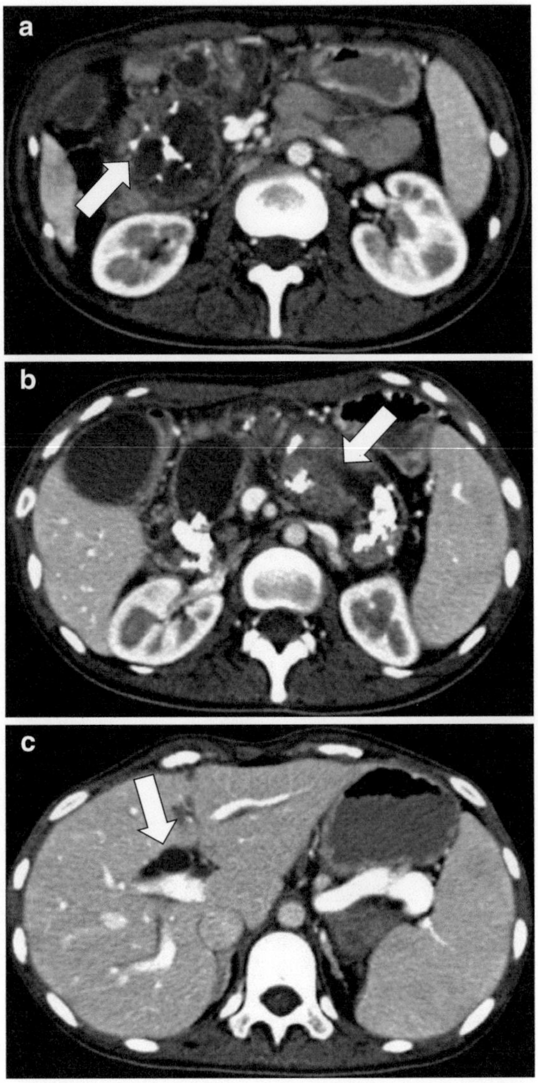

Fig. 7.13 Malignant transformation of chronic pancreatitis on CT. CECT axial (**a**) image shows extensive intraductal calcification and atrophy of the pancreatic parenchyma suggest chronic pancreatitis. An ill-defined low-density mass (*arrows*) adjacent to the pancreatic body (*arrow*) is seen on axial (**b**) image. CECT axial (**C**) image shows Double-duct sign is clearly seen with multiple intraductal calcification (*arrows*) in the dilated pancreatic duct (*arrowheads*)

4.7.2 Pancreatic Intraductal Papillary Mucinous Neoplasm (IPMN)

IPMN is a mucin-producing tumor, arising from the epithelium of the main pancreatic duct or side branches. Histologically, IPMN represents a spectrum of diseases, ranging from benign over borderline to frankly malignant tumors. According to their location, they are classified as main duct, branch duct, and combined type. Main duct type IPMN may show diffuse or segmental dilatation of the main duct due to mucin, typically hyper intense on T_2-WI. A branch duct type is a multilocular cystic lesion, most often in the uncinate process, with communication to the (nondilated) main duct. A combined type will involve the main duct as well as side branches and show massive duct dilatation.

Patients with CP may also present with a dilatation of the main pancreatic duct. dilatation of the main pancreatic duct need to be differentiated from main duct type IPMN (Fig. 7.14a, b). The retention cysts of CP need to be differentiated from branch duct type IPMN (Fig. 7.14c, d)

The follow findings which can help us to differentiate them include (Talamini et al. 2006; Kalaitzakis et al. 2009) (1) patients with IPMN have a different male: female ratio, are older on average, have a lower alcohol intake and smoke fewer cigarettes than both patients with CP. (2) Patients with IPMN, which remains unidentified after pancreaticojejunostomy (PJS), have a

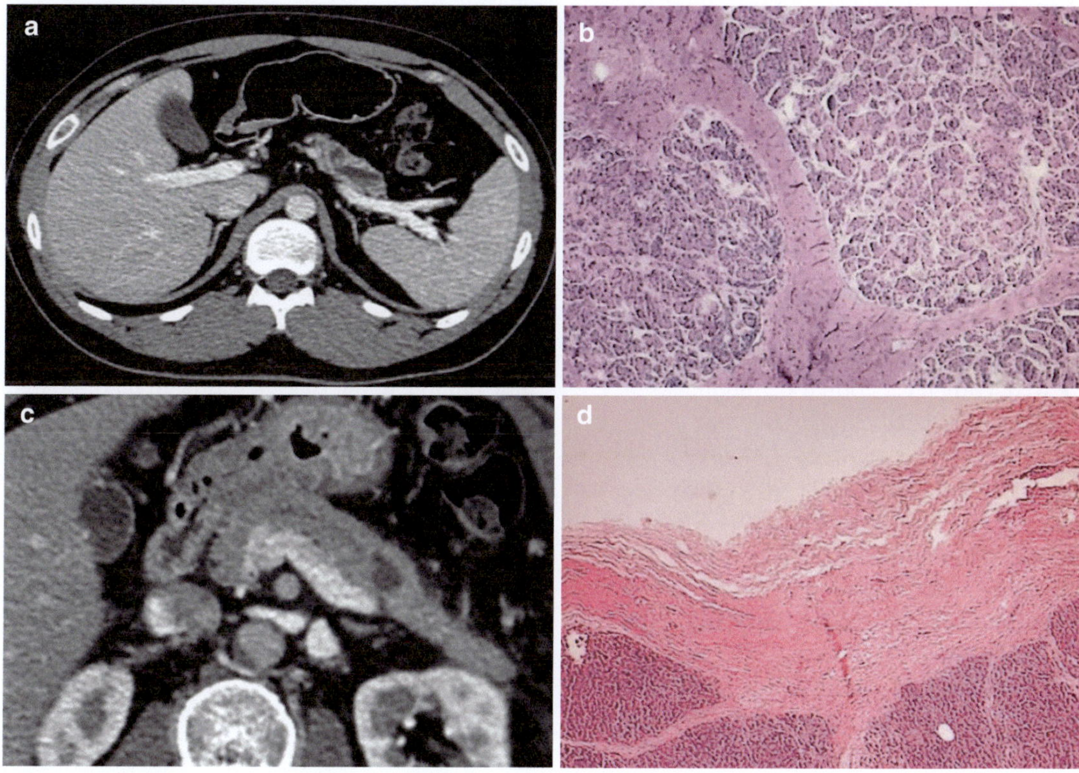

Fig. 7.14 Chronic pancreatitis was misdiagnosed as Pancreatic Intraductal Papillary Mucinous Neoplasm. A 38-year-old male with history of chronic upper back pain. CECT axial (**a**) image shows atrophy of the pancreatic parenchyma and irregular dilatation of the main pancreatic. Histological section (**b**) demonstrates a pancreatic parenchyma with abundant fibrosis (H&E, 20×). A 52-year-old female with history of alcohol abuse. CECT axial (**c**) image shows a small round cystic lesion communicated with main duct. Histological section (**d**) demonstrates bands of thick reactive fibro connective tissue arranged irregularly, creating a cystic cavity (H&E, 20×)

prolonged period of well-being (several years) which is followed by recurrence of pain symptoms (leading to the correct diagnosis and to re-operation). (3) Great care should be taken when diagnosing CP in patients who do not present typical characteristics of the disease, namely age over 50, moderate alcohol intake, non-smokers, women, because there may be concomitant IPMN in such cases which is amenable to appropriate treatment. (4) Most of the patients with IPMN and a previous diagnosis of CP present with endoscopic appearances at onset which are not pathognomonic for IPMN (normal papillary opening, absence of mucus) and ERCP findings indicative of IPMN are only found a posteriori. (5) The different clinical characteristics at onset compared to CP and the anatomopathological data suggest that, in most cases, the IPMN was the cause and not a consequence of the CP.

4.8 Diagnostic Strategy

Transabdominal ultrasound (TUS) is generally used as the first imaging method for patients with suspected CP. The sensitivity reported for TUS in chronic pancreatitis ranges from 49 to 96% (Rosch et al. 2000). This variation reflects the morpho-While the sensitivity of TUS is low for early lesions, it may detect more severe pancreatic changes as well as extrapancreatic alterations such as, for example, bile duct dilatation and fluid collections.

Abdominal computed tomography (CT) scanning has good sensitivity for diagnosing moderate-to-severe CP (Stabile Ianora et al. 2013). However, the early changes associated with CP are more difficult to identify on CT. Diagnostic criteria are similar as for TUS. Yet, compared with TUS, CT is less operator dependent, not compromised by intervening bowel gas, and identifies sensitively pancreatic calcifications. As a rule, sensitivity of CT for CP depends on the severity of the disease and ranges from <60 to 95% (Rosch et al. 2000). Yet, it should be kept in mind that in patients with early stages of CP frequently have normal CT findings.

MRCP has been emphasized that its sensitivity (81–100%), specificity (94–98%), positive (86–93%) and negative (94–98%) predictive values, and diagnostic accuracy (94–97%) are as high as those of ERCP, which makes MRCP a promising alternative to diagnostic ERCP (Merkle and Baillie 2006; Lara et al. 2001; Sai et al. 2008). MRCP is noninvasive, avoids ionizing radiation and contrast administration, and does not routinely require sedation. Moreover, it can provide useful information on the parenchymatous organs in this region in combination with conventional cross-sectional magnetic resonance sequences. Although it has advantages, MRCP also has certain drawbacks. Small duct changes and calcifications are not readily detected, and most importantly, it does not allow simultaneous therapeutic intervention. While ERCP offers a therapeutic option in the same session after the diagnosis is made (e.g., papillotomy, removal of choledocholithiasis, stenting of a biliary stricture), MRCP just offers the diagnosis. Clips, stents, pneumobilia, hemobilia, and ascites might result in artifacts and impede interpretation of the MRCP image. Despite the new technological advances in MRI, its resolution has remained lower than that of ERCP (Keogan and Edelman 2001). Maybe the innovative secretin-stimulated MRCP, which permits the detection of pancreatic flow dynamics and assessment of pancreatic exocrine function, will improve the sensitivity of MRCP in future (Mensel et al. 2014a; Wathle et al. 2014).

ERCP is considered to be the most accurate test for the diagnosis of CP, with sensitivities of 70–90% and specificities of 90–100% (Clark et al. 2016; Gooshe et al. 2015). ERCP is widely considered the gold standard for the morphologic diagnosis and staging of CP. The most commonly used method for staging CP is the Cambridge classification (Milosavljevic et al. 2010). In mild or early disease, side-branch ectasia can be visualized. In more advanced disease, irregularity and dilatation of the main pancreatic duct, as well as strictures, calcifications and cysts may be seen. In ERCP, slight changes are often difficult to detect and variable to interpret. It has been reported that in 30% of patients with small duct disease who have had a normal or near-normal ERCP, an abnormal secretin stimulation test can be found (Gupta and Toskes 2005). Overall, ERCP is useful for those patients in whom other methods failed or are unavailable, in patients with a clinical pattern of recurrent acute pancreatitis, or when a therapeutic intervention is being considered (Safari et al. 2016; Md and Md 2016). The role of ERCP in the evaluation of those patients suspected of having sphincter of Oddi dysfunction as a contributor to acute recurrent pancreatitis or CP continues to be evaluated (Vitale et al. 2009). However, it should be noted that ERCP is invasive and has a substantial risk of complications, in particular acute pancreatitis. In a recent multicenter survey, the overall complication rate was 4% and the procedure-related mortality rate was 0.4% (Bolan and Fink 2003).

The diagnosis of CP at EUS is based on the finding of abnormalities in the pancreatic duct and parenchyma (Stevens 2013). EUS accurately diagnoses CP in most patients with ERCP- or pancreatic-function-test-proven CP. However, they also suggest that 25% of those patients with a normal ERCP and 40% of those with normal pancreatic function tests have an abnormal EUS (Forsmark 2000); at present it is unclear if these patients have CP or if EUS produces false-positive results.

The main indication for EUS-guided fine-needle aspiration (FNA) in the pancreas is to obtain samples from an intrapancreatic mass. EUS is able to detect and target abnormalities of the pancreas that cannot be seen by other imaging procedures. EUS-guided FNA allow the histological analysis of tissue from the pancreas (Sey et al. 2016). The Trucut needle is helpful for diagnosing benign parenchymal diseases of the pancreas, such as autoimmune pancreatitis (Sey et al. 2016; Nayar et al. 2016). Of particular importance is the potential to avoid unnecessary surgery (Chang et al. 1997).

5 ERCP for the Diagnosis of Chronic Pancreatitis

Jin-Huan Lin, Liang-Hao Hu, Lei Xin, Zhuan Liao, and Zhao-Shen Li

5.1 Introduction

The diagnosis of chronic pancreatitis (CP) is based on a combination of clinical, laboratory and imaging findings (Majumder and Chari 2016). Ideally, the most definitive diagnostic criteria for CP should be histologic evidence, but obtaining it on a routine basis is rarely available (Forsmark 2000, 2013). In the clinical practice, ERCP has been generally suggested as the gold standard because of its high sensitivity (70–94%) and specificity (80–100%) of detecting structural abnormalities (Forsmark 2000; Forsmark and Toskes 1995; Etemad and Whitcomb 2001; Adler et al. 2006; Feldman et al. 2015; Shamamian et al. 2009; Nagar and Gorelick 2005) although it is unable to visualize any changes within the parenchyma of the gland and only allows the visualization of the pancreatic ductal system.

5.2 Indications for Diagnostic ERCP

ERCP is usually not used as the first diagnostic tool due to its high cost for the diagnosis and high risk of potential complications after the performance.

Indications for diagnostic ERCP include indefinite diagnosis or differential diagnosis made by other tests, evaluating precisely the ductal changes (location, size and aspect of strictures, pancreatic duct stones, ductal communication of pseudocysts, ductal leaks, etc.) or complications (gastrointestinal or biliary obstruction) caused by CP (Devereaux and Binmoeller 2000), and determining the classification (Sarner and Cotton 1984; Axon et al. 1984; Cremer et al. 1989) of the disease. ERCP can also offer therapy other than diagnosis and identify the underlying cause of CP (anatomic abnormalities such as pancreas divisum, preampullary duodenal wall cysts and posttraumatic pancreatic duct scars) (Brugge 2013; Buxbaum 2012).

5.3 Classical Classification by ERCP

Since the lesion of pancreatic duct is a typical feature of CP, there have been several theories aimed at classifying ductal changes via ERCP, of which the Cambridge Classification and the Morphologic Classification by Cremer et al. are generally accepted.

5.3.1 Cambridge Classification

The Cambridge Classification is the most widely used system for evaluating the severity and distribution of ductal changes on pancreatograms performed by ERCP (Sarner and Cotton 1984; Axon et al. 1984). Severity is graded from normal or equivocal to mild, moderate, or marked changes, and distribution is classified into either local (head, body or tail) or diffuse changes.

Abnormalities in three or more side branches with a normal main pancreatic duct (MPD) are considered as mild changes. When the MPD is also abnormal, moderate changes could be diagnosed. Marked changes are confirmed by the presence of both three or more abnormal side branches and abnormal MPD with one or more additional features (large cavity, duct stricture or obstruction, severe duct dilatation or irregularity, or intraductal filling defects). Besides the severity, changes should also be categorized into local or diffuse according to the proportion of pathological areas.

5.3.2 Morphologic Classification

The location and range of the pathological lesions caused by CP vary greatly from individual to individual; thus a morphologic classification was proposed by Cremer et al. (1989) based on the pancreatograms (Table 7.5). The morphologic changes of CP are divided into four types, namely minor pancreatitis, focal pancreatitis, diffuse pancreatitis and segmental obstructive pancreatitis (Fig. 7.15). Each type has its own characteristic when pancreatography is carried out.

5.4 Application of Diagnostic ERCP

There have been profound differences of diagnostic criteria and algorithms for CP; hence the application of ERCP varies accordingly.

5.4.1 Applying ERCP to Various Diagnostic Systems

The initial efforts for a consensus definition of CP were conducted in Marseille and Rome in 1963, 1984 and 1988 (Sarles 1965; Singer et al. 1985; Sarles et al. 1989). However, it was the Cambridge Classification that first recommended ERCP as one of the diagnostic criteria in 1984 (Sarner and Cotton 1984; Axon et al. 1984), which was recently adopted by the Italian consensus guidelines (Frulloni et al. 2010) and Spanish recommendations (Martinez et al. 2013).

Table 7.5 Morphologic classification of chronic pancreatitis by ERCP (Reprint with permission from Cremer et al. 1989)

Type	Classification	Morphologic changes
I	Minor pancreatitis	MPD is normal or slightly irregular, clubbing or dilatation of secondary ducts
II	Focal pancreatitis	Pancreatitis is confined to the head, body, or tail with macrocystic dilatation of one or more secondary ducts
III	Diffuse pancreatitis	Pancreatitis occurs diffusely with one or more stenoses without upstream dilatation, with or without cyst
IV	Segmental obstructive pancreatitis	Obstruction occurs in the head with global upstream dilatation

MPD main pancreatic duct

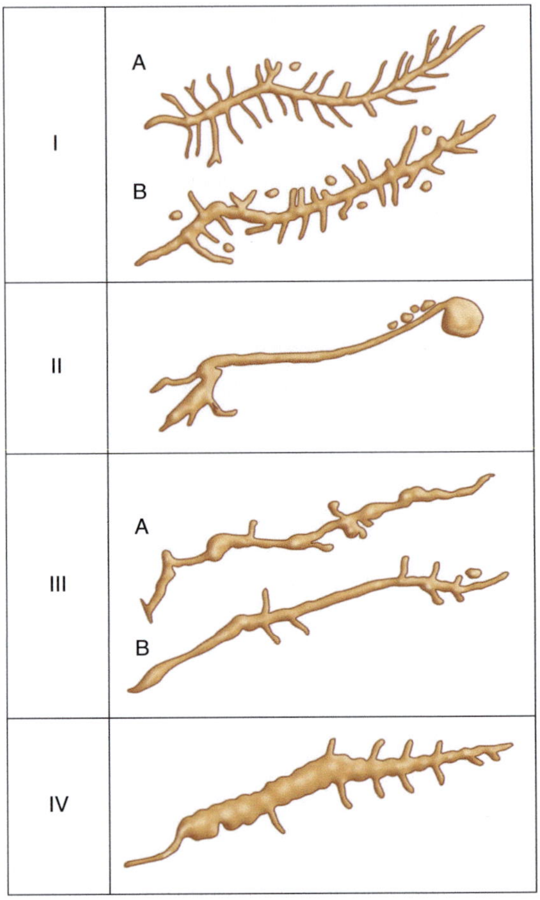

Fig. 7.15 Diagram of morphologic classification of chronic pancreatitis by ERCP (Reprint with permission from Gastrointest Endosc, Cremer et al. 1989)

In 1996, a workshop of experts developed a clinically based classification system for alcoholic chronic pancreatitis (ACP) in Zurich. They employed the Cambridge criteria and categorized moderate or marked changes as definite ACP, and mild changes as probable ACP (Ammann 1997, 1998).

The Japan Pancreas Society grouped their own criteria into definite CP and probable CP, with the ERCP findings different from each other: ERCP may show (a) irregular dilatation of pancreatic duct branches of variable intensity with scattered distribution throughout the entire pancreas or (b) irregular dilatation of the MPD, and branches proximal to complete or incomplete obstruction of the MPD (with pancreatic stones or protein plugs) in definite CP, while the image in those suffering from probable CP would demonstrate irregular dilatation of the MPD alone, intraductal filling defects suggestive of noncalcified pancreatic stones or protein plugs (Homma et al. 1997). Also, the concept of early CP was proposed by the Japanese Society of Gastroenterology in 2009 (Shimosegawa et al. 2010) and the latest revised guidelines in 2015 pointed out that irregular dilatation of more than three duct branches on ERCP is sufficient to confirm early CP (Ito et al. 2016).

However, the Asia-Pacific consensus did not adopt the Japanese criteria and it doubted whether early or less advanced changes of CP could be detectable on ERCP; meanwhile, it listed ductal changes on ERCP as one of the independent diagnostic criteria for CP (Tandon et al. 2002).

By contrast, the role of diagnostic ERCP may be limited by the American Gastroenterological Association because experts considered it not only risky and costly, but also unable to accurately detect minimal or subtle ductal abnormalities which are subject to variability in interpretation and difficulty in identification (Etemad and Whitcomb 2001). Specifically, the American Society for Gastrointestinal Endoscopy recommended that ERCP should be reserved for patients in whom the diagnosis is still unclear after noninvasive pancreatic function testing or other noninvasive (CT, MRI) or less invasive (EUS) imaging studies have been performed (Adler et al. 2006). After then, the guidelines published by the American Pancreatic Association summarized that ERCP could still provide some useful diagnostic information though it is rarely used as a diagnostic modality in CP (Conwell et al. 2014).

Similarly, the German clinical practice guidelines emphasized that only in the case of indefinite diagnosis yielded by all of other imaging methods should ERCP be carried out after the German Society of Digestive and Metabolic Diseases added various imaging modalities into a modified Cambridge Classification and took the changes in the pancreatic parenchyma into consideration (Mayerle et al. 2013; Schreyer et al. 2014). Other grading or classification systems just mentioned ERCP as one of the radiological evidences facilitating the diagnosis (Ramesh 2002; Bagul and Siriwardena 2006).

When it comes to autoimmune pancreatitis (AIP), the diagnostic value of ERCP is highly controversial among several centers (Chari et al. 2006, 2010; Okazaki et al. 2009, 2010; Kamisawa et al. 2010; Otsuki et al. 2008; Shimosegawa et al. 2011; Church et al. 2007; Raina et al. 2009). One of the widely divergent views is that the Japanese consensus guidelines have made ERCP a mandatory diagnostic criterion (Kamisawa et al. 2010) while others only include ERCP as a selective test.

5.4.2 Differentiating CP from Other Diseases by ERCP

It may be useful to perform ERCP for those patients in whom other methods are unavailable, nondiagnostic or make differential diagnosis difficult.

There may be pathological changes in the pancreatic duct in the advanced stage of CP or as a result of pancreatic neoplasms (such as ductal adenocarcinoma and intraductal papillary mucinous neoplasm) that are hard to differentiate, stimulating the utility of ERCP if necessary (Shamamian et al. 2009; Devereaux and Binmoeller 2000; Brugge 2013). On the basis of more pathognomonic changes found in the pancreatic duct, it is possible, with the aid of pancreatic juice collecting, pancreatic duct brushing, intraductal tissue sampling or intraductal pancreatic endoscopy via ERCP, to distinguish correctly between the two disorders in most of the patients (Uhl et al. 2004). Techniques to enhance the accuracy of cytology are in progress after the additional detection of telomerase activity, K-ras mutations, p53 and other biological molecular markers, especially for patients without pancreatic calcifications (Shamamian et al. 2009; Arvanitakis et al. 2004).

ERCP may also be required in the case of AIP when other imaging procedures fail to make a differential diagnosis. An international multicenter study (Sugumar et al. 2011) suggested that four distinct ductal features can be used to differentiate cancer from AIP. Long strictures involving more than one third of the duct length, strictures that do not result in an upstream dilatation of the duct, strictures from which side branches arise and the presence of multiple strictures in the duct are more likely to be caused by AIP than by cancer.

5.5 Limitations of Diagnostic ERCP

Besides other diseases, potential confounding factors for diagnosis include underfilling of the pancreatic duct with contrast medium (Forsmark and Toskes 1995; Forsmark 2000), normal aging effects (Nagai and Ohtsubo 1984; Ross and Forsmark 2001; Ikeda et al. 1994), a recent attack of AP and post-stenting effects (Nagar and Gorelick 2005; Conwell et al. 2014), which can produce changes within the pancreatic duct that mimic those seen in CP. These conditions limit the clinicians' ability to interpret the pancreatogram accurately and may induce false positive results.

Moreover, false negative results could be led by ERCP or other imaging methods because CP can exist not only in the absence of any changes within the pancreatic duct but also with minimal or subtle ductal abnormalities, which are defined as small-duct disease by Forsmark et al. (Forsmark and Toskes 1995; Feldman et al. 2015; Forsmark 2000). Compared with the big-duct disease with substantial abnormalities of the pancreatic structure and function capable of being detected by a wide variety of diagnostic tests, the small-duct disease is much more difficult to be identified, as both imaging studies and functional tests could be normal. Thus, only tests of maximum sensitivity have a chance of making the diagnosis (Nagar and Gorelick 2005).

Another limitation of the diagnostic ERCP is that the extent of morphologic changes does not correlate highly with the clinical presentation and the degree of the organ impairment or its functional status (Forsmark 2013; Sarner and Cotton 1984; Ramesh 2002; Whitcomb et al. 2016). Early histological damage may not involve the pancreatic duct and subtle exocrine or endocrine insufficiency could precede pathognomonic abnormalities of the pancreatic structure visible on routinely performed imaging studies. On the other hand, a group of patients with detectable changes in the MPD have not developed any symptoms during the course of the disease. Therefore, morphological as well as clinical and functional parameters are recommended to be used in a complementary manner to make a comprehensive assessment (Schreyer et al. 2014).

5.6 Summary

In order to minimize the overall cost and risk, diagnostic ERCP is generally considered a second-echelon method to be employed when none of those noninvasive or low-risk tests establishes the diagnosis; besides, the importance of ERCP is further reduced since direct pancreatic function testing (such as hormonal stimulation tests in particular), a valuable complement to the diagnostic algorithm, offers the most sensitivity and allows the identification of earlier or less advanced CP (Forsmark 2000, 2008; Forsmark and Toskes 1995; Ketwaroo et al. 2013; Parsi et al. 2008). However, the test is now only available in a few centers and neither standardized procedures nor normal ranges have been developed between those centers, hampering the wide availability of this promising approach (Forsmark 2000, 2008; Ketwaroo et al. 2013). Actually, ERCP is clearly used more frequently in the clinical practice given the condition that it would effectively make a differential diagnosis, accurately evaluate and classify the severity and distribution of ductal changes, and even efficiently treat the disease at the same time, despite the relatively high cost and risk.

The current paradox of the utility of diagnostic ERCP has stimulated the search for new and hopefully better diagnostic approaches in the future. For example, in addition to conventional endoscopic-based pancreatic function testing, the intraductal secretin stimulation test would collect pancreatic juice directly from the pancreatic duct at the time of ERCP after the administration of secretin alone or followed by cholecystokinin (Conwell et al. 2014; Lieb and Draganov 2008; Paulo et al. 2011; Sze et al. 2014). As a combination of both morphological and functional tests, this method seems to satisfy the need for the future diagnosis of CP.

6 EUS in the Diagnosis of Chronic Pancreatitis

Jian-Wei Zhu, Fei Jiang, and Zhen-Dong Jin

Chronic pancreatitis (CP) is a progressive and irreversible inflammation of the pancreatic gland caused by pathologic impairment that leads to morphological changes of parenchyma and duct, ultimately resulting in morphological alterations and exocrine as well as endocrine dysfunction (Seicean 2010; DiMagno and DiMagno 2010). Its main features are pancreatic fibrosis, inflammatory infiltration, atrophy, calcification, internal and external secretory tissue destruction. The early symptom is abdominal pain, and in advanced stages, patients suffer from diarrhea, weight loss, absorption or malnutrition, diabetes mellitus, and calcification. At present, diagnosis of CP is based on the clinical symptom and imaging examination. Thus most patients are in advanced stage when diagnosis is made. Hence, diagnosis of early stage CP remains a challenge.

Abdominal ultrasonography, CT and Endoscopic retrograde cholangiopancreatography (ERCP) can display parts of CP characteristic changes. But these tests have their own drawbacks. ERCP diagnoses of CP rely on main ductal or side branch change and ductal stone, with high accuracy. But it is not recommended due to the possible and serious complications related to the procedure and the fact that the parenchyma is not visualized (Choueiri et al. 2010). Since the clinical application of endoscopic ultrasonography (EUS) in 80s, it provides a new valuable method for the diagnosis of CP, especially for earlier diagnosis. EUS with high resolution ultrasound probe, allows closely observe the pancreas, so that small changes of the pancreatic parenchyma or duct can be found (Wang et al. 2009b). Compared with other imaging or functional test, EUS may be more earlier or clearly to display subtle changes in parenchyma and duct system, which has higher clinical value in the early diagnosis of CP (Hernandez and Catalano 2010).

6.1 EUS Criteria

6.1.1 Traditional EUS Criteria

Traditional EUS criteria contain nine features, including parenchyma and ductal features (Table 7.6), and the surgical specimens showed that these criteria were related to the histological changes. Eleven diagnostic criteria introduced two additional criteria: pancreas enlargement and pancreatic duct stenosis (Gardner and Levy 2010; Raimondo and Wallace 2004; Bhutani et al. 2009).

The sensitivity and specificity of EUS in the diagnosis of CP were determined by the threshold. Low threshold result in higher sensitivity, which could be used to ruled out CP, but with poor specificity and high risk of over-diagnosis. In converse, high threshold can be used for diagnosis of CP. However, Endoscopic physician found the value of each EUS criteria is unequal in clinical practice (Catalano et al. 1998, 2009; Rajan et al. 2005). Rajan et al. study found the frequency of EUS abnormalities in patients without clinical evidence of CP increases with age, particularly after 60 years of age (Rajan et al. 2005). Their study showed in 120 patients with no history or symptoms of pancreaticobiliary diseases, 28% of the patients had at least one parenchymal and/or ductual

Table 7.6 Nine EUS criteria for CP diagnosis and correlation histologic change

EUS criteria	Histologic correlation
Pancreatic parenchymal criteria	
Hyperechoic foci	Focal fibrosis
Hyperechoic strands	Bridging fibrosis
Lobularity	Lobule fibrosis
Cysts	Cyst/pseudocyst
Pancreatic ductal criteria	
Pancreatic duct dilation	head > 3 mm, body > 2 mm, tail > 1 mm
Pancreatic duct irregularity	Pancreatic duct dilation/stenosis
Hyperechoic pancreatic duct walls	Fibrosis around duct
Visible pancreatic side branches	Side branch ectasia
Intraductal calcifications	Stone

abnormality, which with a trend of increasing abnormality with age. Hyperechoic stranding was the most common finding in all age groups. And no patient had more than three abnormal EUS features. Therefore they thought the threshold number of EUS criteria for the diagnosis of CP is variable and ductal or parenchymal calculi, ductal narrowing, ductal dilatation, or more than three abnormalities appear to be more specific features for the EUS diagnosis of CP at any age.

6.1.2 Rosemont Classification

It is precisely because of the predictive value of each EUS criteria weight EUS is inconsistent, most scholars believe that these criteria need to be optimized utilization. Therefore, in Apr, 2007, a new classification criterion was made in an international consensus meeting which was convened in Rosemont. This system gives a strictly level for each criterion, including Major and minor criterion (Tables 7.7 and 7.8, Figs. 7.16, 7.17, and 7.18) (Catalano et al. 2009).

Table 7.7 Consensus-based parenchymal and ductal features of CP according to the new Rosemont classification (Catalano et al. 2009)

Rank	Feature	Definition	Criteria level	Histologic correlation
Parenchyma features				
1	Hyperechoic foci with shadowing[a]	Echogenic structures ≥2 mm in length and width that shadow	Major A	Parenchymal-based calcifications
2	Lobularity	Well-circumscribed, ≥5 mm structures with enhancing rim and relatively		Unknown
	A. With honeycombing	Contiguous ≥3 lobules	Major B	
	B. Without honeycombing	Noncontiguous lobules	Minor criteria	
3	Hyperchoic foci without shadowing[a]	Echogenic structures foci ≥2 mm in both length and width with no shadowing	Minor criteria	Unknown
4	Cysts[a]	Nechoic, rounded/elliptical structures with or without septations	Minor criteria	Pseudocyst
5	Stranding[b]	Hyperechoic lines of ≥3 mm in length in at least two different directions with respect to the imaged plane	Minor criteria	Unknown
Ductal features				
1	MPD calculi[a]	Echogenic structure(s) within MPD with acoustic shadowing	Major A	Stones
2	Irregular MPD contour	Uneven or irregular outline and ectatic course	Minor criteria	Unknown
3	Dilated side branches	3 or more tubular anechoic structures each measuring ≥1 mm in width, budding from the MPD	Minor criteria	Side-branch ectasia
4	MPD dilation	≥3.5-mm body or ≥1.5-mm tai	Minor criteria	MPD dilation
5	Hyperechoic MPD margin	Echogenic, distinct structure greater than 50% of entire MPD in the body and tail	Minor criteria	Ductal fibrosis

[a]Located in head, body or tail
[b]Located in dorsal of head, body or tail; only located in body or tail

Table 7.8 Rosemont consensus for EUS diagnosis of CP (Catalano et al. 2009)

1. Consistent with CP
(a) 1 major A feature (+)3 ≥ minor features
(b) 1 major A feature (+) 1 major B feature
(c) 2 major A features
2. Suggestive of CP (Diagnosis requires confirmation by additional imaging study (CT, MRI, or ERCP) or pancreatic exocrine function)
(a) 1 major A feature (+) <3 minor features
(b) 1 major B feature (+) ≥3 minor features
(c) ≥5 minor features (any)
3. Indeterminate for CP (Diagnosis requires confirmation by additional imaging study (CT, MRI, or ERCP) or pancreatic exocrine function)
(a) 3–4 minor features, no major features
(b) Major B feature alone or with <3 minor features
4. Normal
≤2 minor features(Excludes cysts, dilated MPD, hyperechoic nonshadowing foci, dilated side branch.), no major features

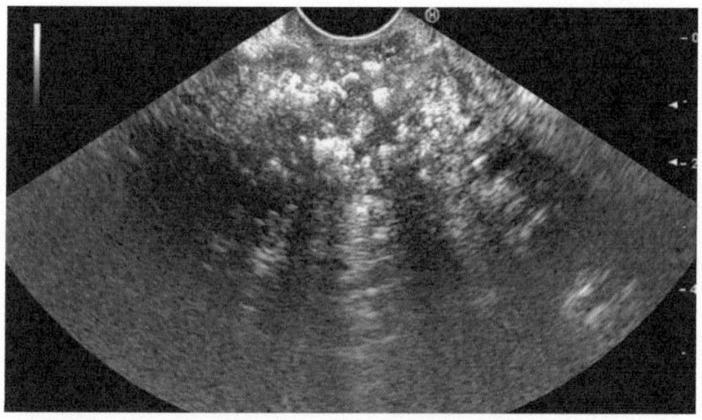

Fig. 7.16 Multiple strong echo foci in the parenchyma of the pancreas with acoustic shadows

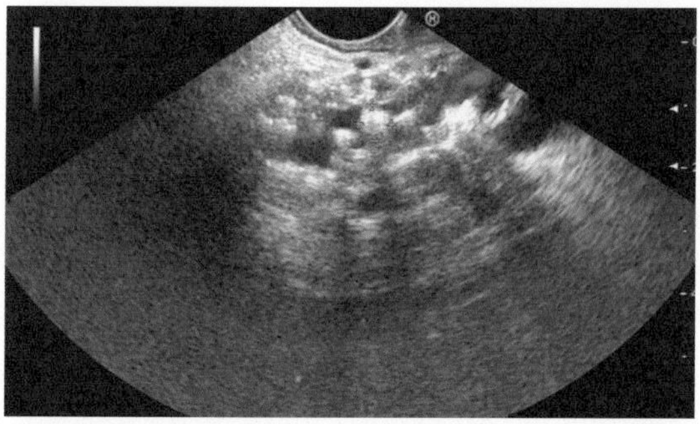

Fig. 7.17 Strong echo with acoustic shadow in main pancreatic duct (stone)

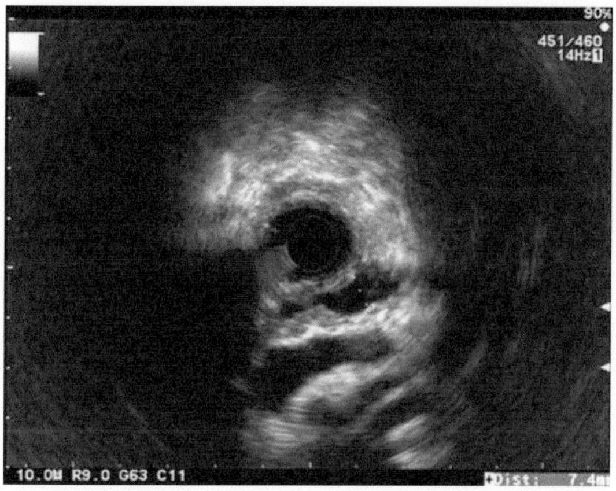

Fig. 7.18 Pancreatic duct distortion and dilation

Since this classification system gives a strictly criteria for EUS based CP diagnostic, it plays an important role in CP diagnosis, especially in early stage (Catalano et al. 2009). But, its significance in diagnosis, treatment, and research of CP is need to be further verified and the criteria should be mortified and improved along with the progress of EUS technology and the deep understanding of the EUS features of various types of CP (Stevens and Parsi 2010; Park and Van Dam 2009). In addition, due to the lack of strict histological comparison, the advantage of EUS in the early stage CP diagnosis has not been fully demonstrated, and factors such as age, body weight, smoking and other factors affect that the EUS based diagnosis still need further study (Gardner and Levy 2010; Stevens 2011).

6.1.3 EUS-Guided Fine Need Aspiration/Biopsy (EUS-FNA/B)

So far, few studies described the value of EUS-FNA for CP diagnosis, due to the possible and severe complications related to the procedure and the lack of a generally agreed histologic definition of CP. Hollerbach et al. (2001) showed compared with EUS, EUS-FNA improves the negative predictive value, but it does not improve the specificity of EUS. Another study showed that in 14 patients with alcohol related CP who underwent EUS guided pancreatic fine needle biopsy (EUS-FNB), adequate tissue samples for histological evaluation were obtained in all cases and infiltration of inflammatory cells was observed in all tissue specimens (Iglesias-Garcia et al. 2006). Biopsies including pancreatic acini were those obtained from patients with mild to moderate EUS changes of CP (up to five EUS criteria). But, biopsy samples from more severe cases (8–10 EUS criteria) were those showing only ductal epithelium with fibrotic components. Therefore although EUS-FNA may be an alternative choice for CP diagnosis and staging, its efficiency and safety for CP diagnosis are remain unclear.

6.1.4 EUS Guided Tru-Cut Biopsy (EUS-TCB)

EUS-TCB is superior to EUS-FNA in obtaining no-surgical modality specimen. A study evaluate the utility and the safety profile of EUS-TCB for the histologic diagnosis of suspected non-focal CP (DeWitt et al. 2005). In this study, 16 patients with suspected CP (> or =3 EUS criteria) underwent transgastric EUS-TCB of the pancreas. EUS-TCB results were as follows: one case of probable CP, two cases of normal pancreas, six cases of non-diagnostic CP, and one case of device malfunction. Complications occurred in two patients. Therefore, the author thought because of potential complications and limited diagnostic yield, this technique is not currently recommended for evaluation of these patients.

6.1.5 EUS and Histologic Correlation

At present, the correlation of EUS features of CP and histologic changes remain undetermined due to the limitation of specimen obtain and no-consensus of histologic diagnosis criteria (Gardner and Levy 2010; Levy and Wiersema 2005). Varadarajulu et al. (2007) found that parenchymal feature of EUS were foci, stranding, and lobulations and ductal feature were dilated or irregular main pancreatic duct, side branches, and hyperechoic duct margins. Four or more EUS criteria provided the best sensitivity, specificity, and accuracy. But in Chong et al. (2007) reported that three or more EUS criteria was thought to provide the best balance of sensitivity and specificity for predicting abnormal histology. In addition, in a recent study (LeBlanc et al. 2014), main pancreatic duct (MPD) dilation and irregularity were found to associated with moderate and severe fibrosis. Lobularity with honeycombing, hyperechoic foci with shadowing, hyperechoic foci without shadowing, MPD dilation, MPD irregularity, and dilated side branches were associated with severe CP. Therefore the importance of pancreatic ductal changes should not be minimized in the evaluation of CP.

6.2 New Techniques Associated to EUS

6.2.1 EUS-Guided Elastography

In recent years, there has been increasing interest in assessing the role of elastography on the evaluation of solid pancreatic tumors, but few studies focus on the management of CP. In 2007, a study was conducted by Janssen J. et al. to investigate the feasibility of EUS elastography of the pancreas (Janssen et al. 2007). They found that EUS elastography could distinguish normal pancreas from CP or pancreatic tumor, but CP and hard tumors cannot be distinguished by elastography. However, another study found there are significant direct linear correlation between the number of EUS criteria of CP and the strain ratio (Iglesias-Garcia et al. 2013). And, the strain ratio varied significantly in different Rosemont classification groups. Therefore, EUS-elastography maybe was an accurate tool for the diagnosis of CP and provided relevant and objective information to support EUS findings. But its role need to be further studied. In the last study, EUS-elastography was used to predict the pancreatic exocrine insufficiency (PEI) of CP patients. It was found that there a direct relationship between strain ratio and the probability of PEI. Strain ratio allows quantification of the probability of PEI in patients with CP (Dominguez-Munoz et al. 2015).

6.2.2 EUS-Guided Contrast Enhancement

The role of contrast enhancement EUS (CE-EUS) in diagnosis of CP has not yet been determined. Most studies focus on the differential diagnosis of pancreatic cancer and focal CP (Saftoiu et al. 2015). However few studies described the CE-EUS feature of CP. One study found CE-EUS enhances the lobular pattern seen by convention EUS in CP patients (Saftoiu et al. 2012). In addition, compared with control, the washout of contrast in CP patients was significantly faster.

6.2.3 Computer Aided Diagnosis (CAD) Based EUS

Although EUS plays an important role in diagnosis of CP, the interpretation of EUS imaging is heavily subjective. EUS images contain medical information regarding textural features that can aid disease diagnosis by using CAD image analysis techniques. Previous studies have demonstrated the ability of EUS imaging with textural feature analyses to improve CP diagnosis (Irisawa et al. 2004; Das et al. 2008). Zhu et al. (2013) combined image analyses with CAD techniques to establish a classification model for EUS imaging to distinguish pancreatic cancer from CP accurately, based on an SVM model, with an accuracy of 96.3%, sensitivity of 93.4% and specificity of 92.2%. In our last study, a new descriptor was introduced for CAD and able to differentiate CP from autoimmune pancreatitis (Zhu et al. 2015).

Conclusion

EUS can be considered as first choices for the morphological diagnosis of CP, as a result of it display small changes of the pancreatic parenchyma or duct. EUS-FNA/B and EUS-TCB could provide specimen for histological diagnosis, but those techniques are not currently recommended for evaluation of this disease due to potential complications and limited diagnostic yield. They are often used for distinguish of CP from pancreatic tumors. New techniques based on EUS provide a new perspective for CP diagnosis. But more studies need to be conducted to evaluate their utility.

References

Adler DG, Lichtenstein D, Baron TH, et al. The role of endoscopy in patients with chronic pancreatitis. Gastrointest Endosc. 2006;63:933–7.

Affronti J. Chronic pancreatitis and exocrine insufficiency. Prim Care. 2011;38(3):515–37.

Albashir S, Bronner MP, Parsi MA, et al. Endoscopic ultrasound, secretin endoscopic pancreatic function test, and histology: correlation in chronic pancreatitis. Am J Gastroenterol. 2010;105:2498–503.

American Diabetes Association. Diagnosis and classification of diabetes mellitus. Diabetes Care. 2014;37(Suppl 1):S81–90.

Ammann RW. A clinically based classification system for alcoholic chronic pancreatitis: summary of an international workshop on chronic pancreatitis. Pancreas. 1997;14:215–21.

Ammann RW. Zurich workshop on alcoholic chronic pancreatitis. Int J Pancreatol. 1998;23:81–2.

Andersen DK. Mechanisms and emerging treatments of the metabolic complications of chronic pancreatitis. Pancreas. 2007;35:1–15.

Andersen DK. The practical importance of recognizing pancreatogenic or type 3c diabetes. Diabetes Metab Res Rev. 2012;28:326–8.

Andersen DK, Andren-Sandberg A, Duell EJ, et al. Pancreatitis-diabetes-pancreatic cancer: summary of an NIDDK-NCI workshop. Pancreas. 2013;42: 1227–37.

Arvanitakis M, Van Laethem JL, Parma J, et al. Predictive factors for pancreatic cancer in patients with chronic pancreatitis in association with K-ras gene mutation. Endoscopy. 2004;36:535–42.

Axon AT, Classen M, Cotton PB, Cremer M, Freeny PC, Lees WR. Pancreatography in chronic pancreatitis: international definitions. Gut. 1984;25:1107–12.

Bagul A, Siriwardena AK. Evaluation of the Manchester classification system for chronic pancreatitis. JOP. 2006;7:390–6.

Balci NC, Smith A, Momtahen AJ, et al. MRI and S-MRCP findings in patients with suspected chronic pancreatitis: correlation with endoscopic pancreatic function testing (ePFT). J Magn Reson Imaging. 2010;31:601–6.

Bhutani MS, Arantes VN, Verma D, et al. Histopathologic correlation of endoscopic ultrasound findings of chronic pancreatitis in human autopsies. Pancreas. 2009;38:820–4.

Bian Y, Wang L, Chen C, et al. Quantification of pancreatic exocrine function of chronic pancreatitis with secretin-enhanced MRCP. World J Gastroenterol:

WJG. 2013;19(41):7177–7182. PMID: 24222963. doi:10.3748/wjg.v19.i41.7177.

Bian Y, Wang L, Chen C, et al. Combination of secretin-enhanced MR cholangiopancreatography and conventional MRI in the diagnosis of chronic pancreatitis. Chin J Radiol. 2014;48(4):294–8.

Bilgin M, Bilgin S, Balci NC, et al. Magnetic resonance imaging and magnetic resonance cholangiopancreatography findings compared with fecal elastase 1 measurement for the diagnosis of chronic pancreatitis. Pancreas. 2008;36:e33–9.

Bolan PJ, Fink AS. Endoscopic retrograde cholangiopancreatography in chronic pancreatitis. World J Surg. 2003;27(11):1183–1191. PMID: 14716502. doi:10.1007/s00268-003-7236-9.

Boninsegna E, Manfredi R, Ventriglia A, et al. Santorinicele: secretin-enhanced magnetic resonance cholangiopancreatography findings before and after minor papilla sphincterotomy. Eur Radiol. 2015;25(8):2437–2444. PMID: 25693665. doi:10.1007/s00330-015-3644-0.

Braganza JM, Lee SH, McCloy RF, McMahon MJ. Chronic pancreatitis. Lancet. 2011;377(9772):1184–97.

Brugge WR. Endoscopic approach to the diagnosis and treatment of pancreatic disease. Curr Opin Gastroenterol. 2013;29:559–65.

Buchler MW, Martignoni ME, Friess H, et al. A proposal for a new clinical classification of chronic pancreatitis. BMC Gastroenterol. 2009;9:93.

Buxbaum J. The role of endoscopic retrograde cholangiopancreatography in patients with pancreatic disease. Gastroenterol Clin North Am. 2012;41:23–45.

Carriere F, Laugier R, Barrowman JA, et al. Gastric and pancreatic lipase levels during a test meal in dogs. Scand J Gastroenterol. 1993;28:443–54.

Catalano MF, Lahoti S, Geenen JE, Hogan WJ. Prospective evaluation of endoscopic ultrasonography, endoscopic retrograde pancreatography, and secretin test in the diagnosis of chronic pancreatitis. Gastrointest Endosc. 1998;48:11–7.

Catalano MF, Sahai A, Levy M, et al. EUS-based criteria for the diagnosis of chronic pancreatitis: the Rosemont classification. Gastrointest Endosc. 2009;69:1251–61.

Ceyhan GO, Bergmann F, Kadihasanoglu M, et al. The neurotropic factor artemin influences the extent of neural damage and growth in chronic pancreatitis. Gut. 2007;56(4):534–44.

Chang KJ, Nguyen P, Erickson RA, et al. The clinical utility of endoscopic ultrasound-guided fine-needle aspiration in the diagnosis and staging of pancreatic carcinoma. Gastrointest Endosc. 1997;45(5):387–93. PMID: 9165320.

Chari ST, Smyrk TC, Levy MJ, et al. Diagnosis of autoimmune pancreatitis: the Mayo Clinic experience. Clin Gastroenterol Hepatol. 2006;4:1010–6.

Chari ST, Kloeppel G, Zhang L, et al. Histopathologic and clinical subtypes of autoimmune pancreatitis: the Honolulu consensus document. Pancreas. 2010;39:549–54.

Chen N, Unnikrishnan IR, Anjana RM, Mohan V, Pitchumoni CS. The complex exocrine-endocrine relationship and secondary diabetes in exocrine pancreatic disorders. J Clin Gastroenterol. 2011;45:850–61.

Chong AK, Hawes RH, Hoffman BJ, et al. Diagnostic performance of EUS for chronic pancreatitis: a comparison with histopathology. Gastrointest Endosc. 2007;65:808–14.

Choueiri NE, Balci NC, Alkaade S, et al. Advanced imaging of chronic pancreatitis. Curr Gastroenterol Rep. 2010;12:114–20.

Chowdhury RS, Forsmark CE. Review article: pancreatic function testing. Aliment Pharmacol Ther. 2003;17:733–50.

Chowdhury R, Bhutani MS, Mishra G, et al. Comparative analysis of direct pancreatic function testing versus morphological assessment by endoscopic ultrasonography for the evaluation of chronic unexplained abdominal pain of presumed pancreatic origin. Pancreas. 2005;31:63–8.

Church NI, Pereira SP, Deheragoda MG, et al. Autoimmune pancreatitis: clinical and radiological features and objective response to steroid therapy in a UK series. Am J Gastroenterol. 2007;102:2417–25.

Clark CJ, Fino NF, Clark N, et al. Trends in the use of endoscopic retrograde cholangiopancreatography for the management of chronic pancreatitis in the United States. J Clin Gastroenterol. 2016;50(5):417–422. PMID: 26890329. doi:10.1097/MCG.0000000000000493.

Conwell DL, Zuccaro G, Purich E, et al. Comparison of endoscopic ultrasound chronic pancreatitis criteria to the endoscopic secretin-stimulated pancreatic function test. Dig Dis Sci. 2007;52:1206–10.

Conwell DL, Lee LS, Yadav D, et al. American Pancreatic Association Practice Guidelines in Chronic Pancreatitis: evidence-based report on diagnostic guidelines. Pancreas. 2014;43:1143–62.

Cremer M, Deviere J, Engelholm L. Endoscopic management of cysts and pseudocysts in chronic pancreatitis: long-term follow-up after 7 years of experience. Gastrointest Endosc. 1989;35:1–9.

Cui Y, Andersen DK. Pancreatogenic diabetes: special considerations for management. Pancreatology. 2011;11:279–94.

Das A, Nguyen CC, Li F, et al. Digital image analysis of EUS images accurately differentiates pancreatic cancer from chronic pancreatitis and normal tissue. Gastrointest Endosc. 2008;67:861–7.

Delhaye M, Van Steenbergen W, Cesmeli E, et al. Belgian consensus on chronic pancreatitis in adults and children: statements on diagnosis and nutritional, medical, and surgical treatment. Acta Gastroenterol Belg. 2014;77:47–65.

Devereaux CE, Binmoeller KF. Endoscopic retrograde cholangiopancreatography in the next millennium. Gastrointest Endosc Clin N Am. 2000;10:117–33.

DeWitt J, McGreevy K, LeBlanc J, et al. EUS-guided Trucut biopsy of suspected nonfocal chronic pancreatitis. Gastrointest Endosc. 2005;62:76–84.

DiMagno MJ, DiMagno EP. Chronic pancreatitis. Curr Opin Gastroenterol. 2010;26:490–8.

Dimagno MJ, Dimagno EP. Chronic pancreatitis. Curr Opin Gastroenterol. 2011;27(5):452–9.

DiMagno EP, Go VL, Summerskill WH. Relations between pancreatic enzyme outputs and malabsorption in severe pancreatic insufficiency. N Engl J Med. 1973;288:813–5.

DiMagno EP, Malagelada JR, Go VL. Relationship between alcoholism and pancreatic insufficiency. Ann N Y Acad Sci. 1975;252:200–7.

Dominguez-Munoz JE, Iglesias-Garcia J, Vilarino-Insua M, et al. 13C-mixed triglyceride breath test to assess oral enzyme substitution therapy in patients with chronic pancreatitis. Clin Gastroenterol Hepatol. 2007;5:484–8.

Dominguez-Munoz JE, Iglesias-Garcia J, Castineira Alvarino M, et al. EUS elastography to predict pancreatic exocrine insufficiency in patients with chronic pancreatitis. Gastrointest Endosc. 2015;81:136–42.

Drenes AM, Krarap AL, Detlefsen S, et al. Pain in chronic pancreatitis: the role of neuropathic pain mechanisms. Gut. 2008;57(11):1616–27.

Dumasy V, Delhaye M, Cotton F, et al. Fat malabsorption screening in chronic pancreatitis. Am J Gastroenterol. 2004;99:1350–4.

Ebert R, Creutzfeldt W. Reversal of impaired GIP and insulin secretion in patients with pancreatogenic steatorrhea following enzyme substitution. Diabetologia. 1980;19:198–204.

Eddes EH, Verkijk M, Gielkens HA, et al. Pancreatic polypeptide secretion in patients with chronic pancreatitis and after pancreatic surgery. Int J Pancreatol. 2001;29:173–80.

Engjom T, Erchinger F, Tjora E, et al. Diagnostic accuracy of secretin-stimulated ultrasonography of the pancreas assessing exocrine pancreatic failure in cystic fibrosis and chronic pancreatitis. Scand J Gastroenterol. 2015;50:601–10.

Erchinger F, Engjom T, Tjora E, et al. Quantification of pancreatic function using a clinically feasible short endoscopic secretin test. Pancreas. 2013;42:1101–6.

Etemad B, Whitcomb DC. Chronic pancreatitis: diagnosis, classification, and new genetic developments. Gastroenterology. 2001;120:682–707.

Ewald N, Bretzel RG. Diabetes mellitus secondary to pancreatic diseases (Type 3c)—are we neglecting an important disease? Eur J Intern Med. 2013;24:203–6.

Feldman M, Friedman LS, Brandt LJ. Sleisenger and Fordtran's gastrointestinal and liver disease—2 volume set: pathophysiology, diagnosis, management. Philadelphia: Saunders; 2015.

Forsmark CE. The diagnosis of chronic pancreatitis. Gastrointest Endosc. 2000;52(2):293–298. PMID: 10922118. doi:10.1067/mge.2000.106889.

Forsmark CE. Pancreatitis and its complications. Totowa: Humana Press; 2005. doi:10.1385/1592598153. ISBN: 978-1-58829-179-0.

Forsmark CE. The early diagnosis of chronic pancreatitis. Clin Gastroenterol Hepatol. 2008;6:1291–3.

Forsmark CE. Management of chronic pancreatitis. Gastroenterology. 2013;144:1282–91.

Forsmark CE, Toskes PP. What does an abnormal pancreatogram mean? Gastrointest Endosc Clin N Am. 1995;5:105–23.

Frulloni L, Lunardi C, Simone R, et al. Identification of a novel antibody associated with autoimmune pancreatitis. N Engl J Med. 2009;361:2135–42.

Frulloni L, Falconi M, Gabbrielli A, et al. Italian consensus guidelines for chronic pancreatitis. Dig Liver Dis. 2010;42(Suppl 6):S381–406.

Gardner TB, Levy MJ. EUS diagnosis of chronic pancreatitis. Gastrointest Endosc. 2010;71:1280–9.

Glaser B, Zoghlin G, Pienta K, Vinik AI. Pancreatic polypeptide response to secretin in obesity: effects of glucose intolerance. Horm Metab Res. 1988;20:288–92.

Gooshe M, Abdolghaffari AH, Nikfar S, et al. Antioxidant therapy in acute, chronic and post-endoscopic retrograde cholangiopancreatography pancreatitis: an updated systematic review and meta-analysis. World J Gastroenterol: WJG. 2015;21(30):9189–9208. PMID: 26290647. doi:10.3748/wjg.v21.i30.9189.

Gupta V, Toskes PP. Diagnosis and management of chronic pancreatitis. Postgrad Med J. 2005;81(958):491–497. PMID: 16085738. doi:10.1136/pgmj.2003.009761.

Gupte AR, Forsmark CE. Chronic pancreatitis. Curr Opin Gastroenterol. 2014;30:500–5.

Haaber AB, Rosenfalck AM, Hansen B, et al. Bone mineral metabolism, bone mineral density, and body composition in patients with chronic pancreatitis and pancreatic exocrine insufficiency. Int J Pancreatol. 2000;27:21–7.

Hernandez LV, Catalano MF. EUS in the diagnosis of early-stage chronic pancreatitis. Best Pract Res Clin Gastroenterol. 2010;24:243–9.

Hoffmeister A, Mayerle J, Beglinger C, et al. S3-Consensus guidelines on definition, etiology, diagnosis and medical, endoscopic and surgical management of chronic pancreatitis German Society of Digestive and Metabolic Diseases (DGVS). Z Gastroenterol. 2012;50:1176–224.

Hollerbach S, Klamann A, Topalidis T, et al. Endoscopic ultrasonography (EUS) and fine-needle aspiration (FNA) cytology for diagnosis of chronic pancreatitis. Endoscopy. 2001;33:824–31.

Homma T, Harada H, Koizumi M. Diagnostic criteria for chronic pancreatitis by the Japan Pancreas Society. Pancreas. 1997;15:14–5.

Iglesias-Garcia J, Vilarino-Insua M, Iglesias-Rey M, et al. Accuracy of the optimized 13C-mixed triglyceride breath test for the diagnosis of steatorrhea in clinical practice. Gastroenterology. 2003;124:1.

Iglesias-Garcia J, Abdulkader I, Larino-Noia J, et al. Histological evaluation of chronic pancreatitis by endoscopic ultrasound-guided fine needle biopsy. Gut. 2006;55:1661–2.

Iglesias-Garcia J, Dominguez-Munoz JE, Castineira-Alvarino M, et al. Quantitative elastography associated with endoscopic ultrasound for the diagnosis of chronic pancreatitis. Endoscopy. 2013;45:781–8.

Ikeda M, Sato T, Morozumi A, et al. Morphologic changes in the pancreas detected by screening ultrasonography in a mass survey, with special reference to main duct dilatation, cyst formation, and calcification. Pancreas. 1994;9:508–12.

Irisawa A, Mishra G, Hernandez LV, et al. Quantitative analysis of endosonographic parenchymal echogenicity in patients with chronic pancreatitis. J Gastroenterol Hepatol. 2004;19:1199–205.

Ito T, Otsuki M, Itoi T, et al. Pancreatic diabetes in a follow-up survey of chronic pancreatitis in Japan. J Gastroenterol. 2007;42:291–7.

Ito T, Ishiguro H, Ohara H, et al. Evidence-based clinical practice guidelines for chronic pancreatitis 2015. J Gastroenterol. 2016;51:85–92.

Janssen J, Schlorer E, Greiner L. EUS elastography of the pancreas: feasibility and pattern description of the normal pancreas, chronic pancreatitis, and focal pancreatic lesions. Gastrointest Endosc. 2007;65:971–8.

Kahl S, Malfertheiner P. The place of endoscopic ultrasound in the diagnosis of chronic pancreatitis. In: Dominguez-Munoz JE, editor. Clinical pancreatology for practising gastroenterologists and surgeons. Oxford: Blackwell Publishing; 2005. p. 246–52.

Kalaitzakis E, Braden B, Trivedi P, et al. Intraductal papillary mucinous neoplasm in chronic calcifying pancreatitis: egg or hen? World J Gastroenterol: WJG. 2009;15(10):1273–5. PMID: 19291831

Kalvaria I, Labadarios D, Shephard GS, et al. Biochemical vitamin E deficiency in chronic pancreatitis. Int J Pancreatol. 1986;1:119–28.

Kamisawa T, Okazaki K, Kawa S, et al. Japanese consensus guidelines for management of autoimmune pancreatitis: III. Treatment and prognosis of AIP. J Gastroenterol. 2010;45:471–7.

Katschinski M, Schirra J, Bross A, et al. Duodenal secretion and fecal excretion of pancreatic elastase-1 in healthy humans and patients with chronic pancreatitis. Pancreas. 1997;15:191–200.

Keller J, Layer P. Human pancreatic exocrine response to nutrients in health and disease. Gut. 2005;54(Suppl 6):1–28.

Keller J, Layer P. Diagnosis of pancreatic exocrine insufficiency in chronic pancreatitis. Exocrine Pancreas Knowledge Base: Pancreapedia; 2015.

Keller J, Aghdassi AA, Lerch MM, et al. Tests of pancreatic exocrine function—clinical significance in pancreatic and non-pancreatic disorders. Best Pract Res Clin Gastroenterol. 2009;23:425–39.

Keller J, Bruckel S, Jahr C, et al. A modified 13C-mixed triglyceride breath test detects moderate pancreatic exocrine insufficiency. Pancreas. 2011;40:1201–5.

Keller J, Meier V, Wolfram KU, et al. Sensitivity and specificity of an abbreviated (13)C-mixed triglyceride breath test for measurement of pancreatic exocrine function. United European Gastroenterol J. 2014a;2(4):288–294. PMID: 25083286. doi:10.1177/2050640614542496.

Keller J, Layer P, Brückel S, et al. 13C-Mixed triglyceride breath test for evaluation of pancreatic exocrine function in diabetes mellitus. Pancreas. 2014b;43:842–8.

Keogan MT, Edelman RR. Technologic advances in abdominal MR imaging. Radiology. 2001;220(2):310–320. PMID: 11477231. doi:10.1148/radiology.220.2.r01au22310.

Ketwaroo G, Brown A, Young B, et al. Defining the accuracy of secretin pancreatic function testing in patients with suspected early chronic pancreatitis. Am J Gastroenterol. 2013;108(8):1360–1366. PMID: 23711627. doi:10.1038/ajg.2013.148.

Knop FK, Vilsboll T, Hojberg PV, et al. Reduced incretin effect in type 2 diabetes: cause or consequence of the diabetic state? Diabetes. 2007;56:1951–9.

Lankisch PG, Schreiber A, Otto J. Pancreolauryl test. Evaluation of a tubeless pancreatic function test in comparison with other indirect and direct tests for exocrine pancreatic function. Dig Dis Sci. 1983;28:490–3.

Lankisch PG, Droge M, Hofses S, et al. Steatorrhoea: you cannot trust your eyes when it comes to diagnosis [letter] [see comments]. Lancet. 1996;347:1620–1.

Lara I, Rodriguez RI, Orillac J. Magnetic resonance cholangiopancreatography: an advanced technique in the diagnosis of biliopancreatic diseases (the first experience in Panama). Rev Med Panama. 2001;26:22–7. PMID: 16161720.

Larsen S, Hilsted J, Tronier B, Worning H. Metabolic control and B cell function in patients with insulin-dependent diabetes mellitus secondary to chronic pancreatitis. Metabolism. 1987;36:964–7.

Larsen S, Hilsted J, Tronier B, Worning H. Pancreatic hormone secretion in chronic pancreatitis without residual beta-cell function. Acta Endocrinol. 1988;118:357–64.

Layer P, Go VL, DiMagno EP. Fate of pancreatic enzymes during small intestinal aboral transit in humans. Am J Physiol. 1986;251:G475–80.

Layer P, Yamamoto H, Kalthoff L, et al. The different courses of early- and late-onset idiopathic and alcoholic chronic pancreatitis. Gastroenterology. 1994;107:1481–7.

Layer P, von der Ohe MR, Holst JJ, et al. Altered postprandial motility in chronic pancreatitis: role of malabsorption. Gastroenterology. 1997;112:1624–34.

LeBlanc JK, Chen JH, Al-Haddad M, et al. Endoscopic ultrasound and histology in chronic pancreatitis: how are they associated? Pancreas. 2014;43:440–4.

Levy MJ, Wiersema MJ. EUS-guided Trucut biopsy. Gastrointest Endosc. 2005;62:417–26.

Lieb JG II, Draganov PV. Pancreatic function testing: here to stay for the 21st century. World J Gastroenterol. 2008;14:3149–58.

Linde J, Nilsson LH, Barany FR. Diabetes and hypoglycemia in chronic pancreatitis. Scand J Gastroenterol. 1977;12:369–73.

Löhr JM, Dominguez-Munoz E, Rosendahl J, et al. Evidence-based guidelines for the diagnosis and therapy of chronic pancreatitis (HaPanEU). UEG J 2017; 5(2):153–99.

Lowenfels AB, Maisonneuve P, Cavallini G, et al. Pancreatitis and the risk of pancreatic cancer. International Pancreatitis Study Group. N Engl J Med. 1993;328(20):1433–1437. PMID: 8479461. doi:10.1056/NEJM199305203282001.

Luaces-Regueira M, Iglesias-Garcia J, Lindkvist B, et al. Smoking as a risk factor for complications in chronic pancreatitis. Pancreas. 2014;43:275–80.

Majumder S, Chari ST. Chronic pancreatitis. Lancet. 2016;387:1957–66.

Mann ST, Stracke H, Lange U, et al. Alterations of bone mineral density and bone metabolism in patients with various grades of chronic pancreatitis. Metabolism. 2003a;52:579–85.

Mann ST, Stracke H, Lange U, et al. Vitamin D3 in patients with various grades of chronic pancreatitis, according to morphological and functional criteria of the pancreas. Dig Dis Sci. 2003b;48:533–8.

Mann ST, Mann V, Stracke H, et al. Fecal elastase 1 and vitamin D3 in patients with osteoporotic bone fractures. Eur J Med Res. 2008;13:68–72.

Martinez J, Abad-Gonzalez A, Aparicio JR, et al. The Spanish Pancreatic Club recommendations for the diagnosis and treatment of chronic pancreatitis: part 1 (diagnosis). Pancreatology. 2013;13:8–17.

Mayerle J, Hoffmeister A, Werner J, et al. Chronic pancreatitis—definition, etiology, investigation and treatment. Dtsch Arztebl Int. 2013;110:387–93.

Md PS, Md UN. Role of ERCP in patients with idiopathic recurrent acute pancreatitis. Curr Treat Options Gastroenterol. 2016;14(3):327–339. PMID: 27371265. doi:10.1007/s11938-016-0096-9.

Meier JJ, Giese A. Diabetes associated with pancreatic diseases. Curr Opin Gastroenterol. 2015;31: 400–6.

Meier JJ, Nauck MA. Is the diminished incretin effect in type 2 diabetes just an epi-phenomenon of impaired beta-cell function? Diabetes. 2010;59:1117–25.

Meier JJ, Breuer TG, Bonadonna RC, et al. Pancreatic diabetes manifests when beta cell area declines by approximately 65% in humans. Diabetologia. 2012;55:1346–54.

Mensel B, Messner P, Mayerle J, et al. Secretin-stimulated MRCP in volunteers: assessment of safety, duct visualization, and pancreatic exocrine function. AJR Am J Roentgenol. 2014a;202(1):102–108. PMID: 24370134. doi:10.2214/AJR.12.10271.

Mensel B, Messner P, Mayerle J, et al. Secretin-stimulated MRCP in volunteers: assessment of safety, duct visualization, and pancreatic exocrine function. Am J Roentgenol. 2014b;202(1):102–108. PMID: WOS:000329113000031. doi:10.2214/ajr.12.10271.

Merkle EM, Baillie J. Exocrine pancreatic function: evaluation with MR imaging before and after secretin stimulation. Am J Gastroenterol. 2006;101(1):137–138. PMID: 16405546. doi:10.1111/j.1572-0241.2006.00400.x.

Milosavljevic T, Kostic Milosavljevic M, Krstic M, et al. Classification of chronic pancreatitis. Dig Dis. 2010;28(2):330–333. PMID: 20814207. doi:10.1159/000319409.

Morselli-Labate AM, Pezzilli R. Usefulness of serum IgG4 in the diagnosis and follow up of autoimmune pancreatitis: a systematic literature review and meta-analysis. J Gastroenterol Hepatol. 2009;24:15–36.

Muniraj T, Aslanian HR, Farrell J, et al. Chronic pancreatitis, a comprehensive review and update. Part II: diagnosis, complications, and management. Dis Mon. 2015;61(1):5–37. PMID: 25681098. doi:10.1016/j.disamonth.2014.12.003.

Nagai H, Ohtsubo K. Pancreatic lithiasis in the aged. Its clinicopathology and pathogenesis. Gastroenterology. 1984;86:331–8.

Nagar AB, Gorelick FS. Pancreatitis and its complications. New York: Human Press; 2005.

Nattermann C, Goldschmidt A, Dancygier H. Endosonography in chronic pancreatitis-a comparison between endoscopic retrograde pancreatography and endoscopic ultrasonography. Endoscopy. 1993;25:565–70.

Navaneethan U, Venkataraman J. Recent advancement in the pathogenesis of pain in chronic pancreatitis: the argument continues. Minerva Gastroenterol Dietol. 2010;56(1):55–63.

Nayar MK, Paranandi B, Dawwas MF, et al. Comparison of the diagnostic performance of 2 core biopsy needles for EUS-guided tissue acquisition from solid pancreatic lesions. Gastrointest Endosc. 2016;85(5):1017–1024. PMID: 27633157. doi:10.1016/j.gie.2016.08.048.

Okazaki K, Kawa S, Kamisawa T, et al. Clinical diagnostic criteria of autoimmune pancreatitis: revised proposal. J Gastroenterol. 2006;41:626–31.

Okazaki K, Kawa S, Kamisawa T, et al. Japanese clinical guidelines for autoimmune pancreatitis. Pancreas. 2009;38:849–66.

Okazaki K, Kawa S, Kamisawa T, et al. Japanese consensus guidelines for management of autoimmune pancreatitis: I. Concept and diagnosis of autoimmune pancreatitis. J Gastroenterol. 2010;45:249–65.

Otsuki M, Chung JB, Okazaki K, et al. Asian diagnostic criteria for autoimmune pancreatitis: consensus of the Japan-Korea Symposium on Autoimmune Pancreatitis. J Gastroenterol. 2008;43:403–8.

Park WG, Van Dam J. Election year fever? Voting on EUS criteria for chronic pancreatitis. Gastrointest Endosc. 2009;69:1262–3.

Parsi MA, Conwell DL, Zuccaro G, et al. Findings on endoscopic retrograde cholangiopancreatography and pancreatic function test in suspected chronic pancreatitis and negative cross-sectional imaging. Clin Gastroenterol Hepatol. 2008;6: 1432–6.

Paulo JA, Lee LS, Wu B, et al. Mass spectrometry-based proteomics of endoscopically collected pancreatic fluid in chronic pancreatitis research. Proteomics Clin Appl. 2011;5:109–20.

Pezzilli R. Chronic pancreatitis: maldigestion, intestinal ecology and intestinal inflammation. World J Gastroenterol. 2009;15(14):1673–6.

Pitchumoni CS. Chronic pancreatitis: pathogenesis and management of pain. J Clin Gastroenterol. 1998;27:101–7.

Rabiee A, Galiatsatos P, Salas-Carrillo R, Thompson MJ, Andersen DK, Elahi D. Pancreatic polypeptide administration enhances insulin sensitivity and reduces the insulin requirement of patients on insulin pump therapy. J Diabetes Sci Technol. 2011;5: 1521–8.

Raimondo M, Wallace MB. Diagnosis of early chronic pancreatitis by endoscopic ultrasound. Are we there yet? JOP. 2004;5:1–7.

Raina A, Yadav D, Krasinskas AM, et al. Evaluation and management of autoimmune pancreatitis: experience at a large US center. Am J Gastroenterol. 2009;104:2295–306.

Rajan E, Clain JE, Levy MJ, et al. Age-related changes in the pancreas identified by EUS: a prospective evaluation. Gastrointest Endosc. 2005;61:401–6.

Ramesh H. Proposal for a new grading system for chronic pancreatitis: the ABC system. J Clin Gastroenterol. 2002;35:67–70.

Rebours V, Vullierme MP, Hentic O, et al. Smoking and the course of recurrent acute and chronic alcoholic pancreatitis: a dose-dependent relationship. Pancreas. 2012;41:1219–24.

Rickels MR, Bellin M, Toledo FG, et al. Detection, evaluation and treatment of diabetes mellitus in chronic pancreatitis: recommendations from PancreasFest 2012. Pancreatology. 2013;13:336–42.

Rosch T, Schusdziarra V, Born P, et al. Modern imaging methods versus clinical assessment in the evaluation of hospital in-patients with suspected pancreatic disease. Am J Gastroenterol. 2000;95(9):2261–2270. PMID: 11007227. doi:10.1111/j.1572-0241.2000.02312.x.

Ross SO, Forsmark CE. Pancreatic and biliary disorders in the elderly. Gastroenterol Clin North Am. 2001;30:531–45.

Roth CG. Fundamentals of body MRI. Philadelphia: Saunders; 2012. p. 135. ISBN: 978-1-4160-5183-1.

Safari MT, Miri MB, Ebadi S, et al. Comparing the roles of EUS, ERCP and MRCP in idiopathic acute recurrent pancreatitis. Clin Med Insights Gastroenterol. 2016;9:35–39. PMID: 27375362. doi:10.4137/CGast. S37927.

Safdi M, Bekal PK, Martin S, et al. The effects of oral pancreatic enzymes (Creon 10 capsule) on steatorrhea: a multicenter, placebo-controlled, parallel group trial in subjects with chronic pancreatitis. Pancreas. 2006;33:156–62.

Saftoiu A, Dietrich CF, Vilmann P. Contrast-enhanced harmonic endoscopic ultrasound. Endoscopy. 2012;44: 612–7.

Saftoiu A, Vilmann P, Dietrich CF, et al. Quantitative contrast-enhanced harmonic EUS in differential diagnosis of focal pancreatic masses (with videos). Gastrointest Endosc. 2015;82:59–69.

Sahai AV, Zimmermann M, Aabakken L, Tarnasky PR, Cunningham JT, Van Velse A, et al. Prospective evaluation of the ability of endoscopic ultrasound to diagnose, exclude, or establish the severity of chronic pancreatitis found by endoscopic retrograde cholagiopancreatography. Gastrointest Endosc. 1998;48:18–25.

Sai JK, Suyama M, Kubokawa Y, et al. Diagnosis of mild chronic pancreatitis (Cambridge classification): comparative study using secretin injection-magnetic resonance cholangiopancreatography and endoscopic retrograde pancreatography. World J Gastroenterol: WJG. 2008;14(8):1218–21. PMID: 18300347.

Sandrasegaran K, Cote GA, Tahir B, et al. The utility of secretin-enhanced MRCP in diagnosing congenital anomalies. Abdom Imaging. 2014;39(5):979–987. PMID: 24748158. doi:10.1007/s00261-014-0131-z.

Sarles H. Proposal adopted unanimously by the participants of the Symposium, Marseilles 1963. Bibl Gastroenterol. 1965;7:7–8.

Sarles H, Adler G, Dani R, et al. The pancreatitis classification of Marseilles-Rome 1988. Scand J Gastroenterol. 1989;24:641–2.

Sarner M, Cotton PB. Classification of pancreatitis. Gut. 1984a;25:756–9.

Sarner M, Cotton PB. Definitions of acute and chronic pancreatitis. Clin Gastroenterol. 1984b;13:865–70.

Schneider A, Hammerstingl R, Heller M, et al. Does secretin-stimulated MRCP predict exocrine pancreatic insufficiency?: a comparison with noninvasive exocrine pancreatic function tests. J Clin Gastroenterol. 2006;40:851–5.

Schneider A, Lohr JM, Singer MV. The M-ANNHEIM classification of chronic pancreatitis: introduction of a unifying classification system based on a review of previous classifications of the disease. J Gastroenterol. 2007;42:101–19.

Schreyer AG, Jung M, Riemann JF, et al. S3 Guideline for chronic pancreatitis—diagnosis, classification and therapy for the radiologist. Rofo. 2014;186: 1002–8.

Seicean A. Endoscopic ultrasound in chronic pancreatitis: where are we now? World J Gastroenterol. 2010;16:4253–63.

Sey MS, Al-Haddad M, Imperiale TF, et al. EUS-guided liver biopsy for parenchymal disease: a comparison of diagnostic yield between two core biopsy needles. Gastrointest Endosc. 2016;83(2):347–352. PMID: 26278654. doi:10.1016/j.gie.2015.08.012.

Shamamian P, Kingman P, Mallen-St J. Imaging of the pancreas: acute and chronic pancreatitis. Berlin: Springer; 2009.

Sherman S, Freeman ML, Tarnasky PR, et al. Secretin (RG1068) Administration increases sensitivity of detection of duct abnormalities by magnetic resonance cholangiopancreatography in patients with pancreatitis. Gastroenterology. 2014. doi: 10.1053/j.gastro.2014.05.035. PMID: 24906040.

Shimosegawa T, Kataoka K, Kamisawa T, et al. The revised Japanese clinical diagnostic criteria for chronic pancreatitis. J Gastroenterol. 2010;45:584–91.
Shimosegawa T, Chari ST, Frulloni L, et al. International consensus diagnostic criteria for autoimmune pancreatitis: guidelines of the International Association of Pancreatology. Pancreas. 2011;40:352–8.
Siegmund E, Löhr JM, Schuff-Werner P. Die diagnostische Validität nichtinvasiver Pankreasfunktionstests-eine Metaanalyse. Z Gastroenterol. 2004;42:1117–28.
Singer MV, Gyr K, Sarles H. Revised classification of pancreatitis. Report of the Second International Symposium on the Classification of Pancreatitis in Marseille, France, March 28–30, 1984. Gastroenterology. 1985;89:683–5.
Song TJ, Kim MH, Moon SH, et al. The combined measurement of total serum IgG and IgG4 may increase diagnostic sensitivity for autoimmune pancreatitis without sacrificing specificity, compared with IgG4 alone. Am J Gastroenterol. 2010;105(7):1655–60.
Stabile Ianora AA, Rubini G, Lorusso F, et al. Chronic pancreatitis: which is the role of 320-row CT for the staging? Recenti Prog Med. 2013;104(7–8):381–386. PMID: 24042412. doi:10.1701/1315.14580.
Steer ML, Waxman I, Freedman S. Chronic pancreatitis. N Engl J Med. 1995;332(22):1482–90.
Stevens T. Update on the role of endoscopic ultrasound in chronic pancreatitis. Curr Gastroenterol Rep. 2011;13:117–22.
Stevens T. Role of endoscopic ultrasonography in the diagnosis of acute and chronic pancreatitis. Gastrointest Endosc Clin N Am. 2013;23(4):735–747. PMID: 24079787. doi:10.1016/j.giec.2013.06.001.
Stevens T, Parsi MA. Endoscopic ultrasound for the diagnosis of chronic pancreatitis. World J Gastroenterol. 2010;16:2841–50.
Stevens T, Parsi MA. Update on endoscopic pancreatic function testing. World J Gastroenterol. 2011;17:3957–61.
Stevens T, Conwell DL, Zuccaro G Jr, et al. A prospective crossover study comparing secretin-stimulated endoscopic and Dreiling tube pancreatic function testing in patients evaluated for chronic pancreatitis. Gastrointest Endosc. 2008;67:458–66.
Sugumar A, Levy MJ, Kamisawa T, et al. Endoscopic retrograde pancreatography criteria to diagnose autoimmune pancreatitis: an international multicentre study. Gut. 2011;60:666–70.
Sze KC, Pirola RC, Apte MV, Wilson JS. Current options for the diagnosis of chronic pancreatitis. Expert Rev Mol Diagn. 2014a;14:199–215.
Talamini G, Bassi C, Falconi M, et al. Early detection of pancreatic cancer following the diagnosis of chronic pancreatitis. Digestion. 1999;60(6):554–61. PMID: 10545726. doi: 7706.
Talamini G, Zamboni G, Salvia R, et al. Intraductal papillary mucinous neoplasms and chronic pancreatitis. Pancreatology. 2006;6(6):626–634. PMID: 17135772. doi:10.1159/000097605.
Tandon RK, Sato N, Garg PK, et al. Chronic pancreatitis: Asia-Pacific consensus report. J Gastroenterol Hepatol. 2002;17:508–18.
Teichmann J, Mann ST, Stracke H, et al. Alterations of vitamin D3 metabolism in young women with various grades of chronic pancreatitis. Eur J Med Res. 2007;12:347–50.
Tetsuo H, Masaru K, Yutaka A, et al. Diagnostic criteria for autoimmune pancreatitis by the Japan pancreas society. J Jpn Pancreas Soc. 2002;17:585–7.
Teuscher AU, Kendall DM, Smets YF, Leone JP, Sutherland DE, Robertson RP. Successful islet autotransplantation in humans: functional insulin secretory reserve as an estimate of surviving islet cell mass. Diabetes. 1998;47:324–30.
Uhl W, Malfertheiner P, Sarr MG. Diseases of the pancreas: acute pancreatitis, chronic pancreatitis, neoplasms of the pancreas. Basel: Karger; 2004.
Vantrappen GR, Rutgeerts PJ, Ghoos YF, et al. Mixed triglyceride breath test: a noninvasive test of pancreatic lipase activity in the duodenum. Gastroenterology. 1989;96:1126–34.
Varadarajulu S, Eltoum I, Tamhane A, et al. Histopathologic correlates of noncalcific chronic pancreatitis by EUS: a prospective tissue characterization study. Gastrointest Endosc. 2007;66:501–9.
Vardanyan M, Rilo HL. Pathogenesis of chronic pancreatitis-induced pain. Discov Med. 2010;9(47):304–10.
Vitale GC, Davis BR, Zavaleta C, et al. Endoscopic retrograde cholangiopancreatography and histopathology correlation for chronic pancreatitis. Am Surg. 2009;75(8):649–53. Discussion 653. PMID: 19725285.
Wang W, Liao Z, Li ZS, et al. Chronic pancreatitis in Chinese children: etiology, clinical presentation and imaging diagnosis. J Gastroenterol Hepatol. 2009a;24(12):1862–8.
Wang LW, Li ZS, Li SD, et al. Prevalence and clinical features of chronic pancreatitis in China: a retrospective multicenter analysis over 10 years. Pancreas. 2009b;38:248–54.
Warshaw AL, Banks PA, Fernández-Del CC. AGA technical review: treatment of pain in chronic pancreatitis. Gastroenterology. 1998;115:765–76.
Wathle GK, Tjora E, Ersland L, et al. Assessment of exocrine pancreatic function by secretin-stimulated magnetic resonance cholangiopancreaticography and diffusion-weighted imaging in healthy controls. J Magn Reson Imaging. 2014;39(2):448–454. PMID: 23649590. doi:10.1002/jmri.24167.
Whitcomb DC, Frulloni L, Garg P, et al. Chronic pancreatitis: an international draft consensus proposal for a new mechanistic definition. Pancreatology. 2016;16:218–24.
Wiersema MJ, Hawes RH, Lehmann GA, Kochmann ML, Sherman S, Kopecky KK. Prospective evalua-

tion of endoscopic ultrasonography and endoscopic retrograde cholangiopancreatography in patients with chronic abdominal pain of suspected pancreatic origin. Endoscopy. 1993;25:555–64.

Yamada. Textbook of gastroenterology. Hoboken: Wiley-Blackwell; 2008.

Zhu M, Xu C, Yu J, et al. Differentiation of pancreatic cancer and chronic pancreatitis using computer-aided diagnosis of endoscopic ultrasound (EUS) images: a diagnostic test. PLoS One. 2013;8:e63820.

Zhu J, Wang L, Chu Y, et al. A new descriptor for computer-aided diagnosis of EUS imaging to distinguish autoimmune pancreatitis from chronic pancreatitis. Gastrointest Endosc. 2015;82:831–6.e831.

Conservative Management of Chronic Pancreatitis

8

Yang-Yang Qian, Zhuan Liao, and Zhao-Shen Li

1 Nutrition and Lifestyle Modification

1.1 Life Style Changes

Continued alcohol consumption can trigger recurrent attacks of acute pancreatitis, and aggressive alcohol intervention can definitely benefit patients from recurrence (Yadav 2011). Immoderate alcohol consumption is also thought as a definite risk factor. Although the incidence and prevalence of CP are low, it increased greatly because of the alcohol consumption and nearly 50% are alcohol related (Yadav et al. 2011). Alcohol impairs cystic fibrosis transmembrane conductance regulator (CFTR) activity and may explain a mechanism for pancreatitis (Park 2016). It was recommended that alcohol cessation improved the course of CP (Gurusamy et al. 2016a). The damage of alcohol can be long lasting as pancreatic functional continuously decreased even after cessation of alcohol use, however the pathological change was slower and less severe (Gullo et al. 1998). Results from observational studies have noticed that smoking is an established risk factor for all forms of pancreatitis and the risk increases in a dose-dependent fashion. When combing cigarette smoking and alcohol consumption, the pathophysiologic effects can be multiplied (Greer et al. 2015). Thus smoking and drinking should be discouraged (Luaces-Regueira et al. 2014). It is reported that smoking cessation can improve the patients' quality of life (Han et al. 2016) and reduce the risk of developing pancreatic calcifications in the first years from the clinical onset of CP (Talamini et al. 2007).

Y.-Y. Qian, M.D. • Z. Liao, M.D. (✉)
Z.-S. Li, M.D. (✉)
Department of Gastroenterology, Changhai Hospital, The Second Military Medical University, Shanghai, China

Shanghai Institute of Pancreatic Diseases, Shanghai, China
e-mail: liaozhuan@smmu.edu.cn; zhaoshenli@hotmail.com

1.2 Diet

CP is a progressive inflammatory disease that leads to fibrosis and different degrees of exocrine and/or endocrine insufficiency. Both may lead to malnutrition over time. The dietary approach is used not only for treatment, but also for prevention of reoccurrence of the condition. Only after total abstinence from alcohol should dietary recommendation be carried out. Generally, a protein diet of 50–75 g is sufficient and well tolerated for an adult and it is better when 30–40% of the energy is absorbed from fats especially vegetable fats. If steatorrhea persists, medium chain triglycerides (MCT) can be given to relieve the symptom as they are directly absorbed across the

Z.-S. Li et al. (eds.), *Chronic Pancreatitis*, DOI 10.1007/978-981-10-4515-8_8

small bowel, but higher doses may be ketogenic and associated with adverse events. Since CP can lead to fat malabsorption, fat soluble vitamins (A, D, E and K), vitamin B12 and other micronutrients should be supplemented as needed. Frequent small meals, low-fat elemental diet composed of purified amino acids but rich in carbohydrates, calories, essential fat-soluble vitamins can benefit patients with CP (Majumder and Chari 2016; Hobbs et al. 2016; Yaghoobi et al. 2016). Survey showed although patients have theoretical knowledge, they seldom implement the diet on a daily basis. So paying more attention to nutritional education for patients suffering from pancreatitis is necessary (Lohr et al. 2013). Of course pancreatic enzyme supplementation with acid suppression therapy is also an essential which will be discussed detailedly later.

2 Pain Management

The pain is usually post-prandial, located in the epigastric abdomen and described as deep, penetrating with radiation to the back. Constant pain can greatly interrupt the quality of life. Cessation of alcohol and smoking may help in symptom relief. In specific situations, endoscopic and surgical interventions may help relieve the symptom, which will be depicted in other chapters. In uncomplicated CP, medical management should be the first line of therapy for pain (Anderson et al. 2016).

2.1 Analgesics

Analgesics are the firstline medical therapy of pain. According to the "pain relief ladder" provided by the WHO, analgesics are typically titrated until obtaining pain relief, but in some situations a top-down approach or combinant medication may also be useful.

Strong opioids, such as morphine, mainly exert their analgesic effects in the central nervous system through different opioid receptors including the μ-receptor, δ-receptor and the κ-receptor (Olesen et al. 2013a). Different opioids have different analgesic effect. Oxycodone was shown to attenuate experimental visceral pain better than morphine in CP patients (Staahl et al. 2007). Opioids can be administrated either orally or transdermally. Transdermal fentanyl might be useful for symptom control in appropriate dose but it is not the ideal first-choice (Niemann et al. 2000). To some extent, tolerance, opioid induced hyperalgesia and narcotic bowel may cause opiate failure and themselves can also result in chronic abdominal pain (Moran et al. 2015).

Cyclooxygenase (COX) is a key enzyme in the synthesis of prostaglandins (PGs) from arachidonic acid leading to pain and inflammation (Bai et al. 2012). Paracetamol (*N*-acetyl-paminophenol) is one of the analgesics recommended for the treatment of mild or moderate pain in CP. Several studies on alcoholic patients proved that the drug can be safely administered at a single dose of 1 g and daily dose of 4 g/24 h while excess dosage would cause hepatic cell damage. CP patients with diagnosed paracematol poisoning may be at high risk of attacked by acute pancreatitis (Siepsiak et al. 2016).

While tramadol has a similar efficacy as morphine in equivalent dose, it seems to have a better side-effect profile (Majumder and Chari 2016). In a double blinded randomized trial, 25 patients with severe chronic pancreatitis were required to take tramadol or morphine for 5 days. Finally less patients on tramadol reported gastrointestinal interference and pain relieving effect of tramadol tended to be beter than morphine on day 4 (Sharma et al. 2014).

Given the neuropathological etiology of pain, the role of neuromodulators in the management of chronic pain has gained great attention. Tricyclic antidepressants (TCAs) and gabaergics, which can modulate the spinal processing of nociceptive signals, are practically being used to control neurogenic pain (Moran et al. 2015). Pregabalin has been applied in various chronic pain disorders and proved to be effective, including post herpetic neuralgia, diabetic neuropathy and neutropathic pain of central origin (Olesen et al. 2013b). A hypothesis-generating study was conduct to provide the evidence that pain relief with pregabalin was associated with increased endogenous inhibitory modulation and antihyperalgesic effects (Bouwense et al. 2015). Side effects were reported more in pregabalin compared to placebo (Gurusamy et al. 2016b).

2.2 Antioxidants

Since the levels of byproducts produced by oxidation are increased in chronic pancreatitis, CP patients can benefit from antioxidant therapy. However, the benefits of antioxidant therapy in the management of CP pain have demonstrated conflicting results. Ahmed and his colleagues (2014) analyzed 12 randomized trials on the effect of antioxidants in CP patients only to find the reported reduction in pain was small thus a strong conclusion whether antioxidants really had a pain relief effect could not be drawn. Zhou et al. (2015) performed a meta-analysis of eight trials including 573 CP patients, and results showed that the intervention of antioxidant use can significantly relieve pain, decrease the patients' need for analgesics and improve pain tolerance in CP patients (Rustag and Njei 2015). Maziar et al. (Gooshe et al. 2015) concluded while there was some evidence to support the pain relieving therapy of antioxidant in AP, its effect on CP and PEP was still doubtful. Recently, Talukdar et al. (2016) carried out a trial with a combination of antioxidant and pregabalin and suggested that the compound exerted significant pain relief effect. Given these controversy in the effect of antioxidants, high quality trials are still needed.

2.3 Pancreatic Enzyme and the Negative Feedback Theory

It is believed that ductal and intereitial hypertension caused by pancreatitic secretion can further increase pancreatic ductal pressure, thus likely leading to pain (Hobbs et al. 2016). But there is no definitive evidence that pancreatic enzyme replacement therapy (PERT) provide general pain relief in CP. Meta-analysis of six double-blinded RCTs from 1983 to 1995 involving 186 patients demonstrated no prominent benefit of PERT in relieving pain caused by CP (Talukdar and Reddy 2013). Jan et al. (D'Haese et al. 2014) evaluated 294 patients with PERT only to find although less patients reported pain recurrence over the 1-year observation period, with confounding effect of other pain-relieving medications, it remained unclear about the effect. Recently, a meta-analysis consisting of five studies conveyed a negative result (Yaghoobi et al. 2016). Of the five studies, only the oldest study using non-enteric-coated enzymes showed improvement in pain score while the other four studies with enteric-coated ones showing opposite results. However, no subgroup data was reported as half of the patients had undergone surgery and it may also have something to do with the use of non-enteric-coated enzyme supplementation which corresponded to the negative feedback theory. However, for initial medical management, oral pancreatic enzyme supplements in adequate dose and with rapid release have been shown to provide some pain relief (Anderson et al. 2016).

3 Pancreatic Exocrine Insufficiency (PEI)

Normally, the amount of postprandial lipase secretion under normal physiologic circumstances can up to 9000–18,000 USP units/min (Trang et al. 2014).The main symptoms of PEI include steatorrhea, a poor coefficient of fat absorption (CFA), and deficiencies in fat-soluble vitamins and essential fatty acids (Aloulou et al. 2015). Traditionally it is believed that pancreas had a large exocrine reserve. As published by Dimagno et al., steatorrhea may not appear until lipase output were deceased to about 10% of normal. However this perspective has been challenged as the perception can lead to disregard for PEI and resultant delay in benefiting CP patients with adequate enzyme therapy (Duggan et al. 2016).

How to implement pancreatic enzyme therapy? The first step is to affirm the etiology of the steatorrhoea. Second, whether nonenteric or enteric coated enzyme needs to be applied. Third is the dosing. The starting dose of enzyme is from 25,000 to 40,000 IU taken with food (Smith et al. 2016). Last but not least, it is the responsibility of physicians to educate their patients about the appropriate way to take enzymes and to verify the effect of enzymes (Berry 2014). One patient may need to take approximately 10,000 USP units of lipase containing enteric coated microbead capsules/tablets per meal and 3000 USP units with snacks (Trang et al. 2014). When symptoms do not improve with PERT, it has been suggested that there is a need to rule out other possible causes, including small intestinal bacterial overgrowth (SIBO) (Capurso et al. 2016).

4 Pancreatic Endocrine Insufficiency

Type 3c diabetes mellitus (T3cDM), also described as pancreatogenic or pancreatogenous diabetes mellitus, refers to diabetes due to disease of the exocrine pancreas. It can be misclassified as T1DM, or more commonly, T2DM. But it is distinct from both. Up to 25% of patients with chronic pancreatitis-related T3cDM were reported to have 'brittle diabetes' with rapid swings in glucose (Duggan et al. 2017) and most people may need insulin therapy. Compared with non-smokers, Smoking can accelerate the development of chronic pancreatitis (~5 years), leading to an increased risk of developing calcifications and endocrine insufficiency (Issa et al. 2014). Since T3cDM are completely different from normal diabetes mellitus and even more difficult to manage due to liable glucose control, routine testing of fasting glucose and HbA1c should be normalized in these patients. In addition to standardized diabetic medications, PERT can help maximize incretin secretion, which is known to protect and proliferate pancreatic beta cells, and early referral to an endocrine specialist is also urged (Gupte and Forsmark 2014). Metformin is often the firstline drug in management of T3cDM, especially in patients who are not overtly malnourished and have mild hyperglycemia (Majumder and Chari 2016). Recently, drugs targeting incretins such as GLP-1 agonists and inhibitors of the incretin-degrading enzyme, dipeptidyl peptidase-4 (DPP-4), have been developed as new treatments for type 2 diabetes mellitus. However, given the uncertain efficacy against T3cDM, the Japanese Society of gastroenterology has proposed the use of these drugs only when the benefits of treatment are considered to surpass the risks. So does sodium/glucose cotransporter 2 (SGLT2) inhibitors (Ito et al. 2015).

In this chapter, we reviewed pharmacological measures for CP. As for CP patients, conservative treatment is still the basic therapeutic strategy. It involves patient education, life style change, nutrition adjustment, "pain relief ladder" and multi-directional approaches for pain management, judicious administration of PERT as well as satisfactory glucose level.

References

Ahmed Ali U, Jens S, Busch OR, et al. Antioxidants for pain in chronic pancreatitis. Cochrane Database Syst Rev. 2014;8:CD008945.

Aloulou A, Schue M, Puccinelli D, et al. Yarrowia lipolytica lipase 2 is stable and highly active in test meals and increases fat absorption in an animal model of pancreatic exocrine insufficiency. Gastroenterology. 2015;149(7):1910–9.e5.

Anderson MA, Akshintala V, Albers KM, et al. Mechanism, assessment and management of pain in chronic pancreatitis: recommendations of a multidisciplinary study group. Pancreatology. 2016;16(1):83–94.

Bai H, Chen X, Zhang L, et al. The effect of sulindac, a non-steroidal anti-inflammatory drug, attenuates inflammation and fibrosis in a mouse model of chronic pancreatitis. BMC Gastroenterol. 2012;12:115.

Berry AJ. Pancreatic enzyme replacement therapy during pancreatic insufficiency. Nutr Clin Pract. 2014;29(3):312–21.

Bouwense SA, Olesen SS, Drewes AM, et al. Pregabalin and placebo responders show different effects on central pain processing in chronic pancreatitis patients. J Pain Res. 2015;8:375–86.

Capurso G, Signoretti M, Archibugi L, et al. Systematic review and meta-analysis: small intestinal bacterial overgrowth in chronic pancreatitis. United European Gastroenterol J. 2016;4(5):697–705.

D'Haese JG, Ceyhan GO, Demi IE, et al. Pancreatic enzyme replacement therapy in patients with exocrine pancreatic insufficiency due to chronic pancreatitis. Pancreas. 2014;43(6):834–41.

Duggan SN, Ni Chonchubhair HM, Lawal O, et al. Chronic pancreatitis: a diagnostic dilemma. World J Gastroenterol. 2016;22(7):2304–13.
Duggan SN, Ewald N, Kelleher L, et al. The nutritional management of type 3c (pancreatogenic) diabetes in chronic pancreatitis. Eur J Clin Nutr. 2017;71(1):3–8.
Gooshe M, Abdolghaffari AH, Nikfar S, et al. Antioxidant therapy in acute, chronic and post-endoscopic retrograde cholangiopancreatography pancreatitis: an updated systematic review and meta-analysis. World J Gastroenterol. 2015;21(30):9189–208.
Greer JB, Thrower E, Yadav D. Epidemiologic and mechanistic associations between smoking and pancreatitis. Curr Treat Options Gastroenterol. 2015;13(3):332–46.
Gullo L, Barbara L, Labo G. Effect of cessation of alcohol use on the course of pancreatic dysfunction in alcoholic pancreatitis. Gastroenterology. 1998;95(4):1063–8.
Gupte AR, Forsmark CE. Chronic pancreatitis. Curr Opin Gastroenterol. 2014;30(5):500–5.
Gurusamy KS, Pallari E, Hawkins N, et al. Management strategies for pancreatic pseudocysts. Cochrane Database Syst Rev. 2016a;4:CD011392.
Gurusamy KS, Lusuku C, Davidson BR. Pregabalin for decreasing pancreatic pain in chronic pancreatitis. Cochrane Database Syst Rev. 2016b;2:CD011522.
Han S, Kheder J, Bocelli L, et al. Smoking cessation in a chronic pancreatitis population. Pancreas. 2016;45(9):1303–8.
Hobbs PM, Johnson WG, Graham DY. Management of pain in chronic pancreatitis with emphasis on exogenous pancreatic enzymes. World J Gastrointest Pharmacol Ther. 2016;7(3):370–86.
Issa Y, Bruno MJ, Bakker OJ, et al. Treatment options for chronic pancreatitis. Nat Rev Gastroenterol Hepatol. 2014;11(9):556–64.
Ito T, Ishiguro H, Ohara H, et al. Evidence-based clinical practice guidelines for chronic pancreatitis 2015. Jpn Soc Gastroenterol. 2015;51:85–92.
Lohr JM, Haas SL, Lindgren F, et al. Conservative treatment of chronic pancreatitis. Dig Dis. 2013;31(1):43–50.
Luaces-Regueira M, Iglesias-Garcia J, Lindkvist B, et al. Smoking as a risk factor for complications in chronic pancreatitis. Pancreas. 2014;43(2):275–80.
Majumder S, Chari ST. Chronic pancreatitis. Lancet. 2016;387(10031):1957–66.
Moran RA, James T, Pasricha PJ. Pancreatic pain. Curr Opin Gastroenterol. 2015;31(5):407–15.
Niemann T, Madsen LG, Larsen S, et al. Opioid treatment of painful chronic pancreatitis. Int J Pancreatol. 2000;27(3):235–40.
Olesen SS, Juel J, Graversen C, et al. Pharmacological pain management in chronic pancreatitis. World J Gastroenterol. 2013a;19(42):7292–301.
Olesen SS, Graversen C, Bouwense SA, et al. Quantitative sensory testing predicts pregabalin efficacy in painful chronic pancreatitis. PLoS One. 2013b;8(3):e57963.
Park WG. Clinical chronic pancreatitis. Curr Opin Gastroenterol. 2016; 32(5):1.
Rustag T, Njei B. Antioxidant therapy for pain reduction in patients with chronic pancreatitis a systematic review and meta analysis. Pancreas. 2015;44(5):812–8.
Sharma V, Rana SS, Bhasin DK. Medical management of pain in chronic pancreatitis. Trop Gastroenterol. 2014;35(4):205–11.
Siepsiak M, Szalek E, Karbownik A, et al. Pharmacokinetics of paracetamol in patients with chronic pancreatitis. Pharmacol Rep. 2016;68(4):733–6.
Smith RC, Smith SF, Wilson J, et al. Summary and recommendations from the Australasian guidelines for the management of pancreatic exocrine insufficiency. Pancreatology. 2016;16(2):164–80.
Staahl C, Dimcevski G, Andersen SD, Thorsgaard N, et al. Differential effect of opioids in patients with chronic pancreatitis: an experimental pain study. Scand J Gastroenterol. 2007;42(3):383–90.
Talamini G, Bassi C, Falconi M, et al. Smoking cessation at the clinical onset of chronic pancreatitis and risk of pancreatic calcifications. Pancreas. 2007;35:320–6.
Talukdar R, Reddy DN. Pain in chronic pancreatitis: managing beyond the pancreatic duct. World J Gastroenterol. 2013;19(38):6319–28.
Talukdar R, Lakhtakia S, Nageshwar Reddy D, Rao GV, et al. Ameliorating effect of antioxidants and pregabalin combination in pain recurrence after ductal clearance in chronic pancreatitis: results of a randomized, double blind, placebo-controlled trial. J Gastroenterol Hepatol. 2016;31(9):1654–62.
Trang T, Chan J, Graham DY. Pancreatic enzyme replacement therapy for pancreatic exocrine insufficiency in the 21(st) century. World J Gastroenterol. 2014;20(33):11467–85.
Yadav D. Recent advances in the epidemiology of alcoholic pancreatitis. Curr Gastroenterol Rep. 2011;13(2):157–65.
Yadav D, Timmons L, Benson JT, et al. Incidence, prevalence, and survival of chronic pancreatitis: a population-based study. Am J Gastroenterol. 2011;106(12):2192–9.
Yaghoobi M, McNabb-Baltar J, Bijarchi R, et al. Pancreatic enzyme supplements are not effective for relieving abdominal pain in patients with chronic pancreatitis: meta-analysis and systematic review of randomized controlled trials. Can J Gastroenterol Hepatol. 2016;2016:8541839.
Zhou D, Wang W, Cheng X, et al. Antioxidant therapy for patients with chronic pancreatitis: a systematic review and meta-analysis. Clin Nutr. 2015;34(4):627–34.

Endoscopic Management of Chronic Pancreatitis

9

Boon Eu Andrew Kwek, Tiing Leong Ang, and Amit Maydeo

1 Introduction

Chronic pancreatitis is an on-going inflammatory process of the pancreas that causes morphological changes, leading to pain or functional loss (Etemad and Whitcomb 2001). Abdominal pain is the most common presentation, affecting 85–90% of patients, and leads to a diminished quality of life (Braganza et al. 2011; Pezizilli and Fantini 2005). The various structural complications of chronic pancreatitis include pancreatic ductal stones, ductal strictures, distal biliary strictures and pseudocysts. While endoscopic therapy (endotherapy) is an established modality in treating these complications, other causes of pain including pancreatic cancer, duodenal stenosis and gastroparesis should be excluded.

In this chapter, we discuss the current status of endotherapy for patients with pancreatic ductal stones, pancreatic ductal strictures, benign biliary strictures and pseudocysts. In addition, we also discuss the role of endosonography-guided celiac plexus block when abdominal pain due to chronic pancreatitis is intractable.

B.E.A. Kwek, M.B.B.S., M.R.C.P (✉)
T.L. Ang, M.B.B.S., F.R.C.P
Department of Gastroenterology and Hepatology, Changi General Hospital, 2 Simei St 3, Singapore 529889, Singapore
e-mail: andrew_kwek@cgh.com.sg

A. Maydeo, M.B.B.S., M.D.
Baldota Institute of Digestive Sciences, Global Hospital, 35, D.E. Borges Road, Hospital Avenue, Parel, Mumbai, Maharashtra 400012, India

2 Pancreatic Ductal Stones

Ductal stones are a pathognomonic feature in patients with chronic pancreatitis. In 50–90% of patients, stones are detected at presentation. Although common, they are generally regarded as a consequence rather than the cause of chronic pancreatitis (Maydeo et al. 2007; Ammann et al. 1988). Endoscopic therapy to remove pancreatic ductal stones should be considered if the patient has abdominal pain. By removing the downstream ductal obstruction, pancreatic juice outflow would be improved, leading to a reduction in ductal hypertension which is a contributary pain factor.

2.1 Pre-endotherapy Assessment and Patient Selection

The selection of patients for endotherapy requires assessment of the stone distribution, density and morphology. This may be performed using a fluoroscopy machine with a rotatable arm. In addition, ductal anatomy and associated strictures or variants may be best evaluated with magnetic resonance cholangiopancreatography (MRCP) (Fig. 9.1a, b).

Z.-S. Li et al. (eds.), *Chronic Pancreatitis*, DOI 10.1007/978-981-10-4515-8_9

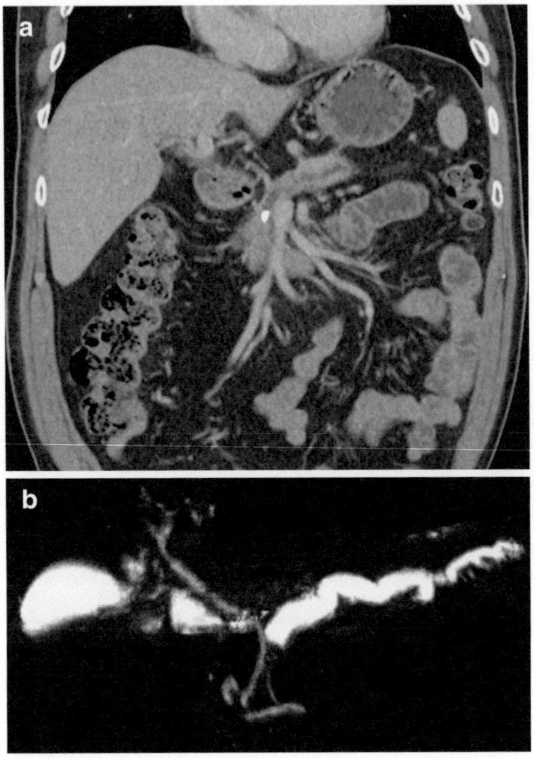

Fig. 9.1 (**a**) Computed Tomography of a patient with a calcific stone at the pancreatic genu. (**b**) Magnetic resonance cholangiopancreatography of the same patient with ductal stone at the genu, upstream ductal dilation and a convoluted downstream ventral pancreatic duct

Table 9.1 Factors favouring successful pancreatic ductal stone clearance by endotherapy

1.	Three or less stones
2.	Location of stones at pancreatic head and/or body
3.	Absence of stricture downstream to the stone
4.	Stone size of 10 mm or less
5.	Absence of impacted stones

Predictive factors favouring successful stone clearance by endotherapy are reported in Table 9.1 (Sherman et al. 1991).

2.2 Role of Pre-endotherapy Extracorporeal Shockwave Lithotripsy (ESWL)

ESWL should be performed for patients who have stones that are more than 5 mm in diameter. With successful ESWL, aiming for pulverisation of stones to granular powder form, complete ductal clearance rates would be improved. The lithotriptor machines frequently used for ESWL of renal stones are also used for pancreatic ductal stones.

Commonly used settings include shockwaves of up to a maximum of 5000 shocks per session, at an intensity of 5–6 (15,000–16,000 kv) on a scale of 1–6, with a frequency of 90–100 shocks/min (Tandan et al. 2010; Hu et al. 2015). Patients usually require sedation and analgesia during the procedure; at our unit, patients are given patient-controlled analgesia using intravenous fentanyl. An experienced ESWL technician will be able to localise and target the radio-opaque pancreatic ductal stones for effective fragmentation in about 90% of patients, with the majority requiring less than three sessions (Tandan et al. 2010; Nguyen-Tang and Dumonceau 2010).

Although generally well-tolerated, complications of ESWL include skin ecchymosis and pain (Tandan et al. 2010). A large series showed an overall post-ESWL complication rate of 6.7%, with pancreatitis being the most common (4.4%) (Li et al. 2014). Other complications include infection, *steinstrasse*, perforation, bleeding and pancreatic fistula. *Steinstrasse* or "stone street" presents with an acute abdominal pain secondary to stone fragments incarceration at the major papilla, causing pancreatic drainage obstruction. This may occur in up to 1% of patients (Hu et al. 2015).

2.3 Endotherapy

Within a few days of the ESWL session, endotherapy is performed to remove the stone fragments and to ensure good ductal drainage. Selective cannulation of the pancreatic duct is achieved by aiming for the 1–2 o'clock position of the major papilla. Contrast instillation allows for delineation of the ductal morphology and anatomy (Fig. 9.2). The guidewire may then be maneuvred safely to reach the distal upstream pancreatic duct, with particular attention to avoid forceful wire manipulation should it enter a side branch. This reduces the risk of side branch injury causing leakage of pancreatic juice and subsequent pancreatitis.

Pancreatic sphincterotomy is then performed to facilitate easy access of instruments and removal of stone fragments. Stone fragments may then be removed by trawling with wire-guided balloon or basket. Subsequently, a pancreatic ductal stent may then be inserted if a stricture is present or if some stone fragments remain.

Although there has been no consensus on the use of prophylactic antibiotics, some endoscopists would prescribe a short-course of oral fluoroquinolone. Follow-up procedures are then performed at 3-month intervals to assess for ductal improvement, with a stent-free trial commenced when ductal clearance and pancreatic outflow is satisfactory.

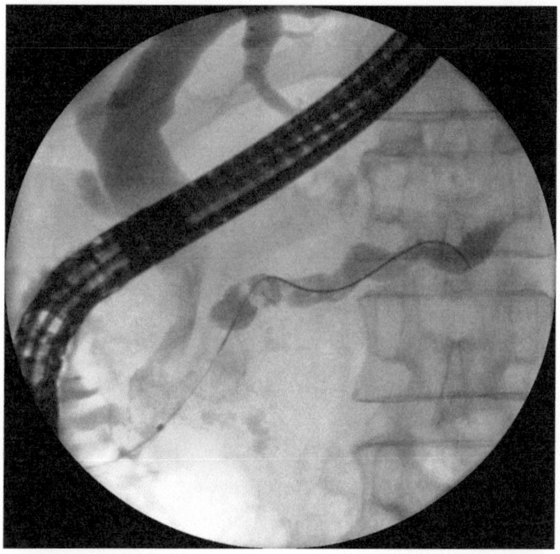

Fig. 9.2 Pancreatography of a patient with chronic pancreatitis, with a dilated pancreatic duct and stones in the head and body regions. There is relative narrowing of the distal common bile duct due to chronic pancreatitis, with upstream ductal dilation

ESWL and endotherapy provide pain relief in 60–85% of patients. Table 9.2 summarises selected series in the last two decades. Subsequent to initial endotherapy, repeated sessions may be required in 20% of patients and surgery in up to 25% of patients (Dumonceau et al. 2012). Complications include bleeding, luminal perforation, pancreatitis and pancreaticobiliary sepsis (Tandan et al. 2010, 2013; Hu et al. 2015; Tadenuma et al. 2005; Delhaye et al. 1992, 2004; Brand et al. 2000; Costamagna et al. 1997; Sauerbruch et al. 1992).

2.4 ESWL Alone

In some patients, ESWL alone may be sufficient to achieve ductal decompression. Ohara et al. reported successful ductal clearance in 24 of 32 patients (75%), with subsequent pain relief in 79% of patients over 44 months (Ohara et al. 1996). Dumonceau et al. conducted a randomized study comparing ESWL alone and ESWL with endotherapy in 55 patients (Dumonceau et al. 2007). At 2 years follow-up, pain relief was seen in 38% and 45%, respectively. When effective, a shorter hospital stay

Table 9.2 Pain relief after ESWL and endotherapy for chronic calcific pancreatitis

Author	Year	N	Ductal clearance (%)	Pain relief (%)	Follow-up duration
Hu et al. (2015)	2015	214	72.4	95.3	18.5 months
Tandan et al. (2013)	2013	(a) 364	100	(a) 68.7	(a) 24–60 months
		(b) 272		(b) 60.3	(b) >60 months
Tandan et al. (2010)	2010	1006	93	84	6 months
Tadenuma et al. (2005)	2005	117	56	63	6.5 years
Delhaye et al. (2004)	2004	56	86	66.1	14.4 years
Brand et al. (2000)	2000	48	75	82	7 months
Costamagna et al. (1997)	1997	35	74	71.9	26.8 months
Delhaye et al. (1992)	1992	122	59	85	14 months
Sauerbruch et al. (1992)	1992	24	71	83.3	24 months

and lower treatment cost may be possible by the approach of ESWL without ERCP.

3 Main Pancreatic Duct Strictures

MPD (main pancreatic duct) strictures occur due to a previous embedded stone or the necro-inflammatory process surrounding the duct. Insertion of a pancreatic duct stent leads to ductal decompression and pain relief. This is best seen in patients with strictures located within the head of pancreas and associated with upstream ductal dilation (Cremer et al. 1991). Other predictors of good outcome after MPD stenting include absence of pancreas divisum and non-alcoholic aetiology of chronic pancreatitis (Cremer et al. 1991; Eleftherladis et al. 2005).

Endotherapy for MPD strictures include pancreatic sphincterotomy, stricture dilation and ductal stenting with a temporary stent. While pancreatic sphincterotomy alone may improve ductal drainage in patients with juxtapapillary strictures, most other strictures would need some form of dilation as they are usually very tight and fibrotic (Fig. 9.3a–c). When dilation with radial expansion balloons or dilator bougies fail, the Soehendra stent retriever may be used as a boring tool for difficult strictures (Ziebert and DiSario 1999).

Itoi et al. described a novel technique using wire-guided snare forceps to incise a refractory stricture. Although successful in the two described cases, the risk of severe complications of perforation, bleeding and pancreatic parenchymal injury is present (Itoi et al. 2010).

Stents may be inserted in a single or multiple fashion. The types of available stents include plastic or self-expanding metallic stents. The overall aim is to eventually remove the stents and confirm the resolution of the stricture via pancreatography. If a dominant stricture persists, the patient is unlikely to be pain-free without continual stenting. A dominant stricture is defined as presence of at least one of the following features: upstream MPD dilation of ≥6 mm in diameter; prevention of contrast

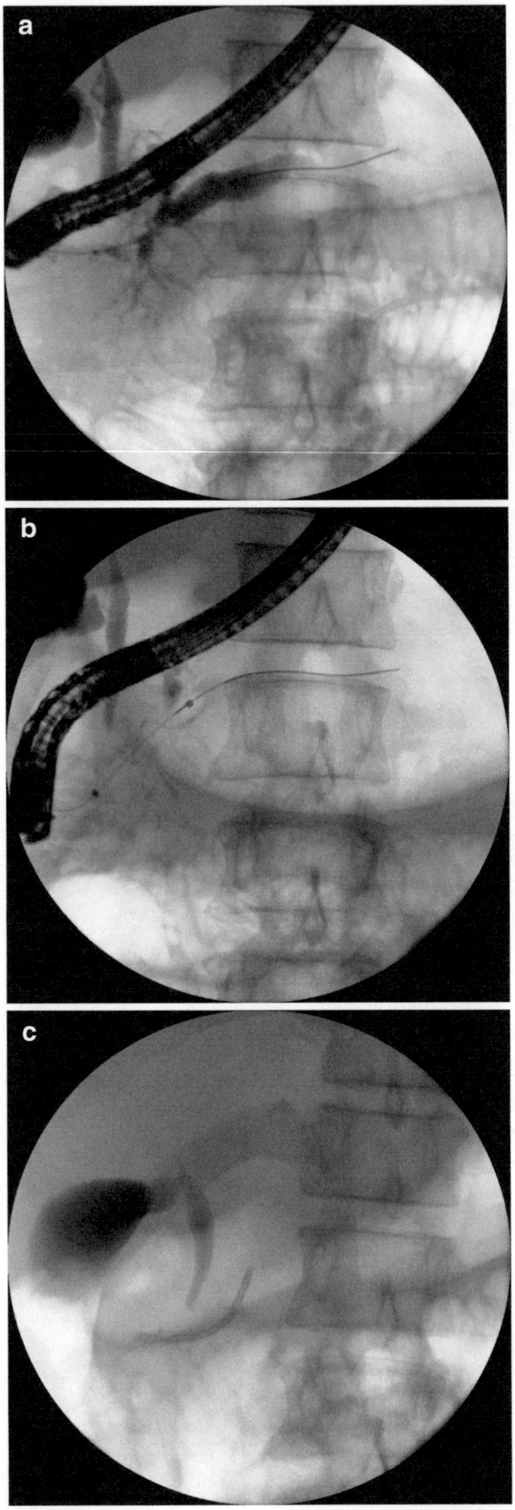

Fig. 9.3 (**a**) Pancreatography showing a tight pancreatic duct stricture at the head region. (**b**) Balloon dilation of the stricture. (**c**) Plastic stent insertion with drainage of the pancreatic duct

medium outflow alongside a 6-Fr catheter inserted upstream from the stricture; or abdominal pain during continuous infusion of a naso-pancreatic catheter inserted upstream from the stricture with 1L saline for 12–24 h (Dumonceau et al. 2012). Practically, we perform three-monthly assessments for stricture resolution; observing for good contrast outflow, smooth passage of a 7-Fr catheter within the duct and diminished focal narrowing. Once these are confirmed, we remove the stents and observe the patient clinically in the coming months.

MPD stenting is successful in 85–98% of patients, with immediate pain relief in 65–95% (Dumonceau et al. 2012). Over a follow-up period of 14–58 months, pain relief is seen in 32–68%. Surgery may still be required in 4–26% of patients, due to non-response to treatment or complications (Eleftherladis et al. 2005; Vitale et al. 2004; Binmoeller et al. 1995). Complications occur in 6–39% of patients, including mild pancreatitis (most common), stent migration and pancreatic sepsis (Dumonceau et al. 2012; Eleftherladis et al. 2005; Vitale et al. 2004; Binmoeller et al. 1995).

3.1 Plastic Stent

The outcomes from selected series of plastic stent insertion for MPD strictures are summarised in Table 9.3. Plastic stents of varying diameters of 7-, 8.5-, or 10-Fr may be used in a single or multiple fashion. When multiple stents are successfully inserted, a higher rate of stricture resolution is seen (Costamagna et al. 2006).

3.2 Self-Expandable Metal Stent

Self-expandable metal stents (SEMS) have larger diameters than plastic stents and may provide a more durable stricture dilation effect. This was studied using covered SEMS in 13 patients by Park et al. (2008). While the covering membrane reduces stent dysfunction from tissue in-growth and allows for future removal, stent migration was a frequent complication, occurring in five patients (38%). Other complications include mild pancreatitis and cholestatic liver dysfunction. To overcome the problem of stent migration, a specially-designed covered SEMS (Niti-S Pancreatic Stent [bumpy type], Taewoong Medical, Seoul, South Korea) was deployed in 32 patients (Moon et al. 2010). All the stents were easily removed at 3 months, with resolution of strictures. However, three patients developed recurrent strictures, requiring repeat stenting in two patients and surgery in one.

4 Comparison of Endoscopic Therapy with Surgery for Chronic Obstructive Pancreatitis

The most common surgical procedure for pancreatic ductal drainage is the modified Puestow operation or lateral pancreaticojejunostomy. Two randomized controlled trials compared endoscopic therapy and surgery for patients with painful chronic calcific pancreatitis. Table 9.4 summarizes the results of these studies (Díte et al. 2003; Cahen et al. 2007, 2011).

Table 9.3 Plastic stenting for main pancreatic duct strictures

Author	Year	N	Initial pain relief (%)	Stent duration	Sustained pain relief after stent removal (%)	Follow-up duration
Costamagna et al. (2006)	2006	19[a]	100	7 months	84	38 months
Eleftherladis et al. (2005)	2005	100	100	23 months	62	69 months
Vitale et al. (2004)	2004	89	83	5 months	68	43 months
Binmoeller et al. (1995)	1995	93	74	15.7 months	65	58 months

[a]Multiple stents approach: each patient had a median number of three stents, with diameters ranging from 8.5- to 11.5-Fr

Table 9.4 Randomized controlled trials of endoscopic therapy and surgery for painful obstructive chronic pancreatitis

Author	Year	N	Pain relief		Comments
			Initial	Long-term	
Díte et al. (2003)	2003	E: 36	Complete pain relief; 1 year	Complete pain relief; 5 years	1. Endotherapy group patients did not receive ESWL; potentially reducing the optimal benefits of endotherapy
		S: 36	E: 51.6%	E: 15%	2. Protocol excluded cumulative stenting or repeat endotherapy sessions for recurrent symptoms, thus reducing the maximum potential of endotherapy
			S: 42.1%	S: 33.8%; p = 0.002	3. Statistical significance was seen in "complete pain relief" outcome only
Cahen et al. (2007, 2011)	2007	E: 19	Complete or partial relief; 2 years	Complete or partial relief; 79 months	1. There was a lower than usual overall technical success rate (53%) in the endotherapy group, perhaps due to the high proportion (84%) of patients who had pancreatic duct strictures
	2011	S: 20	E: 32%	E: 38%	2. In the long term, additional drainage procedure was required in 68% of patients in the endotherapy group and 5% of patients in the surgical group
			S: 75%; p = 0.003	S: 80%; p = 0.042	3. 47% of patients in the endotherapy group eventually underwent surgery

E endotherapy
S surgery

These results show that endotherapy and surgery has similar early benefits for pain relief but in the long-term, surgery provides more durable pain relief. However, as surgery has significant morbidity and mortality (18%–53% and 0%–5%, respectively, for resections, and 0%–4% mortality for MPD drainage) (Dumonceau et al. 2012), an individualized approach should be considered in the discussion with patients.

Endotherapy may reduce the need for surgical procedures, act as a bridge to surgery, or predict the response to surgical drainage. However, in patients with pancreatic stones or strictures prominently located at the tail region, surgery may be the better initial approach due to the lower success rate of endotherapy to address diseases in the distal upstream region (Dumonceau et al. 2012).

5 Benign Biliary Strictures

Distal common bile duct strictures from inflammation-induced periductal fibrosis occur in up to 46% of patients with chronic calcific pancreatitis (Adler et al. 2006; Abdallah et al. 2007). Indications for biliary drainage are summarised in Table 9.5 (Dumonceau et al. 2012). Careful evaluation (e.g. brush cytology, endoscopic ultrasound or intraductal ultrasound) should be performed to exclude a malignant aetiology of the stricture. Various studies report biliary stenting with either a single plastic stent or multiple side-by-side plastic stents, or with covered SEMS.

5.1 Plastic Stent

Usually, the plastic biliary stents are inserted for a duration of at least a year and exchanged at 3–4 months intervals to avoid problems of stent clogging and cholangitis. In patients with recurrent or persistent biliary stricture, surgical drainage should be considered. Patients with pancreatic head calcifications do poorly with biliary stenting, with the need for repeat endotherapy or surgery (Kahl et al. 2003).

While the technical success of biliary stent insertion is more than 90% in most cases, the long-term success from a single biliary stent insertion is generally poor, ranging from 10 to 32%, after a stent duration of 9–21 months. In some series, up to 49% of patients required surgical drainage (Dumonceau et al. 2012). However, Vitale et al. reported a high long-term success rate (80%) of the single biliary stent approach in a group of patients with a low prevalence of chronic calcific pancreatitis (Vitale et al. 2000).

The multiple side-by-side biliary stents approach have better long-term success rates, ranging from 44 to 92%, after a stent duration of 14–21 months. However, up to 13% may still require surgical drainage (Dumonceau et al. 2012).

Table 9.5 Indications for biliary drainage in benign biliary stricture secondary to chronic pancreatitis

1.	Presence of symptoms
2.	Presence of secondary biliary cirrhosis
3.	Presence of biliary stones
4.	Progression of biliary stricture
5.	Asymptomatic elevation of serum alkaline phosphatase (>2–3 times the upper limit of normal values)
6.	Asymptomatic elevation of serum bilirubin for longer than 1 month

5.2 SEMS

The use of the wider diameter covered SEMS for a period of 3–6 months is associated with long term success rates of 50–80% (Dumonceau et al. 2012). Problems with stent migration is reduced when the partially covered SEMS is used instead of the fully covered SEMS (Cahen et al. 2008; Behm et al. 2009). However, when compared with other causes of benign biliary strictures, chronic pancreatitis is associated with a lower success rate for stricture resolution despite the use of SEMS (Poley et al. 2012).

While biliary stenting provide immediate improvement of jaundice in most patients, long-term ductal patency after stent removal remains a significant issue in most patients with chronic calcific pancreatitis. In patients with poor compliance to regular stent exchanges, endotherapy may not be advisable due to the significant septic complications that may occur. Also, although promising, SEMS placement remains investigational and no comparison studies between insertion of SEMS, plastic stents or surgical drainage have been concluded.

6 Pancreatic Pseudocysts

Pancreatic pseudocyst (PP), an amylase-rich fluid collection surrounded by a wall of fibrous granulation tissue, is due to disruption of the MPD or its side branches from acute pancreatitis, pancreatic trauma or chronic pancreatitis (Banks et al. 2013; Bradley 1993). PP occurs in 20–40% of patients with chronic pancreatitis, with low rate of spontaneous resolution (0–9%) in this setting

(Andrén-Sandberg and Dervenis 2004a, b). Indications for treatment include the presence of infection, an enlarging PP and symptoms related to the PP (abdominal pain, gastric outlet obstruction, early satiety, weight loss or jaundice).

The pancreatic duct should be evaluated to address factors predisposing to pseudocyst recurrence, namely ductal disruptions, stones and strictures. Ductal evaluation may be performed with MRCP or ERCP. Pancreatic ductal disruption is seen in 40–60% of patients with peripancreatic fluid collections, with better treatment outcomes when a bridging stent is inserted (Trevino et al. 2010).

6.1 Drainage of PP

Simple cyst aspiration alone is limited by a high recurrence rate (70%). Longer-term drainage may be achieved by percutaneous, endoscopic or surgical approaches. While percutaneous catheter drainage has a success rate of 84% and a recurrence rate of 7%, it is frequently complicated by the development of pancreatic-cutaneous fistulas (Gumaste and Dave 1991; Spivak et al. 1998; Boggi et al. 1999).

Endoscopic drainage is usually performed by puncturing the PP transmurally under EUS guidance to avoid inadvertent puncture of blood vessels that may occur during the direct puncture method. It is important to ascertain the presence of a defined wall enclosing the fluid collection, to reduce the risk of fluid leakage and secondary peritonitis. The puncture site may be dilated with dilator catheters or balloons. While cystotome access is an option, the needle-knife cautery method is discouraged due to significant risks of perforation or pseudocyst rupture. Following dilation of the puncture site, at least two double-pigtail stents are placed. These stents should only be removed after at least 2 months, if cross-sectional imaging confirms the resolution of the PP (Eleftherladis et al. 2005). In smaller PPs (<50 mm), transpapillary drainage may be sufficient (Dumonceau et al. 2012). Cystduodenostomy approach has higher long-term success rate than cystogastrostomy (83.1% vs. 64.0%), which may be related to a longer fistula patency (Dumonceau et al. 2012). While endoscopic drainage may have a high initial technical success rate of 97%, a significant number require alternative therapy for persistent or recurrent PP formation, reducing its overall success rate to 71% in a series of 92 patients (Cahen et al. 2005).

In a randomised controlled trial, surgical drainage had similar success, complications and reintervention rates compared to endoscopic drainage. However, the less invasive endoscopic approach had shorter length of stay, better scores for physical and mental health, and lower costs (Varadarajulu et al. 2013). This was similar to an earlier comprehensive review by Rosso et al., that reported an endoscopic drainage success rate of over 80–90%, similar morbidity to surgical approach (13.3% vs. 16.0%; endoscopy vs. surgery) and similar long-term PP recurrence rate (10.7% vs. 9.8%; endoscopy vs. surgery). However, mortality rate was higher in the surgical group (0.2% vs. 2.5%) (Rosso et al. 2003).

Endoscopic drainage-related morbidity and mortality rates are 13.0% and 0.3%, respectively (Dumonceau et al. 2012). Significant complications include bleeding, perforation and infection. When detected, pseudocyst associated pseudoaneurysms should be treated via angiographic embolisation prior to attempting endoscopic drainage of the PP. Antibiotic prophylaxis should also be given.

The use of short covered SEMS with lumen-apposing bilateral flanges for PP drainage has reported efficacy in numerous series (Itoi et al. 2012; Shah et al. 2015; Talreja et al. 2008; Gornals et al. 2013) (Fig. 9.4a–c). Its advantages include a single-step deployment, low stent migration rate with its flanges, and improved access and drainage with its wider diameter. Shah et al. reported technical success in 30 of 33 patients (91%) with PPs or walled-off pancreatic necrosis (WON) (Shah et al. 2015). Failure was attributed to limited operator experience at study

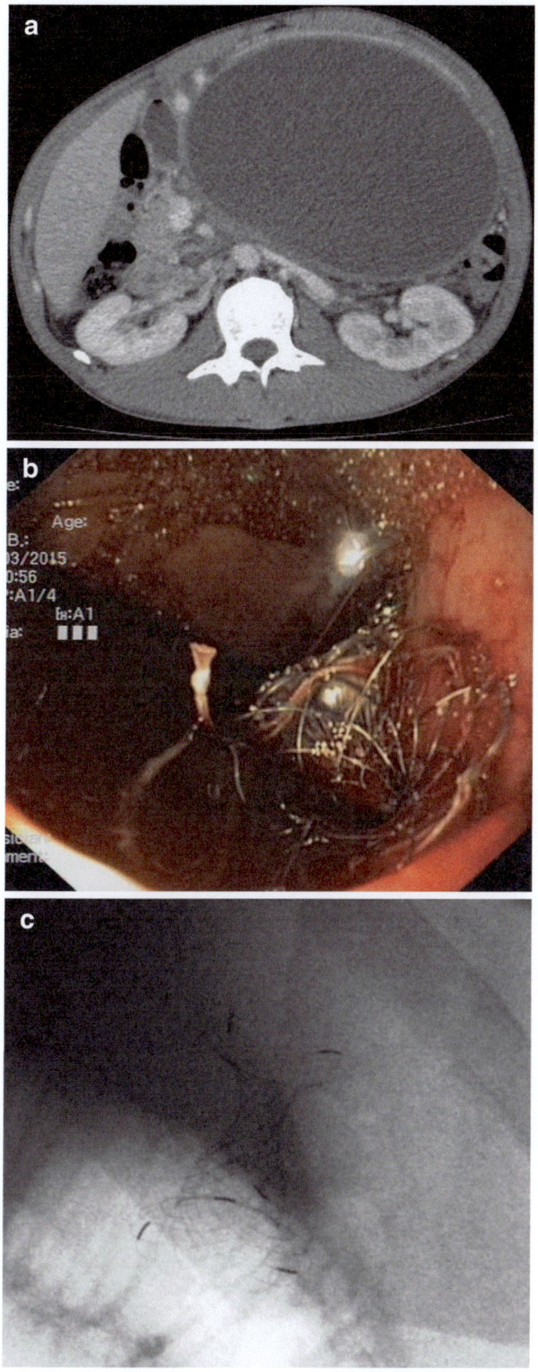

Fig. 9.4 (**a**) Computed Tomography of a patient with a large pancreatic pseudocyst. (**b**) Endoscopic view of pseudocyst drainage using a lumen-apposing SEMS. (**c**) X-ray view of the SEMS

onset and one device malfunction. Overall, PP and WON resolution was achieved in 28 patients (85%). Complications were seen in 5 of 33 patients (15.2%); access-site infection, stent migration, back pain, fever with prolonged hospitalisation and abdominal pain requiring endoscopy. Future comparative trials are required to determine the relative efficacy and cost-effectiveness of the lumen-apposing SEMS and the double-pigtail plastic stents methods.

7 Endosonography-Guided Celiac Plexus Block

EUS-guided celiac plexus block (CPB) may be considered in patients with persistent pain despite adequate medical therapy, including the use of opioid and non-opioid analgesics. Alcohol and tobacco cessation, psychosocial support to reduce opioid dependence, and pancreatic enzyme and antioxidant supplementation are important adjuncts. In EUS-guided CPB, a mixture of corticosteroid and local anaesthetic is injected into the coeliac plexus to disrupt the afferent pain signals.

In comparison with other approaches (CT-, fluoroscopy- or ultrasound-guided), EUS-guided celiac plexus block has better pain relief, lower cost and is the preferred choice of the patient (Gress et al. 1999; Santosh et al. 2009). Also, the EUS-guided approach avoids the potential neurological risks of paraplegia associated with the posterior transcutaneous approach.

Success rates range from 50 to 60%, although recent data showed pain relief in up to 76% after the first procedure in 248 patients (Puli et al. 2009; Kaufman et al. 2010; Sey et al. 2015). However, pain relief is transient and most patients require repeated sessions. The median duration of response after the first session was 10 weeks (Sey et al. 2015). Another study showed an initial pain response in 55% which reduced to 10% after 24 weeks (Gress et al. 2001). Also, a meta-analysis reported lower median pain relief duration of 11–37 days post procedure, although persistent benefit was seen in some patients for up to 48 weeks (Kaufman et al. 2010). In patients who had more than one EUS-guided CPB procedure, predictors of pain relief after subsequent blocks were older age and presence of pain relief after the first procedure (Sey et al. 2015).

Complications of this procedure include transient diarrhea secondary to sympathetic denervation, hypotension, pancreatitis and local infections. These may occur in up to one-third of patients (Kaufman et al. 2010), and usually resolve with supportive management of intravenous fluids, anti-diarrhoeal agents or prophylactic antibiotics.

8 Endoscopic Therapy and Exocrine/Endocrine Insufficiency

While abdominal pain is the main indication for pancreatic endotherapy, the outcome of endotherapy on exocrine or endocrine insufficiency are inconclusive. Longitudinal studies show that despite endotherapy, pancreatic function generally deteriorates with time. In a study with 636 patients, the number of patients with diabetes mellitus nearly doubled (75–139 patients) during a long-term follow-up of more than 5 years (Tandan et al. 2013). However, the number of patients with steatorrhoea remained relatively the same during that period.

However, Inui et al. reported post-endotherapy improvement in both endocrine and exocrine functions in 24.3% and 38% of patients, respectively (Inui et al. 2005). In addition, Tadenuma et al. showed greater deterioration of exocrine function over time in patients with incomplete stone removal than those who had complete removal (Tadenuma et al. 2005). Moreover, in those who had complete stone removal, a smaller proportion required insulin at long-term follow-up compared to those who had incomplete stone removal; 13.5% versus 39.4%. Thus, pancreatic function appears to improve in some patients but well-designed studies are necessary to specifically investigate the effect of endotherapy on exocrine and endocrine functions.

9 Summary

Endotherapy provides pain relief in patients with obstructive ductal disease from stones and strictures, and alleviates symptoms in those with biliary strictures and pancreatic pseudocysts. Although surgery has more durable outcomes, endotherapy is less invasive than surgery, with lower morbidity and mortality rates. New approaches with new endoscopic tools and accessories continue to improve the outcomes of endotherapy. In addition, when pain is persistent, the celiac plexus block may provide good relief via a minimally invasive method.

References

Abdallah AA, Krige JE, Bornman PC. Biliary tract obstruction in chronic pancreatitis. HPB (Oxford). 2007;9:421–8.

Adler DG, Lichtenstein D, Baron TH, et al. The role of endoscopy in patients with chronic pancreatitis. Gastrointest Endosc. 2006;63:933–7.

Ammann RW, Muench R, Otto R, et al. Evolution and regression of pancreatic calcification in chronic pancreatitis. A prospective long-term study of 107 patients. Gastroenterology. 1988;95:1018–28.

Andrén-Sandberg A, Dervenis C. Pancreatic pseudocysts in the 21st century. Part I: classification, pathophysiology, anatomic considerations and treatment. JOP. 2004a;5:8–24.

Andrén-Sandberg A, Dervenis C. Pancreatic pseudocysts in the 21st century. Part II: natural history. JOP. 2004b;5:64–70.

Banks PA, Bollen TL, Dervenis C, et al. Classification of acute pancreatitis--2012: revision of the Atlanta classification and definitions by international consensus. Gut. 2013;62:102–11.

Behm B, Brock A, Clarke BW, et al. Partially covered self-expandable metallic stents for benign biliary strictures due to chronic pancreatitis. Endoscopy. 2009;41:547–51.

Binmoeller KF, Jue P, Seifert H, et al. Endoscopic pancreatic stent drainage in chronic pancreatitis and a dominant stricture: long-term results. Endoscopy. 1995;27:638–44.

Boggi U, Di Candio G, Campatelli A, Pietrabissa A, Mosca F. Nonoperative management of pancreatic pseudocysts. Problems in differential diagnosis. Int J Pancreatol. 1999;25:123–33.

Bradley EL 3rd. A clinically based classification system for acute pancreatitis. Summary of the International Symposium on Acute Pancreatitis, Atlanta, Ga, September 11 through 13, 1992. Arch Surg. 1993;128:586–90.

Braganza JM, Lee SH, McCloy RF, McMahon MJ. Chronic pancreatitis. Lancet. 2011;377:1184–97.

Brand B, Kahl M, Sidhu S, et al. Prospective evaluation of morphology, function, and quality of life after extracorporeal shockwave lithotripsy and endoscopic treatment of chronic calcific pancreatitis. Am J Gastroenterol. 2000;95:3428–38.

Cahen D, Rauws E, Fockens P, et al. Endoscopic drainage of pancreatic pseudocysts: long-term outcome and procedural factors associated with safe and successful treatment. Endoscopy. 2005;37:977–83.

Cahen DL, Gouma DJ, Nio Y, et al. Endoscopic versus surgical drainage of the pancreatic duct in chronic pancreatitis. N Engl J Med. 2007;356:676–84.

Cahen DL, Rauws EA, Gouma DJ, Fockens P, Bruno MJ. Removable fully covered self-expandable metal stents in the treatment of common bile duct strictures due to chronic pancreatitis: a case series. Endoscopy. 2008;40:697–700.

Cahen DL, Gouma DJ, Laramée P, et al. Long-term outcomes of endoscopic vs surgical drainage of the pancreatic duct in patients with chronic pancreatitis. Gastroenterology. 2011;141:1690–5.

Costamagna G, Gabbrielli A, Mutignani M, et al. Extracorporeal shock wave lithotripsy of pancreatic stones in chronic pancreatitis: immediate and medium-term results. Gastrointest Endosc. 1997;46:231–6.

Costamagna G, Bulajic M, Tringali A, et al. Multiple stenting of refractory pancreatic duct strictures in severe chronic pancreatitis: long-term results. Endoscopy. 2006;38:254–9.

Cremer M, Deviere J, Delhaye M, et al. Stenting in severe chronic pancreatitis; results of medium term follow-up in 76 patients. Endoscopy. 1991;23:171–6.

Delhaye M, Vandermeeren A, Baize M, Cremer M. Extracorporeal shockwave lithotripsy of pancreatic calculi. Gastroenterology. 1992;102:610–20.

Delhaye M, Arvanitakis M, Verset G, Cremer M, Devière J. Long-term clinical outcome after endoscopic pancreatic ductal drainage for patients with painful chronic pancreatitis. Clin Gastroenterol Hepatol. 2004;2:1096–106.

Díte P, Ruzicka M, Zboril V, Novotný I. A prospective, randomized trial comparing endoscopic and surgical therapy for chronic pancreatitis. Endoscopy. 2003;35:553–8.

Dumonceau JM, Costamagna G, Tringali A, et al. Treatment for painful calcified chronic pancreatitis: extracorporeal shock wave lithotripsy versus endoscopic treatment: a randomised controlled trial. Gut. 2007;56:545–52.

Dumonceau JM, Delhaye M, Tringali A, et al. Endoscopic treatment of chronic pancreatitis: European Society of Gastrointestinal Endoscopy (ESGE) Clinical Guideline. Endoscopy. 2012;44:784–800.

Eleftherladis N, Dinu F, Delhaye M, et al. Long-term outcome after pancreatic stenting in severe chronic pancreatitis. Endoscopy. 2005;37:223–30.

Etemad B, Whitcomb DC. Chronic pancreatitis: diagnosis, classification, and new genetic developments. Gastroenterology. 2001;120:682–707.

Gornals JB, De la Serna-Higuera C, Sánchez-Yague A, et al. Endosonography-guided drainage of pancreatic fluid collections with a novel lumen-apposing stent. Surg Endosc. 2013;27:1428–34.

Gress F, Schmitt C, Sherman S, Ikenberry S, Lehman G. A prospective randomized comparison of endoscopic ultrasound- and computed tomography-guided celiac plexus block for managing chronic pancreatitis pain. Am J Gastroenterol. 1999;94:900–5.

Gress F, Schmitt C, Sherman S, et al. Endoscopic ultrasound-guided celiac plexus block for managing abdominal pain associated with chronic pancreatitis: a prospective single center experience. Am J Gastroenterol. 2001;96:409–16.

Gumaste UV, Dave PB. Pancreatic pseudocyst drainage—the needle or the scalpel? J Clin Gastroenterol. 1991;13:500–5.

Hu LH, Ye B, Yang YG, et al. Extracorporeal shock wave lithotripsy for Chinese patients with pancreatic stones—a prospective study of 214 cases. Pancreas. 2016;45(2):298–305.

Inui K, Tazuma S, Yamaguchi T, et al. Treatment of pancreatic stones with extracorporeal shock wave lithotripsy results of a multicenter survey. Pancreas. 2005;30:26–30.

Itoi T, Sofuni A, Itokawa F, et al. Transpapillary incision of refractory circumscript pancreatic duct stricture using wire-guided snare forceps. World J Gastroenterol. 2010;16(12):1541–4.

Itoi T, Binmoeller KF, Shah J, et al. Clinical evaluation of a novel lumen apposing metal stent for endosonography-guided pancreatic pseudocyst and gallbladder drainage (with videos). Gastrointest Endosc. 2012;75:870–6.

Kahl S, Zimmermann S, Genz I, et al. Risk factors for failure of endoscopic stenting of biliary strictures in chronic pancreatitis: a prospective follow-up study. Am J Gastroenterol. 2003;98:2448–53.

Kaufman M, Singh G, Das S, et al. Efficacy of endoscopic ultrasound-guided celiac plexus block and celiac plexus neurolysis for managing abdominal pain associated with chronic pancreatitis and pancreatic cancer. J Clin Gastroenterol. 2010;44:127–34.

Li BR, Liao Z, Du TT, et al. Risk factors for complications of pancreatic extracorporeal shock wave lithotripsy. Endoscopy. 2014;46:1092–100.

Maydeo A, Soehendra N, Reddy N, Bhandari S. Endotherapy for chronic pancreatitis with intracanalar stones. Endoscopy. 2007;39:653–8.

Moon SH, Kim MH, Park DH, et al. Modified fully covered selfexpandable metal stents with antimigration features for benign pancreatic duct strictures in advanced chronic pancreatitis, with a focus on the safety profile and reducing migration. Gastrointest Endosc. 2010;72:86–91.

Nguyen-Tang T, Dumonceau JM. Endoscopic treatment in chronic pancreatitis, timing, duration and type of intervention. Best Pract Res Clin Gastroenterol. 2010;24:281–98.

Ohara H, Hoshino M, Hayakawa T, et al. Single application extracorporeal shock wave lithotripsy is the first choice for patients with pancreatic duct stones. Am J Gastroenterol. 1996;91:1388–94.

Park DH, Kim MH, Moon SH, et al. Feasibility and safety of placement of a newly designed, fully covered self-expandable metal stent for refractory benign pancreatic ductal strictures: a pilot study (with video). Gastrointest Endosc. 2008;68:1182–9.

Pezizilli R, Fantini L. Chronic pancreatitis: assessing the quality of life. J Pancreas. 2005;6:406–9.

Poley JW, Cahen DL, Metselaar HJ, et al. A prospective group sequential study evaluating a new type of fully covered self-expandable metal stent for the treatment of benign biliary strictures (with video). Gastrointest Endosc. 2012;75:783–9.

Puli SR, Reddy JB, Bechtold ML, Antillon MR, Brugge WR. EUS-guided celiac plexus neurolysis for pain due to chronic pancreatitis or pancreatic cancer pain: a meta-analysis and systematic review. Dig Dis Sci. 2009;54:2330–7.

Rosso E, Alexakis N, Ghaneh P, et al. Pancreatic pseudocyst in chronic pancreatitis: endoscopic and surgical treatment. Dig Surg. 2003;20:397–406.

Santosh D, Lakhtakia S, Gupta R, et al. Clinical trial: a randomized trial comparing fluoroscopy guided percutaneous technique vs. endoscopic ultrasound guided technique of coeliac plexus block for treatment of pain in chronic pancreatitis. Aliment Pharmacol Ther. 2009;29:979–84.

Sauerbruch T, Holl J, Sackmann M, Paumgartner G. Extracorporeal lithotripsy of pancreatic stones in patients with chronic pancreatitis and pain: a prospective follow up study. Gut. 1992;33:969–72.

Sey MSL, Schmaltz L, Al-Haddad MA, et al. Effectiveness and safety of serial endoscopic ultrasound–guided celiac plexus block for chronic pancreatitis. Endosc Int Open. 2015;3:E56–9.

Shah RJ, Shah JN, Waxman I, et al. Safety and efficacy of endoscopic ultrasound-guided drainage of pancreatic fluid collections with lumen-apposing covered self-expanding metal stents. Clin Gastroenterol Hepatol. 2015;13(4):747–52.

Sherman S, Lehman GA, Hawes RH, et al. Pancreatic ductal stones: frequency of successful endoscopic removal and improvement in symptoms. Gastrointest Endosc. 1991;37:511–7.

Spivak H, Galloway JR, Amerson JR, et al. Management of pancreatic pseudocysts. J Am Coll Surg. 1998;186:507–11.

Tadenuma H, Ishihara T, Yamaguchi T, et al. Long-term results of extracorporeal shockwave lithotripsy and endoscopic therapy for pancreatic stones. Clin Gastroenterol Hepatol. 2005;3:1128–35.

Talreja JP, Shami VM, Ku J, et al. Transenteric drainage of pancreatic-fluid collections with fully covered self-expanding metallic stents (with video). Gastrointest Endosc. 2008;68:1199–203.

Tandan M, Reddy DN, Santosh D, et al. Extracorporeal shock wave lithotripsy and endotherapy for pancreatic calculi-a large single center experience. Indian J Gastroenterol. 2010;29:143–8.

Tandan M, Reddy DN, Talukdar R, et al. Long-term clinical outcomes of extracorporeal shockwave lithotripsy in painful chronic calcific pancreatitis. Gastrointest Endosc. 2013;78:726–33.

Trevino JM, Tamhane A, Varadarajulu S. Successful stenting in ductal disruption favorably impacts treatment outcomes in patients undergoing transmural drainage of peripancreatic fluid collections. J Gastroenterol Hepatol. 2010;25:526–31.

Varadarajulu S, Bang JY, Sutton BS, et al. Equal efficacy of endoscopic and surgical cystogastrostomy for pancreatic pseudocyst drainage in a randomized trial. Gastroenterology. 2013;145:583–90.e1.

Vitale GC, Reed DN, Nguyen CT, et al. Endoscopic treatment of distal bile duct stricture from chronic pancreatitis. Surg Endosc. 2000;14:227–31.

Vitale GC, Cothron K, Vitale EA, et al. Role of pancreatic duct stenting in the treatment of chronic pancreatitis. Surg Endosc. 2004;18:1431–4.

Ziebert JJ, DiSario JA. Dilation of refractory pancreatic duct strictures: the turn of the screw. Gastrointest Endosc. 1999;49:632–5.

Surgical Treatment of Chronic Pancreatitis

10

Sui-Zhi Gao and Gang Jin

1 Introduction

Surgical treatment is one important part of clinical management for chronic pancreatitis (CP), the goals of which can roughly be divided into three categories: to remit or eliminate pain; to retain pancreatic tissues as much as possible and to treat complications. Nevertheless, surgical approaches could not slow the disease progression or restore normal secretion functions. Therefore, surgeons should strictly follow surgical indications.

2 Indications

Currently, the consensus opinion on surgical indications can be stated as follows: Surgeries should be considered when (1) abdominal pain is intractable; (2) there are severe complications, such as jaundice due to common bile duct obstruction, duodenal stenosis, portal vein stenosis combined with portal vein hypertension, pancreatic necrosis or pancreatic fistula; (3) pancreatic malignancy is suspected (Yin et al. 2012; Forsmark 2013).

3 Surgical Procedures

Overall, CP lesions include pancreatic duct stenosis or dilation and pancreatic masses of different pathological patterns, promoting drainage and resection as two main surgical approaches. Meanwhile, when patients suffer from CP combined with bile duct disease, operation treatment for the abnormal biliary system, including timely cholecystectomy and biliary tract exploration, should not be neglected. Currently, commonly applied surgical methods for CP are three types: drainage (decompression), resection and neurectomy (Ni et al. 2015). Depending on pathogenesis of disease and lesion sites, targeted procedures ought to be correctly selected.

4 Decompression and Drainage

The procedure is the firstline surgical treatment for patients with dilated main pancreatic duct (≥7 mm) (Büchler and Warshaw 2008) and no inflammatory masses at the pancreatic head (Parekh and Natarajan 2015). Nowadays, while the causes of pain from CP remain controversial,

S.-Z. Gao, M.D.
Department of Pancreatic Surgery, Changhai Hospital, The Second Military Medical University, Shanghai, China

G. Jin, M.D. (✉)
Department of Pancreatic Surgery, Changhai Hospital, The Second Military Medical University, Shanghai, China

Chinese Institute of Pancreatic Diseases, Shanghai, China
e-mail: jingang@sohu.com

Z.-S. Li et al. (eds.), *Chronic Pancreatitis*, DOI 10.1007/978-981-10-4515-8_10

it probably has something to do with the combination of pancreatic duct obstruction and parenchymal hypertension, leading to ischemia and accumulation of H^+ (Poulsen et al. 2013). As for this, several procedures have developed.

1. DuVal procedure
   In order to reduce high pressure in main pancreatic duct, in 1954, DuVal and Zollinger et al. performed the pancreatic tail resection along with splenectomy and pancreaticojejunostomy of the residual pancreatic end and jejunum. However, this anastomotic method will bring about countercurrent of pancreatic juice, and inconspicuous decompression will sustain in a long run. Therefore, DuVal procedure is almost abandoned in clinical practice.
2. Duodenal papilla plasty
   In 1956, Doubilet reported duodenal papilla plasty, during which operation duodenal was incised and then duodenal papilla together with orifices of pancreatic duct was shaped. But when the main duct dilates like beads (that is multiple narrow), both of the methods could not attain perfect drainage effect.
3. Side-to-side pancreaticojejunostomy
   As the two procedure are less effective on decompression, Puestow and Gillesby developed a technique that combining a longitudinal incision of the pancreatic duct and a pancreaticojejunostomy with the pancreatic tail and spleen resection. The Puestow procedure can be applied to multiple strictures pancreatolithiasis but it also bring patients severe trauma. Shortly thereafter, Partington and Rochelle modified this procedure by extensively opening the duct to clear stones and then performing only a side-to side pancreaticojejunostomy without a distal pancreatectomy. The procedure preserves substantial pancreatic parenchyma, which is important for maintaining pancreatic function (Issa et al. 2014), therefore, it is the most widely applied CP decompression procedure in clinic. However, Puestow procedure and Partington procedure are not indicated in patients with an inflammatory mass in the head of the pancreas, small duct disease, hereditary chronic pancreatitis, and idiopathic pancreatitis who do not have marked dilated ducts (Parekh and Natarajan 2015). Once patients have the conditions mentioned above, Partington procedure could not have adequate drainage at the pancreatic head, thus resection or combined procedures are recommended.

5 Pancreatectomy

As for CP patients with less dilated duct and fibrotic pancreatic tissues, especially calcified ones, pancreatectomy should be taken. On the basis of pathological region and extent, the resection is classified as follows.

1. Pancreatoduodenectomy or pylorus-preserving pancreatoduodenectomy
   Since the classical pancreatoduodenectomy (PD) and Pylorus-preserving pancreatoduodenectomy (PPPD) were respectively proposed in 1946 and 1978, they have increasingly been used in the treatment of patients with CP with the continuous improvement in their safety. PD and PPPD are applied to CP patients with no dilated ducts, especially to those whose lesions locating in pancreatic head and unciform process, with a low surgical mortality rate and a high long-term pain relief rate (Büchler and Warshaw 2008; Jimenez et al. 2000).
2. Duodenum-preserving pancreatic head resection
   In 1972, Beger performed the first duodenum-preserving pancreatic head resection (DPPHR), also called the Beger procedure. The neck of the pancreas is separated over the portal vein, and the head and uncinate process are subtotally excised preserving the duodenum and the intrapancreatic bile duct. The advantage of Beger procedure is long-term pain relief with the preservation of pancreatic body and tail, the physiologic function of the stomach, duodenum, and common bile duct. It is a safe and effective procedure in some patients with an expanded inflammatory mass in the head of the pancreas associated pain in CP. In 1987, Frey modified the procedure into

side to side pancreaticojejunostomy incorporated with a local resection of pancreatic head, which is a combination of DPPHR and drainage. When CP patients have pancreatic duct obstruction and small inflammatory masses at the pancreatic head, the Frey procedure can be considered. Compared with the standard resections such as the Whipple operation, Beger and Frey operations can get a better global quality of life (Yin et al. 2012) and a lower postoperative morbidity (Farkas et al. 2006). Therefore, these tend to better the outcome following organ-preserving surgery compared to the traditional operations. The Berne procedure is to aim at the condition of portal hypertension in certain patients with CP (Gloor et al. 2001), involving a local pancreatic head resection, without complete removal of the pancreas and without lateral pancreaticojejunostomy. Moreover, Izbicki et al. developed the Hamburg procedure specialized for patients with "small duct" pancreatitis (pancreatic duct diameter < 3 mm) (Kutup et al. 2010). The key point of the operation is to resect ventral pancreas in a V shape and perform a Roux-en-Y anastomosis, in order to adequately drainage the second and third pancreatic branches.

3. Distal pancreatectomy
   A distal pancreatectomy (DP) can be applied in patients with normal proximal pancreatic tissues and main pancreatic duct stenosis, with a reported hospital mortality of 0–3.8% and a morbidity of 15–31% (Sakorafas et al. 2001). Besides, normal duct but with hydatoncus in pancreatic tail is indication for DP. The procedure can safely preserve spleen and delay the attack of diabetes mellitus.
4. Total pancreatectomy
   As total pancreatectomy heavily destroys pancreatic endocrine and exocrine functions, it is only chosen when lesion involves the whole pancreas or abdominal pain sustains after conducting limited pancreatectomy as well as drainage. Several studies reported this procedure successfully reduced pain under stable glycemic control and improved quality of life (Wilson et al. 2015a, b), but long-term prognosis should be further studied. Moreover, to restore the endocrine function, total pancreatectomy should be conducted with the combination of islet autologous transplantation and selection criteria remain to be fulfilled (Bellin et al. 2015). In view of the high postoperative ulcer incidence and severe metabolic disorders, TP should only be considered once other surgical treatment options proved to be useless or unlikely to improve symptoms (Bramis et al. 2012).

6 Neurectomy

The innervation of pancreas include: pancreatic sympathetic nerve from celiac plexus or other plexus accompanied with arteries; pancreatic head plexus, from right abdominal ganglia and superior mesenteric plexus; pancreatic tail plexus, from left abdominal ganglia. Splanchnicectomy and celiac ganglionectomy can be selectively carried out according to the pain location. Although the procedure has a reported favorable shortdated pain relief, it is rarely used in clinical practice with worsened outcome over time (Issa and Ali 2014; Baghdadi et al. 2008).

7 Postoperative Complications

Early postoperative complications with CP patients include postoperative bleeding, pancreatic fistula, intestinal fistula and infections. The morbidity rate has been decreased these years due to improved surgery skills. However, for patients who undergo the pancreatectomy, insufficient endocrine function is common after operation, causing frequently occurrence of IIIc diabetes and diarrhea. As some studies reported, the cumulative incidence of new-onset diabetes millitus after distal pancreatectomy was fairly high (De Bruijn and van Eijck 2015) and the incidence depended on the preexisting disease, pancreatic resection range and follow-up time. Besides, to some extent, the removal position is correlated with the insufficient endocrine or exocrine functions. Generally speaking, proximal pancreatectomy makes negative effect on exocrine function, but distal pancreatectomy reduces endocrine function.

The surgical procedures for CP patients are various, with no single procedure suitable for every patient, and the outcome of operation remains individual-specific. To achieve optimal surgical results, surgeons should sufficiently evaluate the patient's clinical features, auxiliary examination results, and history of treatments to develop an individualized surgical option. Besides, preoperative diseases or customs, such as alcohol addiction, which will affect postoperative morbidity, must be solved to attain satisfying operation effect.

References

Baghdadi S, Abbas MH, Albouz F, et al. Systematic review of the role of thoracoscopic splanchnicectomy in palliating the pain of patients with chronic pancreatitis. Surg Endosc. 2008;22(3):580–8.

Bellin MD, Gelrud A, Arreazarubin G, et al. Total pancreatectomy with islet autotransplantation: summary of an NIDDK workshop. Ann Surg. 2015;261(1):21–9.

Bramis K, Gordon-Weeks AN, Friend PJ, et al. Systematic review of total pancreatectomy and islet autotransplantation for chronic pancreatitis. Br J Surg. 2012;99(6):761–6.

Büchler MW, Warshaw AL. Resection versus drainage in treatment of chronic pancreatitis. Gastroenterology. 2008;134(5):1605–7.

De Bruijn KM, van Eijck CH. New-onset diabetes after distal pancreatectomy: a systematic review. Ann Surg. 2015;261(5):854–61.

Farkas G, Leindler L, Daróczi M, et al. Prospective randomized comparison of organ-preserving pancreatic head resection with pylorus-preserving pancreaticoduodenectomy. Langenbecks Arch Surg. 2006;391(4):338–42.

Forsmark CE. Management of chronic pancreatitis. Gastroenterology. 2013;144(6):1282–91.

Gloor B, Friess H, Uhl W, et al. A modified technique of the Beger and Frey procedure in patients with chronic pancreatitis. Dig Surg. 2001;18(1):21–5.

Issa Y, Ali UA. Preoperative opioid use and the outcome of thoracoscopic splanchnicectomy in chronic pancreatitis: a systematic review. Surg Endosc. 2014;28(2):405–12.

Issa Y, Bruno MJ, Bakker OJ, et al. Treatment options for chronic pancreatitis. Nat Rev Gastroenterol Hepatol. 2014;11(9):556–64.

Jimenez RE, Fernandez-Del CC, Rattner DW, et al. Outcome of pancreaticoduodenectomy with pylorus preservation or with antrectomy in the treatment of chronic pancreatitis. Ann Surg. 2000;231(3):293–300.

Kutup A, Vashist Y, Kaifi JT, et al. For which type of chronic pancreatitis is the "Hamburg procedure" indicated? J Hepatobiliary Pancreat Sci. 2010;17(6):758–62.

Ni Q, Yun L, Roy M, et al. Advances in surgical treatment of chronic pancreatitis. World J Surg Oncol. 2015;13(1):1–6.

Parekh D, Natarajan S. Surgical management of chronic pancreatitis. Indian J Surg. 2015;77(5):121–33.

Poulsen JL, Olesen SS, Malver LP, et al. Pain and chronic pancreatitis: a complex interplay of multiple mechanisms. World J Gastroenterol. 2013;19(42):7282–91.

Sakorafas GH, Sarr MG, Rowland CM, et al. Postobstructive chronic pancreatitis: results with distal resection. Arch Surg. 2001;136(6):643–8.

Wilson GC, Sutton JM, Smith MT, et al. Total pancreatectomy with islet cell autotransplantation as the initial treatment for minimal-change chronic pancreatitis. HPB. 2015a;17(3):232–8.

Wilson GC, Sutton JM, Smith MT, et al. Completion pancreatectomy and islet cell autotransplantation as salvage therapy for patients failing previous operative interventions for chronic pancreatitis. Surgery. 2015b;158(4):879–80.

Yin Z, Sun J, Yin D, et al. Surgical treatment strategies in chronic pancreatitis: a meta-analysis. Arch Surg. 2012;147(10):961–8.

11 Special Types of Chronic Pancreatitis

Atsushi Masamune, Atsushi Kanno, Tooru Shimosegawa, Prachand Issarapu, Sumit Paliwal, Seema Bhaskar, Giriraj Ratan Chandak, Maisam Abu-El-Haija, and Aliye Uc

1 Autoimmune Pancreatitis

Atsushi Masamune, Atsushi Kanno, and Tooru Shimosegawa

Abbreviations

AIP	Autoimmune pancreatitis
CP	Chronic pancreatitis
CT	Computed tomography
ERP	Endoscopic retrograde pancreatography
EUS-FNA	Endoscopic ultrasound-guided fine needle aspiration
GEL	Granulocytic epithelial lesion
ICDC	International Consensus Diagnostic Criteria
IDCP	Idiopathic duct-centric chronic pancreatitis Ig, immunoglobulin
LPSP	Lymphoplasmacytic sclerosing pancreatitis
miRNA	microRNA
MPD	Main pancreatic duct
NOS	Not otherwise specified
OOI	Other organ involvement
PSL	Prednisolone

Prachand Issarapu and Sumit Paliwal contributed equally to this work.

A. Masamune, M. D., Ph.D. (✉) • A. Kanno
T. Shimosegawa
Division of Gastroenterology, Tohoku University Graduate School of Medicine,
1-1 Seiryo-machi, Aoba-ku, Sendai 980-8574, Japan
e-mail: amasamune@med.tohoku.ac.jp

P. Issarapu • S. Paliwal • S. Bhaskar
G.R. Chandak (✉)
Genomic Research on Complex Diseases (GRC Group), CSIR-Centre for Cellular and Molecular Biology, Hyderabad, Telangana 500007, India
e-mail: chandakgrc@ccmb.res.in; chandakgrc@gmail.com

M. Abu-El-Haija
Division of Gastroenterology, Hepatology and Nutrition, Cincinnati Children's Hospital Medical Center, Cincinnati, OH, USA

A. Uc, M.D. (✉)
Division of Pediatric Gastroenterology, Stead Family Department of Pediatrics, University of Iowa Children's Hospital, Iowa City, IA, USA

Stead Family Department of Pediatrics, The University of Iowa Carver College of Medicine, BT1120-C, 200 Hawkins Drive, Iowa City, IA 52242, USA
e-mail: aliye-uc@uiowa.edu

Z.-S. Li et al. (eds.), *Chronic Pancreatitis*, DOI 10.1007/978-981-10-4515-8_11

Abstract Autoimmune pancreatitis (AIP) is a relatively rare type of pancreatitis with a hypothesized autoimmune mechanism. AIP has several distinct clinical, serological, and morphological characteristics. Diffuse enlargement of the pancreas and irregular narrowing of the main pancreatic duct are typical imaging findings of AIP. AIP frequently presents with obstructive jaundice and increased serum immunoglobulin G4 (IgG4). AIP has two distinct phenotypes: type 1 and type 2 AIP. Histologically, lymphoplasmacytic sclerosing pancreatitis is characteristic of type 1 AIP, whereas idiopathic duct-centric chronic pancreatitis with granulocytic epithelial lesions is characteristic of type 2 AIP. Type 1 AIP is now regarded as a pancreatic manifestation of systemic IgG4-related disease and is often associated with extra-pancreatic lesions such as IgG4-related sclerosing cholangitis. AIP can be diagnosed according to the International Consensus Diagnostic Criteria based on pancreatic parenchymal imaging, ductal imaging, serology, other organ involvement, histology, and response to steroids (optional). AIP patients respond dramatically to corticosteroid therapy and corticosteroid has been established as a standard therapy for the treatment of AIP patients. The requirement of maintenance therapy has been controversial. For patients who are either intolerant of corticosteroids or have multiple relapses, there are other treatment options, including corticosteroid-sparing immunomodulators and B-cell depletion therapy using rituximab, which might be alternative treatment options. Overall, the prognosis of AIP is good. It is controversial whether AIP patients have an increased risk for cancer. Obviously, long-term follow-up will be required to clarify the outcomes of AIP patients.

1.1 Introduction

Autoimmune pancreatitis (AIP) is a relatively rare type of pancreatitis with a hypothesized autoimmune mechanism. It was first described by Sarles et al. (1961) as a subtype of idiopathic chronic pancreatitis (CP) in 1961. AIP was proposed as a clinical entity in 1995 (Yoshida et al. 1995). Yoshida et al. (1995) reported that this type of pancreatitis had several unique clinical, serological, and morphological features including increased serum γ-globulin or immunoglobulin (Ig) G levels; diffuse enlargement of the pancreas and narrowing of the main pancreatic duct (MPD); biliary stenosis; good response to steroids; and lymphoplasmacytic sclerosing pancreatitis (LPSP) on histology. Thereafter, extensive research has been conducted in this field over two decades and AIP has been established as a unique disease entity (Kamisawa et al. 2013; Hart et al. 2015b; Okazaki and Uchida 2015). In this chapter, we mainly review the diagnosis and management of AIP.

1.2 Epidemiology

AIP is a relatively rare disease. There have been few epidemiological studies to estimate the prevalence and incidence of patients with AIP. The latest nationwide epidemiological survey in Japan estimated the total number of AIP patients who visited hospitals in 2011 as 5745, which meant a prevalence rate of 4.6 per 100,000 persons (Kanno et al. 2015a). Among them, newly diagnosed AIP was estimated to be 1801, corresponding to an incidence rate of 1.4 per 100,000 persons. AIP mostly occurs in the middle-aged to elderly. In this Japanese survey, the mean age of the AIP patients was 66.3 peaking at 70–79 years in men and 60–69 years in women. The male-to-female sex ratio was 3.2.

1.3 Clinical Presentations

In an international, multicenter study of 1064 patients with AIP (Hart et al. 2013a), the most common symptom of AIP patients was painless jaundice, followed by pancreatitis/abdominal pain and abnormal imaging such as diffuse pancreatic enlargement and mass, and pancreatic dysfunction. AIP patients may have symptoms due to extrapancreatic involvement of IgG4-related disease such as salivary gland enlargement (Kamisawa et al. 2015).

1.4 Imaging

Diffuse enlargement of the pancreas with loss of the normal lobulated contour is the classical appearance of AIP on cross-sectional imaging. Typically, enhancement is decreased during the early phase and delayed in the late phase due to inflammation. A low attenuating rim, termed capsule-like rim, is known to be highly characteristic of AIP (Fig. 11.1a).

Typical pancreatograhic findings are long (>1/3 length of the MPD) or multiple strictures without marked dilatation of the upstream MPD, but with side branches arising from strictured segments (Fig. 11.1b).

1.5 Serum Markers

Hamano et al. (2001) reported that serum IgG4 was useful to diagnose AIP with high sensitivity and specificity in 2001. In the latest nationwide epidemiological survey in Japan (Kanno et al. 2015a), serum IgG4 was elevated in 739/855 (86.4%) patients with a mean value of 533 mg/dL. Anti-nuclear antibodies were positive in 263/785 (33.5%) patients, 486/862 (56.4%) patients had high levels of IgG, and rheumatoid factors were positive in 125/576 (21.7%) patients. Although elevated IgG4 is characteristic of type 1 AIP, an elevation of IgG4 is also seen in 5% of the normal population and in 10% of pancreatic cancer patients (Sah and Chari 2011). Therefore, IgG4 is not a specific diagnostic marker for definitive AIP, but, when combined with other features of AIP, it can be of great value to diagnose AIP.

Other serum specific biomarkers of AIP, especially those predicting disease relapse, have not yet been identified. Candidate markers include microRNA (miRNA) (Ciesla et al. 2011). MiRNA is a small noncoding RNA, 20–23 bases in length. MiRNA orchestrates multiple biological processes by targeting hundreds of target mRNAs through the 3′ untranslated region sequences, resulting in reduced expression of the target genes (Farazi et al. 2011). MiRNAs also exist within serum protected by stable structures such as the microvesicles or exosomes (Kosaka et al. 2010). Based on these unique characteristics, serum miRNAs have potential as novel biomarkers. Hamada et al. (2015) reported that hsa-miR-150-5p and hsa-miR-30-3p were commonly up-regulated in the serum of AIP patients compared to the samples of controls, chronic pancreatitis, and pancreatic cancer. The pathological roles of the up-regulated miRNAs remain to be clarified.

1.6 Histology

LPSP is a characteristic histological feature of type 1 AIP (Kamisawa et al. 2013; Hart et al. 2015a; Okazaki and Uchida 2015). Type 2 AIP is

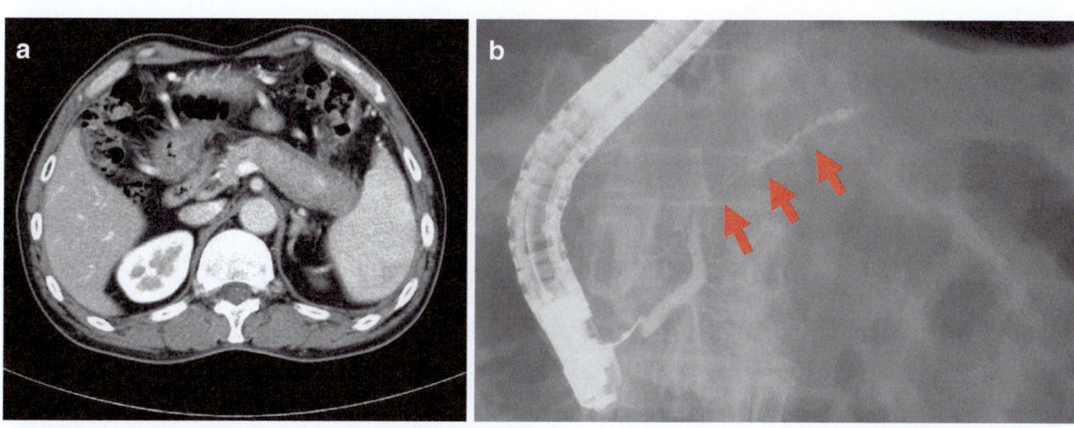

Fig. 11.1 Imaging findings of pancreatic parenchyma and duct in type 1 AIP. (**a**) Computed tomography image showing diffuse swelling of the pancreas accompanied by a low-density capsule-like rim. (**b**) Diffusely irregular narrowing of the main pancreatic duct on endoscopic retrograde pancreatography

characterized by idiopathic duct-centric chronic pancreatitis (IDCP) or granulocytic epithelial lesions (GEL): the infiltration and accumulation of neutrophils in the epithelium of pancreatic ducts accompanied by ductal destruction (Notohara et al. 2003). ICDC currently requires that the histological specimens be acquired by endoscopic ultrasound (EUS) -trucut biopsy or operation (Shimosegawa et al. 2011). EUS-guided fine-needle aspiration (EUS-FNA) is not included in the ICDC as a method for the histological evaluation because it is difficult to obtain adequate specimens for histopathological analysis (Shimosegawa et al. 2011). However, several reports have suggested that EUS-FNA is useful to diagnose AIP. Kanno et al. (2015b) reported that AIP could be histologically diagnosed according to ICDC in 20/25 (80%) patients using EUS-FNA with a 22-G needle (Fig. 11.2). Kanno et al. (2016) further validated their findings by a prospective multicenter study. They showed that 45/78 (57.7%) patients could be diagnosed with LPSP (levels 1 or 2) according to ICDC.

1.7 Other Organ Involvement (OOI)

It has been increasingly recognized that type 1 AIP is a pancreatic manifestation of systemic IgG4-related disease (Umehara et al. 2012; Kamisawa et al. 2015). Extra-pancreatic involvements include IgG4-related sclerosing cholangitis (Fig. 11.3a), retroperitoneal fibrosis, dacryoadenitis/sialadenitis (Fig. 11.3b), and interstitial nephritis. Type 2 AIP is frequently accompanied by inflammatory bowel diseases in about 30% of cases (Kamisawa et al. 2013; Hart et al. 2015a; Okazaki and Uchida 2015). ^{18}F-fluorodeoxyglucose positron emission tomography is useful for detecting extra-pancreatic lesions as well as pancreatic ones (Fig. 11.3c).

1.8 Diagnosis Criteria for AIP

1.8.1 History

The world's first diagnostic criteria for AIP were proposed by the Japan Pancreas Society (JPS) in 2002 (Members of the Criteria Committee for Autoimmune Pancreatitis of the Japan Pancreas Society 2002). The criteria consisted of three diagnostic items, (1) imaging findings (mandatory), (2) serological and (3) pathological findings. The 2002 criteria defined the length of MPD narrowing as more than 1/3 of the whole pancreas on endoscopic retrograde pancreatography (ERP) to avoid misdiagnosis of pancreatic cancer as AIP. Therefore, localized-type AIP could not be diagnosed according to the 2002 JPS criteria. The 2002 JPS criteria were revised in 2006 (Okazaki et al. 2006). In this revision, the length of MPD narrowing was eliminated and IgG4 was incorporated as a serological item.

Thereafter, diagnostic criteria were proposed worldwide including in Korea (Kim et al. 2006) and the United States (Chari et al. 2006). Additional diagnostic features, including various appearances on computed tomography (CT),

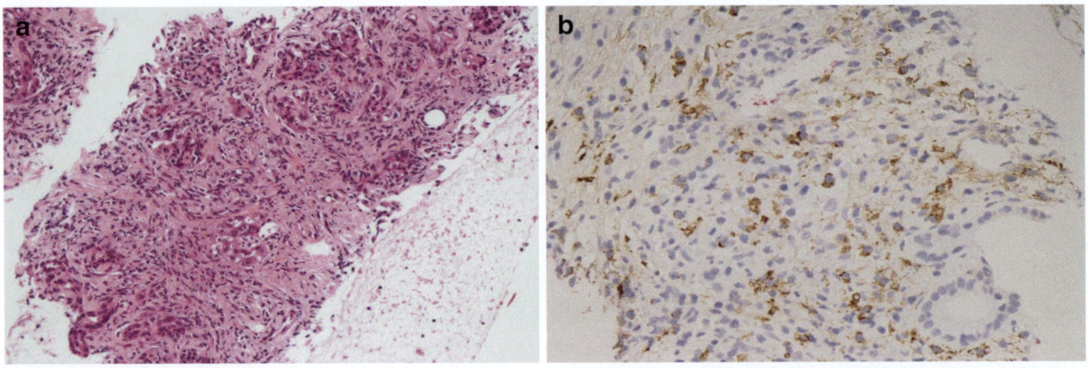

Fig. 11.2 Biopsy specimens obtained by EUS-FNA using a 22-G needle. (**a**) Infiltration of plasma cells and lymphocytes with fibrosis (storiform fibrosis) (H&E, X100). (**b**) Immunostaining for IgG4 showing infiltration of IgG4-positive plasma cells (X100)

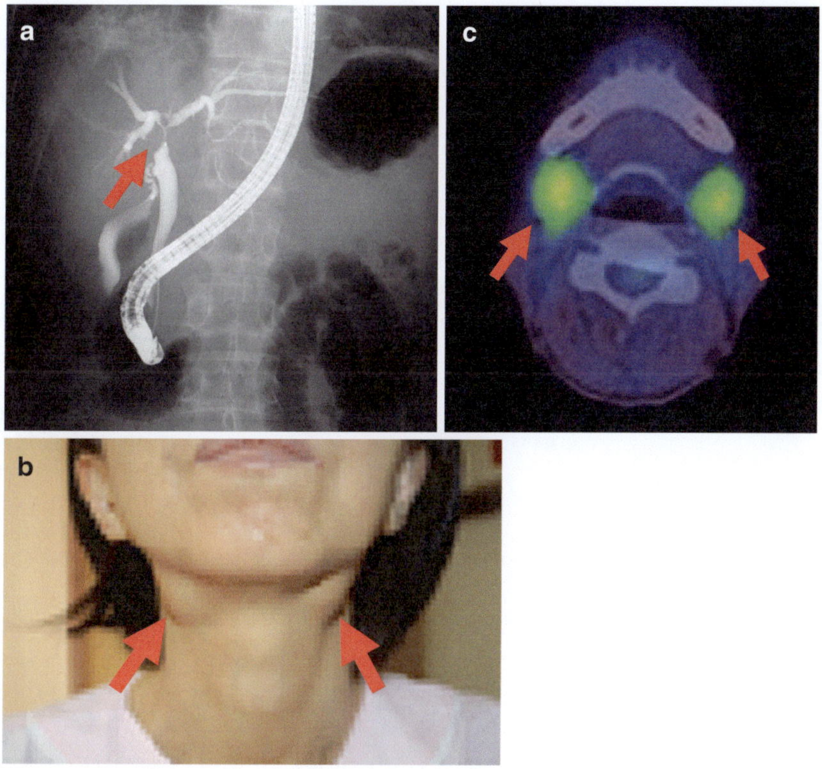

Fig. 11.3 Other organ involvement. (**a**) Endoscopic retrograde cholangiopancreatography showing strictures of the bile duct in the hilar hepatic lesions (*red arrow*). (**b**) Swelling of the submandibular glands (*red arrows*). (**c**) ^{18}F-FDG uptake by the submandibular glands is shown on ^{18}F-fluorodeoxyglucose positron emission tomography (*red arrows*)

OOI and response to steroids were incorporated in these diagnostic criteria. The diagnostic criteria in the United States, namely HISORt criteria, were revised in 2009. The revised HISORt criteria covered both LPSP and IDCP/GEL (Chari et al. 2009). However, the lack of common diagnostic criteria for AIP was a large obstacle for international comparative studies.

In 2009, experts in this field discussed the consensus on the diagnostic criteria for AIP in Honolulu, Hawaii. It was agreed that the clinical phenotypes associated with LPSP and IDCP/GEL should be distinguished, but, the terminology was controversial. Most experts agreed that LPSP and IDCP/GEL should be referred to as type 1 and type 2 AIP, respectively, but others objected to the use of the term 'autoimmune' to describe IDCP (Chari et al. 2010). During the next year, there was further discussion in Fukuoka, Japan, and, finally, the ICDC for AIP were proposed (Shimosegawa et al. 2011). The ICDC took global differences in clinical practice into consideration to be used worldwide to safely diagnose AIP without misdiagnosing pancreatic cancer as AIP.

1.8.2 Overview of the ICDC

In the ICDC, AIP is diagnosed according to the parenchymal imaging (P), ductal imaging on ERP (D), serology (S), other organ involvement (OOI), histology of the pancreas (H), and response to steroid (Rt; optional). Each cardinal feature is categorized as level 1 or level 2 according to the reliability for diagnosis.

AIP is classified into two subtypes: type 1 related to LPSP and type 2 related to IDCP/GEL. Type 1 and type 2 AIP are diagnosed according to the independent diagnostic criteria. Table 11.1 summarizes the level 1 and level 2 criteria for type 1 AIP in ICDC. If imaging findings of the pancreatic parenchyma yield typical findings (diffuse enlargement with

Table 11.1 Level 1 and Level 2 criteria for type 1 AIP in ICDC

	Criterion	Level 1	Level 2
P	Parenchymal imaging	**Typical**:	**Indeterminate (including atypical**[a]**)**:
		Diffuse enlargement with delayed enhancement (sometimes associated with rim-like enhancement)	Segmental/focal enlargement with delayed enhancement
D	Ductal imaging (ERP)	Long (>1/3 length of the main pancreatic duct) or multiple strictures without marked upstream dilatation	Segmental/focal narrowing without marked upstream dilatation (duct size, <5 mm)
S	Serology	IgG4 >2 X upper limit of normal value	IgG4, 1–2 X upper limit of normal value
OOI	Other organ involvement	**(a) or (b)**	**(a) or (b)**
		(a) Histology of extrapancreatic organs	**(a) Histology of extrapancreatic organs including endoscopic biopsies of bile duct**[b]:
		Any three of the following:	Both of the following:
		1. Marked lymphoplasmacytic infiltration with fibrosis and without granulocytic infiltration	1. Marked lymphoplasmacytic infiltration without granulocytic infiltration
		2. Storiform fibrosis	2. Abundant (>10 cells/HPF) IgG4 positive cells
		3. Obliterative phlebitis	
		4. Abundant (>10 cells/HPF) IgG4-positive cells	
		(b) Typical radiological evidence	**(b) Physical or radiological evidence**
		At least one of the following:	At least one of the following:
		1. Segmental/multiple proximal (hilar/intrahepatic) or proximal and distal bile duct stricture	1. Symmetrically enlarged salivary/lacrimal glands
		2. Retroperitoneal fibrosis	2. Radiologic evidence of renal involvement described in association with AIP
H	Histology of the pancreas	**LPSP (core biopsy/resection)**	**LPSP (core biopsy)**
		At least three of the following:	Any two of the following
		1. Periductal lymphoplasmacytic infiltrate without granulocytic infiltration	1. Periductal lymphoplasmacytic infiltrate without granulocytic infiltration
		2. Obliterative phlebitis	2. Obliterative phlebitis
		3. Storiform fibrosis	3. Storiform fibrosis
		4. Abundant (>10 cells/HPF) IgG4-positive cells	4. Abundant (>10 cells/HPF) IgG4-positive cells
		Diagnostic steroid trial	
Response to steroid (Rt)[c]		Rapid (≦2 weeks) radiologically demonstrable resolution or marked improvement in pancreatic/extra-pancreatic manifestations	

[a]Atypical: Some AIP cases may show low-density mass, pancreatic ductal dilatation or distal atrophy. Such atypical imaging findings in patients with obstructive jaundice and/or pancreatic mass are highly suggestive of pancreatic cancer. Such patients should be managed as pancreatic cancer unless there is strong collateral evidence for AIP and a thorough workup for cancer is negative

[b]Endoscopic biopsy of duodenal papilla is a useful adjunctive method because ampulla is often involved pathologically in AIP

[c]Diagnostic steroid trial should be conducted carefully by pancreatologists with caveats only after negative workup for cancer including endoscopic ultrasound-guided fine-needle aspiration

delayed enhancement), type 1 AIP can be definitively diagnosed if there are any non-D level 1/level 2 findings (Table 11.2). If pancreatic imaging findings were indeterminate (segmental or focal enlargement with delayed enhancement), two or more level 1 (+level 2D) findings are required to diagnose type 1 AIP definitively. If the core biopsy specimens or resected pancreatic tissues indicate LPSP, definitive type 1 AIP can be diagnosed based on the histological findings alone.

Table 11.3 summarizes the level 1 and level 2 criteria for type 2 AIP. Histological examination is required for a diagnosis of type 2 AIP. The

Table 11.2 Diagnosis of definitive and probable type 1 AIP using ICDC

Diagnosis	Primary basis for diagnosis	Imaging evidence	Collateral evidence
Definitive type 1 AIP	Histology	Typical/indeterminate	Histologically confirmed LPSP (level 1 H)
	Imaging	Typical	Any non-D level 1/level 2
		Indeterminate	Two or more from level 1 (+level 2 D[a])
	Response to steroid	Indeterminate	Level 1 S/OOI + Rt or level 1 D + level 2 S/OOI/H + Rt
Probable type 1 AIP		Indeterminate	Level 2 S/OOI/H + Rt

[a]Level 2 D is counted as level 1 in this setting
ICDC International Consensus Diagnostic Criteria, *AIP* autoimmune pancreatitis, *LPSP* lymphoplasmacytic sclerosing pancreatitis

Table 11.3 Level 1 and level 2 criteria for type 2 AIP

	Criterion	Level 1	Level 2
P	Parenchymal imaging	**Typical:**	**Indeterminate (including atypical[a]):**
		Diffuse enlargement with delayed enhancement (sometimes associated with rim-like enhancement)	Segmental/focal enlargement with delayed enhancement
D	Ductal imaging (ERP)	Long (>1/3 length of the main pancreatic duct) or multiple strictures without marked upstream dilatation	Segmental/focal narrowing without marked upstream dilatation (duct size <5 mm)
OOI	Other organ involvement		Clinically diagnosed inflammatory bowel disease
H	Histology of the pancreas (core biopsy/resection)	**IDCP:**	
		Both of the following:	Both of the following:
		1. Granulocytic infiltration of duct wall (GEL) with or without granulocytic acinar inflammation	1. Granulocytic and lymphoplasmacytic acinar infiltrate
		2. Absent or scant (0–10 cells/HPF) IgG4-positive cells	2. Absent or scant (0–10 cells/HPF) IgG4-positive cells
		Diagnostic steroid trial	
Response to steroid (Rt)[b]		Rapid (<2 weeks) radiologically demonstrable resolution or marked improvement in manifestations	

[a,b]See Table 11.1

Table 11.4 Diagnosis of definitive and probable type 2 AIP using ICDC

Diagnosis	Imaging evidence	Collateral evidence
Definitive type 2 AIP	Typical/indeterminate	Histologically confirmed IDCP or Clinical IBD + Level 2 H + Rt
Probable type 2 AIP	Typical/indeterminate	Level 2 H/clinical inflammatory bowel disease + Rt

AIP autoimmune pancreatitis, *IDCP* idiopathic duct-centric chronic pancreatitis

Table 11.5 Diagnosis of AIP-not otherwise specified using ICDC

Diagnosis	Imaging evidence	Collateral evidence (case with only D1/2)
AIP-not otherwise specified	Typical/indeterminate	D1/2 + Rt

level 1 histological findings of GEL are sufficient for a definitive diagnosis of type 2 AIP (Table 11.4). Alternatively, in the case of level 2 histological findings, definitive type 2 AIP can be made if the patient has inflammatory bowel disease and responds to steroids.

Cases that have level 1 or level 2 ductal imaging findings and respond to steroids, without other cardinal features of AIP, are diagnosed as AIP-not otherwise specified (AIP-NOS). These cases should be carefully followed up, because other diseases are possible (Table 11.5).

1.9 Comparison of the Clinical Presentations of Type 1 and Type 2 AIP

Hart et al. (2013a) reported an international collaborative study of 1064 patients with AIP (978 (91.9%) type 1 AIP and 86 (8.1%) type 2 AIP) diagnosed according to the ICDC. Patients with type 2 AIP were diagnosed at younger ages than those with type 1 AIP (average: 61.4 years in type 1 AIP subjects and 39.9 years in type 2 subjects). The proportion of males was higher in type 1 AIP patients (77%) than in type 2 patients (55%). The proportion of patients with type 2 AIP was significantly higher in Europe (12.9%) than in Asia (3.7%). Remission could be induced in almost all cases with type 1 and type 2 AIP. Relapses were more common in patients with type 1 AIP (30.9%) than in those with type 2 AIP (9.3%). Hart et al. (2015a) also reported the clinical features of 43 patients with type 2 AIP (31 definitive and 12 probable cases) treated at the Mayo Clinic in the United States. Twenty five out of the 43 (58.1%) patients developed acute pancreatitis, 12/43 (27.9%) patients had recurrent pancreatitis, and 15/43 (34.9%) patients had pancreatic mass/obstructive jaundice. The cumulative relapse rate was 10.6% at 3 years (median follow-up period of 2.9 years). In Japan, Notohara et al. (2015) compared the clinical features of patients with type 1 AIP and type 2 AIP in Japan. They showed that type 2 AIP patients were younger and had more frequent abdominal pain and increased serum pancreatic enzymes than those with type 1 AIP. Obstructive jaundice, elevated serum IgG and IgG4, the presence of autoantibodies, association of IgG4-related diseases including sclerosing cholangitis, diabetes mellitus, and imaging findings of extrapancreatic biliary dilatation and intrapancreatic biliary strictures were more common in patients with type 1 AIP than in type 2 AIP.

1.10 Treatments

Both type 1 and type 2 AIP patients respond well to corticosteroids. In an international multicenter study, 681/684 (99.6%) patients with type 1 AIP and 48/52 (92.3%) patients with type 2 AIP achieved clinical remission by the initial treatment with corticosteroid (Hart et al. 2013a). In a multicenter study from Japan, the remission rate was higher in corticosteroid-treated AIP patients than in those with no treatment (98% vs. 74%, $P < 0.001$) (Kamisawa et al. 2009). Based on these observational studies, corticosteroid has been established as the standard therapy for the treatment of AIP patients (Hart et al. 2013a; Kamisawa et al. 2009; Pannala and Chari 2009; Kamisawa et al. 2014), and a rapid response to the corticosteroid treatment is included in the ICDC (Shimosegawa et al. 2011). Known risk factors for disease relapse include proximal biliary involvement (Ghazale et al. 2008; Hart et al. 2013a) and presentation with diffuse pancreatic enlargement (Sah et al. 2010; Kubota et al. 2011).

The requirement of maintenance therapy has been controversial. Maintenance therapy is not common in the United States and Europe, due to the concern of serious corticosteroid-related complications caused by increased cumulative amounts of corticosteroid (Ghazale et al. 2008; Pannala and Chari 2009). One standard protocol is the administration of oral prednisolone (PSL) for 4 weeks followed by tapering by 5 mg each week until being discontinued after 11 weeks (Ghazale et al. 2008). In addition, nearly half of the patients do not relapse even without maintenance therapy, and relapsed cases respond well to the re-administration of corticosteroid (Ghazale et al. 2008). However, many patients who achieved remission relapsed soon after the cessation of corticosteroid treatment. In a Pittsburg study, 9 out of 15 (60%) patients who achieved complete remission developed relapses within 8–12 weeks after the corticosteroid cessation (Raina et al. 2009). In Japan, long-term maintenance therapy with low-dose corticosteroid is preferred and recommended in the Japanese guidelines (Kamisawa et al. 2014). In a multicenter study from Japan, 10/38 (26%) cases relapsed during maintenance treatment with PSL at more than 5 mg/day, and this was significantly lower than the relapse rate of 14/26 (54%) patients who discontinued the therapy (Kamisawa et al. 2010). Very recently, Masamune et al. (2016) reported a randomized controlled trial of long-term maintenance corticosteroid therapy in Japan. They showed that long-term maintenance corticosteroid therapy for 3 years (maintenance therapy group) significantly decreased relapses in AIP patients compared with those who discontinued the therapy at 26 weeks (cessation group). Seven out of 30 (23.3%) patients in the maintenance therapy group developed relapses, whereas 11 out of 19 (57.9%) patients in the cessation group relapsed within 3 years. The relapse rate over 3 years was significantly higher in the cessation group than that in the maintenance therapy group ($P = 0.011$). No serious steroid-associated complications such as serious infection requiring discontinuation of PSL administration were observed. Although this study had several limitations including its small sample size, the results suggested that long-term low-dose maintenance corticosteroid therapy would be an option to decrease relapses.

For patients who are either intolerant of corticosteroids or have multiple relapses, there are other treatment options including corticosteroid-sparing immunomodulators and B-cell depletion therapy using rituximab to avoid increased cumulative amounts of corticosteroid (Hart et al. 2013b).

1.11 Prognosis

Overall, the prognosis of AIP is good. The 5-year survival rates for AIP patients were similar to those of the age- and sex-matched US population (Sah et al. 2010). Exocrine and endocrine functions in the pancreas might be recovered by steroids in the short-term (Nishimori et al. 2006; Ko et al. 2010), but the long-term preservation of these functions remains to be determined. A portion of AIP patients develop pancreatic calcification or CP (Maruyama et al. 2013). One remaining important issue is whether patients with AIP have an increased risk for pancreatic cancer (Hart et al. 2014). In the 2011 nationwide survey in Japan (Kanno et al. 2015a), malignant tumors were found in 109 out of 923 (11.8%) AIP patients during a mean follow-up period of 4.8 years, but only seven cases were pancreatic cancer (Kanno et al.

2015a). Gastric cancer (21 patients) and colorectal cancer (16 patients) were the most common malignant tumors. One explanation for the relatively high frequency of malignancy in AIP patients is that most AIP patients are middle-aged to elderly. Hirano et al. (2014) reported that cancer risk is not higher in AIP patients than in the general population. It was also suggested that AIP might have an aspect of paraneoplastic syndrome, because the incidence of cancer was increased within the first year after the diagnosis of AIP (Shiokawa et al. 2013). Obviously, long-term follow-up will be required to address this issue.

Acknowledgements *Financial Supports*: Supported in part by the Ministry of Health, Labour, and Welfare of Japan.

Conflict of Interest: None declared.

2 Evolution of Phenotypic and Genetic Profile of Tropical Calcific Pancreatitis

Prachand Issarapu, Sumit Paliwal, Seema Bhaskar, and Giriraj Ratan Chandak

Abstract Historically, tropical calcific pancreatitis (TCP) was defined as a juvenile form of chronic calcific, non-alcoholic pancreatitis with younger age of onset, presence of large intraductal calculi, accelerated course of the disease and, high risk of developing diabetes and pancreatic cancer. The clinical features of TCP have evolved over the past few decades with relatively older age of onset and a milder form of the disease. In addition, the proportion of cases presenting with imaging abnormalities like calcification, ductal dilation and glandular atrophy is variably reported. This may be related to the technological advances that allow early detection of the disease, as well as to better awareness about the disease. Etiology of TCP is still obscure. The proposed causal role of malnutrition and cassava toxicity has been refuted; instead, role of micronutrient deficiencies is being investigated. Over last two decades, there has been great emphasis on understanding the genetic basis of chronic pancreatitis (CP) including TCP. As a result, several susceptibility genes including cationic and anionic trypsinogens, serine protease inhibitor kazal type I, cathepsin B, chymotrypsin C, carboxypeptidase A1, claudin 2 and others have been discovered. Results from our studies have supported the notion that there exists genetic and mutational diversity between TCP in Indians and CP in Western populations. Overall results suggest that TCP is a complex multifactorial disease and further exhaustive studies are required to dissect the role of individual factors as well as understand their cumulative effect in the disease pathophysiology.

2.1 Introduction

Tropical calcific pancreatitis (TCP) was first described more than half a century ago as a rapidly progressing disease with onset in childhood and adolescence, recurrent abdominal pain, marked ductal dilation, presence of unusually large calculi and pronounced malnourishment. Majority of such cases were reported from Southern India. Over the last two decades, there has been a noticeable change in the clinical presentation of the disease. This has forced the researchers to re-evaluate the underlying causes. Consequently, while many of the earlier presumptions have been challenged, several new evidences are emerging. For instance, instead of macronutrient deficiency, role of micronutrient deficiencies is being investigated. Additionally, genetic and molecular studies have taken the center stage to understand the pathobiology. In this chapter, we discuss the evolution of the phenotypic presentation of TCP and role of emerging genetic risk factors associated with the disease. Majority of the data cited/presented represents the work originating from India.

2.2 Phenotypic Perspectives

2.2.1 The Past

Kini in 1938 first presented a case of chronic pancreatitis with multiple pancreatic calculi from India (Kini 1938). Zuidema, in 1950s described young diabetic patients who were often malnourished and also showed fibrosis and calcification of the pancreas (Zuidema 1955, 1959). Later, several similar observations from Southern India, Uganda, Nigeria and other parts of Africa, Brazil, Bangladesh, Sri Lanka and Thailand were reported (Shaper 1960; Kinnear 1963; Mngola 1982; Dani et al. 1986; Azad Khan et al. 1991; Illangovekara 1995; Vannasaeng et al. 1998). However, the largest series of studies conducted by Geevarghese describing young patients with malnutrition, pancreatic calculi and diabetes brought attention to this peculiar condition (Geevarghese 1968). The close association of these reports with the tropical parts of the world led to the origin of term 'Tropical Calcific/Chronic Pancreatitis (TCP)'. It was identified as a juvenile form of chronic calcific, non-alcoholic pancreatitis with distinctive features like younger age of onset, presence of large intraductal calculi, accelerated course of the disease and high susceptibility to developing diabetes. Since then several terminologies such as juvenile pancreatitis, chronic calcific pancreatitis, fibrocalculous pancreatitis, tropical pancreatitis etc., have been in use. In the simplest words, tropical pancreatitis was described by Geevarghese as a disease with "*Pain in childhood, diabetes in puberty and death at the prime of life*" (Geevarghese 1968).

During 1970s, TCP patients particularly from Southern India were often malnourished children, adolescents or occasionally, young adults with a cyanotic hue of the lips, bilaterally enlarged parotid glands, a pot belly and sometimes pedal edema (Balakrishnan 1987; Balakrishnan et al. n.d.). These features formed a 'classic picture' of diagnosing TCP. In the absence of sophisticated diagnostic methodologies, it was possible for gastroenterologists to make 'spot diagnosis' while walking around the hospital wards based on these striking features (Balakrishnan et al. n.d.). They were such glaringly obvious that this clinical phenotype with plain abdomen X-ray showing pancreatic intraductal calculi would clinch the diagnosis. Notably, unlike alcoholic calcific/chronic pancreatitis (ACP) cases of the West, these patients did not have any history of alcohol abuse or smoking. Later imaging studies using endoscopic retrograde cholangiopancreatography (ERCP) and ultrasonography showed clear-cut distinction between TCP and ACP (Balakrishnan et al. 1985). Formation of large, discrete, intraductal dense calculi were observed in TCP whereas ACP had small speckled parenchymal calculi with irregular, indefinite margins. The extent of ductal dilation, pancreatic calculi, and pancreatic atrophy were also more in TCP compared with other forms of chronic pancreatitis (Moorthy et al. 1992). Moreover, majority of the patients invariably developed diabetes which was later termed as Fibrocalculous Pancreatic Diabetes (FCPD) (Mohan et al. 1998). The histopathology and immunochemistry of the pancreas in these subjects showed atrophy of the exocrine pancreatic tissue and reduced number of islets (Govindarajan et al. 2001). Collectively, insulin positivity in islets was reduced that directly correlated with serum C-peptide levels and inversely with the duration of diabetes (Yajnik et al. 1990). The series of patients reported by Geevarghese were indeed cases of FCPD (Geevarghese 1968).

In brief, the following features distinguished TCP from other forms of chronic pancreatitis: (a) early age of onset; (b) malnourished patients; (c) presence in tropics; (d) non-alcoholism; (e) chronic abdominal pain; (f) manifestation of main pancreatic duct with ductal dilatation; (g) large pancreatic calculi primarily in the head region; (h) insulin-dependent but ketosis resistant diabetes; (i) absence of family history of pancreatitis; (j) no other discernible cause of CP.

2.2.2 The Present

The 'classical picture' of TCP has undergone a significant change over the years. Compared with the patients of 1980s, the age of onset and presentation is almost a decade older now, but it is significantly earlier than ACP (Balakrishnan et al. 2006, 2008; Bhasin et al. 2009; Rajesh et al. 2014a). Additionally, there is heterogeneity in macroscopic features observed in the pancreas of these patients. Reports from Southern India observe calcification in 90% of patients (Balakrishnan et al. n.d.; Rajesh et al. 2014a) whereas those form Northern India suggest it to range from 40 to 80% (Bhasin et al. 2009; Bhatia n.d.; Midha et al. 2010). Development of calculi (60–70%), dilated pancreatic duct (55–65%), and atrophy of the gland (30–40%) have been observed as the major imaging modalities (Balakrishnan et al. 2008). The proportion of FCPD cases has also reduced substantially from 1.6% of all diabetic patients during the early 1990s to 0.2% during the period 2006–2010, whereas the prevalence of diabetes secondary to ACP has remained unchanged (Papita et al. 2012). Moreover, during the above periods of study, while FCPD patients have shown a trend of delay in the age at diagnosis, diabetes secondary to ACP now develops at an earlier age (Papita et al. 2012).

Recent reports have put forward the following diagnostic measures to define TCP: age at onset below 30 years, a body mass index (BMI) lower than 18.5 kg/m^2, absence of any other causes of pancreatitis, and presence of diabetes (Balakrishnan et al. 2008; Midha et al. 2010). Only 4–6% of patients fulfill the above criteria and can be classified as having TCP (Balakrishnan et al. 2008; Midha et al. 2010). These reports have thus questioned the existence of TCP and emphasize on using the term idiopathic chronic pancreatitis (ICP) instead. However, several of these points have been debated (Paliwal et al. 2011). To begin with, using BMI as a diagnostic measure for classification of CP is questionable because a BMI < 18.5 kg/m^2 indicates underweight status and not malnourishment. Moreover, prospective case-control studies to evaluate cause and effect relation of malnutrition with CP/TCP report that only 15–20% of cases are underweight/malnourished prior to the onset of the disease and majority of patients lost weight afterwards (Midha et al. 2008; Sathiaraj et al. 2010). A study where Bonnet monkeys were fed with protein-poor carbohydrate-rich diet reported occurrence of ductal changes, with mucoid metaplasia and parenchymal atrophy (Sandhyamani et al. 1999). Further, the animals predominantly developed inflammatory and vascular changes in the pancreas and showed cardiac changes; pancreatic lesions were similar to those typically seen in FCPD. Nevertheless, pancreatic calculi were not seen. Putting all these together it is more likely that malnutrition is an aftereffect and not a cause. It is speculated that with the growing economy, there has been improvement in the nutritional status that is reflected in the phenotype, i.e. normal BMI and late presentation (Balakrishnan 2011).

Over time, several other factors including cassava/cyanogens toxicity, oxidative stress and trace element deficiency have been proposed to be involved in the etiopathogenesis of TCP. Cassava (tapioca, *Manihot esculenta*) consumption is quite common in some parts of world including Kerala in Southern India, from where a large number of TCP cases have been reported. It has long been considered as one of the major causal factors for TCP. In theory, excessive consumption of cassava could cause TCP because cassava is 87.5% carbohydrate with negligible protein, vitamin or mineral content. It contains toxic harmful metabolites such as cyanogenic glycosides, detoxification of which requires sulphur containing amino acids methionine and cysteine amino acid reserve (Rosling 1987). Later, hypothesis of cassava as the sole causal factor for TCP was rejected because, (1) all who consumed cassava did not develop TCP (Girish et al. 2011a), (2) TCP was also observed in places where cassava was not consumed (Balakrishnan et al. 2008; Garg and Tandon 2004); and, (3) rat model studies did not observe diabetes or pancreatitis on long-term cassava consumption (Mathangi et al. 2000). Though, now the community has rejected the causal role of cassava but the involvement of environmental toxins in disease pathophysiology cannot be denied as they could be playing a co-factor role rather than being involved in direct causation.

Micronutrient deficiencies are common in CP and might be participating in the pathogenesis via oxidative stress. An early study from Southern India (Braganza et al. 1993) has shown that culinary practices that reduce the biological availability of ascorbic acid and beta-carotene may expose the pancreas to oxidative stress and thereby to the changes leading to development of TCP at an early age. Increased oxidative detoxification has been linked with chronic pancreatitis. This study also implicated the role of xenobiotic stress in the etiopathogenesis of TCP. Further studies from Southern India also report increased lipid peroxidation and reduced antioxidant status both in TCP and ACP (Girish et al. 2011b, 2012). This is an extension to the previous observation that wherein zinc deficiency was proposed to play a significant role in CP (Girish et al. 2009). Folate deficiency has also been reported in CP including TCP (Rajesh et al. 2010).

Studies have categorized ICP into early-onset (≤30 years) and late-onset (>30 years) and there are reservations over the idea of considering those belonging to early-onset category to be similar to TCP (Bhasin et al. 2009; Rajesh et al. 2014a). There are opinions that change in phenotype of TCP is due to modifications in diet and lifestyle that have occurred over a couple of decades (Balakrishnan 2011). It is further argued that, "to deny retrospectively that there was no entity of TCP is historically incorrect" (Balakrishnan 2011). Recent reports also suggest an increased tendency of alcohol consumption and smoking even in cases of TCP (Balakrishnan et al. 2006; Rajesh et al. 2014a). Consequentially, TCP is now displaying phenotypic similarity to ICP and is also being edged out by ACP. Indeed, studies from Southern India (Balakrishnan et al. n.d.; Rajesh et al. 2014b) report a sharp increase in proportion of ACP cases from a lowly 3% during the 1980s to approximately 33% over the last decade, whereas those from Northern India observe a parallel existence of ACP or slight predominance of TCP/ICP (Bhasin et al. 2009; Midha et al. 2010).

2.3 Genetic Risk Factors

Familial clustering of TCP is well documented (Mohan et al. 1989; Kambo et al. 1989; Pitchumoni 1970). One of the earliest studies reported familial aggregation in nearly 8% of TCP patients (Mohan et al. 1989). It provided evidence of vertical transmission or horizontal distribution of the disease, which hinted at the involvement of genetic factors in pathogenesis of TCP. Ours and others' attempts to fine map genetic risk factors for TCP have revealed that genes regulating both "Trypsin-Central" and "Trypsin-independent" pathways contribute to its pathogenesis. The major factors contributing to these pathways are discussed below.

2.3.1 Trypsin-Central Pathway

Observations made more than a century ago by Chiari, a German pathologist engendered the belief that pancreatitis is an autodigestive disease caused due to inappropriate activation of digestive enzymes within the pancreas itself (Chiari 1896). Interestingly, early intracellular trypsinogen activation was noted consistently in several animal models of pancreatitis studied over the past few decades (Hofbauer et al. 1998; Lerch and Gorelick 2000; Dawra et al. 2011). The discovery of *PRSS1* c.365G>A (p.R122H) association with hereditary pancreatitis further supported the trypsin-central paradigm of pancreatitis (Whitcomb et al. 1996a). This led pancreatitis researchers to investigate mechanisms of intracellular trypsinogen activation. Subsequent focus was thus on trypsin itself or other genes that regulate its activity. The major trypsin-central candidate genes studied in CP including TCP so far are: cationic trypsinogen (*PRSS1,* MIM276000), anionic trypsinogen (*PRSS2,* MIM601564), Serine Protease Inhibitor Kazal Type I (*SPINK1,* MIM167790), Cathepsin B (*CTSB,* MIM116810) and Chymotrypsin C (*CTRC,* MIM601405).

Trypsinogen genes (*PRSS1* and *PRSS2*)

Several coding mutations in *PRSS1* (particularly p.A16V, p.N29I and p.R122H) are known to be associated with CP in Europeans (Whitcomb et al. 1996a). Ours and other groups have attempted to affirm this association in TCP. However, neither mutations in *PRSS1* predicting susceptibility to CP in Western populations have been identified in TCP patients (Chandak et al. 2002, 2004). Mutations in *PRSS2* were investigated presuming the disease mechanism akin to that of *PRSS1*. Previous research by various groups ruled out any causal role for *PRSS2* in ICP and TCP (Idris et al. 2005; Chen et al. 1999). The protective role of p.G191R *PRSS2* mutation, identified in Europeans (Witt et al. 2006) has also not been replicated in Indians (Mahurkar et al. 2009). Additionally, no copy number mutations in *PRSS1/PRSS2* have been found in TCP patients (Masson et al. 2008a). More recently, the sole genome wide association study (GWAS) in individuals of European descent identified a strong association of *PRSS1-PRSS2* loci variant rs10273639 with both sporadic and alcohol-related CP (ACP) (Whitcomb et al. 2012). The results, however, could be replicated only with ACP in another European study (Derikx et al. 2015). It was argued that non-replication of results with non-alcoholic CP (NACP) was primarily due to mixture of patients with different etiologies in the GWAS. Interestingly, using TCP as a model of NACP, we have been able to replicate the association of rs10273639 [OR (95%CI) = 0.72 (0.61–0.85); $P = 3.5 \times 10^{-5}$] (Paliwal et al. 2016). Moreover, this variant was found to be in perfect linkage disequilibrium ($r^2 = 1.0$) with another regulatory variant rs4726576 which has been identified to be the causal variant (Boulling et al. 2015). Nevertheless, the frequency of the risk allele ($AF_c = 0.27$) was found to be significantly lower in Indians compared with the Europeans (CEU; $AF_c = 0.59$; $P < 1 \times 10^{-4}$) indicating a swap in major and minor allele between the two populations (Fig. 11.4). The same is reflected in the haplotype carrying the risk allele at rs10272629/rs4726576 in *PRSS1*. The prevalence of *PRSS1* lowering allele in Indians is consistent with other reports that the content of digestive enzymes such as trypsin, chymotrypsin etc. in pancreatic juice of Indians is 2–4 times lower compared with Europeans (Balakrishnan et al. 1988). It may thus be speculated that low levels of cationic trypsinogen undermines central role of trypsinogen in the pathophysiology of TCP.

Serine Protease Inhibitor Kazal Type I (*SPINK1*)

SPINK1 encodes the pancreatic secretory trypsin inhibitor (PSTI), also synthesized in acinar cells of the exocrine pancreas. It has long been considered as a line of defense against premature intrapancreatic activation of trypsin due to its ability to inhibit upto 20% of the potential trypsin activity. Following the initial discovery (Witt et al. 2000),

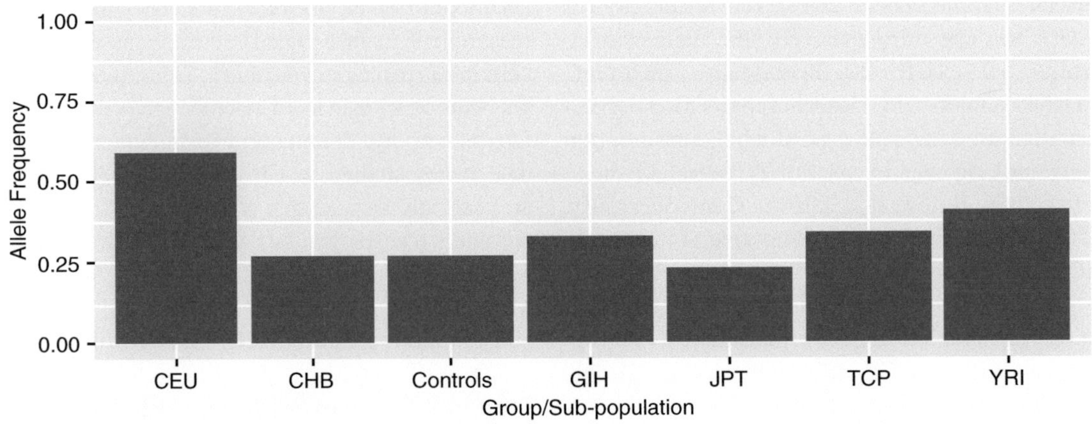

Fig. 11.4 Risk allele frequency of *PRSS1* rs10273639 in various groups/sub-populations including TCP patients and controls. *TCP* Tropical calcific pancreatitis, *GIH* Gujarati Indians in Houston, *CEU* Utah residents with ancestry from northern and western Europe, *CHB* Han Chinese in Beijing, China, *JPT* Japanese in Tokyo, Japan, *YRI* Yoruba in Ibadan, Nigeria

multiple studies worldwide have reported identification and association of several mutations in *SPINK1* with various forms of chronic pancreatitis including TCP (Chandak et al. 2002, 2004; Bhatia et al. 2002; Chowdhury et al. 2002; Hassan et al. 2002; Schneider et al. 2002). Most common of these is the c.101G>A (p.N34S) variant. More recently the role of *SPINK1* promoter variants in pathophysiology of ICP together with TCP has also been assessed (Boulling et al. 2011). A rare loss-of-function variant c.-142T>C that disrupts the HNF1 binding site thereupon leading to reduced *SPINK1* expression was identified exclusively in two TCP patients. A second rare variant c.-215G>T observed in three TCP patients however did not show any effect on *SPINK1* expression. These results point to the fact that risk variants in *SPINK1* promoter are rare and thus p.N34S *SPINK1* remains the predominant risk predictor for TCP.

Cathepsin B (*CTSB*)

Human cathepsin B, a member of the peptidase C1 family, is a 339 amino acid long cysteine protease. It predominantly localizes to the lysosomes and plays an pivotal role in intracellular degradation and turnover of proteins. About three decades ago, a role for lysosomal enzymes was speculated in the pathophysiology of pancreatitis (Steer et al. 1984). This idea stemmed from an earlier observation wherein cathepsin B was shown to be capable of activating trypsinogen (Greenbaum and Hirshkowitz 1961). Results from several subsequent studies further supported the thought (Kukor et al. 2002; Szilágyi et al. 2001). Further, evidence also existed that supramaximal stimulation directs redistribution of lysosomal enzymes leading to their co-localization with digestive enzyme zymogens within intra-acinar cytoplasmic vacuoles (Saluja et al. 1987). Above observations presented CTSB as a strong candidate gene for pancreatitis. Indeed, in a study involving 306 TCP patients and 330 controls, we revealed a unique association of p. L26V *CTSB* polymorphism with TCP (OR = 2.09, 95%CI: 1.55–2.81; P = 0.013) (Mahurkar et al. 2006). Besides p.L26V variant, polymorphism p.S53G also had a significantly dissimilar distribution in p.N34S *SPINK1* carriers and non-carriers (Mahurkar et al. 2006). These variants reside in the pro-peptide region and were proposed to lead to CTSB mis-localization to zymogen granules thus resulting in premature trypsinogen activation. However, the functional validation is still awaited. Lately, a study with moderate sample size of 150 cases and 150 controls from North India failed to replicate the previous association (Singh et al. 2014). The minor allele frequency of 0.33% in controls observed in this study is surprisingly much lesser than that of 30% reported earlier, which raises doubt on the veracity of the results.

Chymotrypsin C (*CTRC*)

Human chymotrypsin C, a 268 amino acid long serine protease that is secreted from the pancreas and has a chymotrypsin-like protease activity is shown to regulate trypsin (ogen) activity with high specificity in calcium-dependent manner (Nemoda and Sahin-Tóth 2006). A few recent reports have documented that in humans, CTRC proteolytically regulates auto-activation of trypsinogens via two independent and seemingly conflicting mechanisms (Nemoda and Sahin-Tóth 2006; Szmola and Sahin-Tóth 2007). Considering the focal role of premature intracellular activation of cationic trypsinogen in pancreatitis, impairment of the CTRC-dependent regulation of trypsinogen was hypothesized to be critical in the pathophysiology of CP. Two studies involving individuals of Indian origin reported the association of CTRC variants with CP including TCP (Rosendahl et al. 2008; Derikx et al. 2009). Nevertheless, both the studies focused on specific region of the gene in a small number of subjects. Our study (Paliwal et al. 2013) in a large, ethnically matched case-control cohort, predominantly comprising TCP patients, had interesting observations. Unlike European CP patients wherein c.738_761del24 (p.K247_R254del) and c.760C>T (p.R254W) were the key mutations, non-synonymous variants c.217G>A (p.A73T) [OR (95% CI) = 9.48(2.19–41.03); P = 2.5 × 10^{-4}] and c.703G>A (p.V235I) [OR (95% CI) = 7.60(2.52–25.71); P = 1 × 10^{-5}] were the major risk predictors for TCP. Functionally, p.A73T exhibits its pathogenicity by eliciting ER stress whereas p.V235I variant reduced the activity and secretion of the protein (Szmola and Sahin-Tóth 2010; Beer et al. 2013). In addition, for synonymous variant c.180C>T heterozygous subjects had an increased risk of TCP compared with the individuals harboring wild allele [OR (95% CI) = 2.44 (1.81–3.30); P = 2.9×10^{-9}] and the risk magnified manifold for individuals homozygous for risk allele [OR (95% CI) = 10.09 (2.98–34.22); P = 5.7×10^{-6}]. Interestingly, the repertiore of CTRC mutations identified in TCP patients was altogether different from that reported in Western CP patients, providing further stress to the earlier evidence of genetic and mutational heterogeneity in TCP.

2.3.2 Trypsin-Independent Pathways

Carboxypeptidase A1 (*CPA1*)

Biochemical data presented in a recent study led to the proposition that CTRC is likely a physiological co-activator of pro-carboxypeptidase A1 (proCPA1) and pro-carboxypeptidase A2 (proCPA2) (Szmola et al. 2011). Next to trypsinogens, proCPA1 is the most abundant protein in pancreatic juice comprising over 10% of the total protein. In view of this, a large multinational collaborative study lately analyzed the involvement of *CPA1* in chronic pancreatitis. The genetic and functional data demonstrated the global role of *CPA1* variants in the pathogenesis of CP including TCP (Witt et al. 2013). However, the spectrum of mutations observed in different populations was heterogeneous. In TCP patients of Indian origin, three novel non-synonymous variants (p.D32H, p.R169H and p.Y308H) identified were present solely in patients whereas the frequency of p.A208T was similar between patients and controls. Apparent activities of p. D32H, p.R169H and p.Y308H variants were 79%, 24% and 3% respectively of the wild protein, whereas their respective relative secretion levels were 75%, 23% and 17% of the native protein. This supports the earlier presumption that the mutational spectrum in various CP-associated genes is different in TCP than in other types of CP in the Western world.

Pancreatic Stone Protein (*Reg1a*)

Pancreatic calcification occurs in majority of CP cases. Human Reg protein accounts for nearly 10–14% of total protein content in pancreatic juice. It was previously identified as a major component of protein matrix of calculi in patients with ACP and hence termed as pancreatic stone protein (PSP) (De Caro et al. 1979). Conflicting reports exist for its role in the process of calcification. *In vitro* observations that it is able to delay the crystal nucleation process as well as inhibit the growth of preformed calcium carbonate crystals led to the proposition that PSP could act as a crystal growth inhibitor in the normally supersaturated pancreatic juice (Multigner et al. 1983). Prior reports of reduced PSP concentration in the pancreatic juice of CP patients supported this hypothesis (Giorgi et al. 1989). However, later reports challenged the idea by demonstrating that PSP does not interact specifically with calcium carbonate crystals (De Reggi et al. 1998). Further, it was argued that pancreatic juice of CP patients instead may have higher levels of smaller PSP isoforms like pancreatic thread protein (PTP) that tend to precipitate because they are insoluble at the physiological pH (Cerini et al. 1999). These observations made Reg1A an interesting candidate gene. The fact that Reg proteins are also associated with pancreatic islet regeneration, diabetogenesis and amelioration of surgical diabetes (Watanabe et al. 1994) in animal models compelled earlier researchers to look at its role in FCDP (Boonyasrisawat et al. 2002; Hawrami et al. 1997). These studies conducted on a limited number of samples, however, could not gather any evidence in support. Our study on relatively larger sample size also failed to detect any association with TCP or FCPD suggesting that polymorphisms in *Reg1A* are unlikely to contribute to the pathogenesis of pancreaticolithogenesis in TCP (Mahurkar et al. 2007).

Glycoprotein 2 (*GP2*)

Several preliminary studies in various species reported that a single glycoprotein of 75–92 kDa represents bulk (>25–30%) of the zymogen granule membrane protein (MacDonald and Ronzio 1972; Paquet et al. 1982; LeBel and Beattie

1984a, b). This glycoprotein, GP2, was identified as an integral membrane. It is attached to the cytoplasmic leaflet of the membrane via a glycosyl phosphatidylinositol linkage and is susceptible to release from the membrane by the enzyme phosphatidylinositol-specific phospholipase C (Tsujii-Hayashi et al. 2002). GP2 has been reported to be the most abundant protein in the pancreatic acinar cells and is not detected in the endocrine pancreas. Almost 50% of the protein is soluble in granule content and is derived from the membrane–bound precursor as a result of shedding after arrival the zymogen granule (Havinga et al. 1985). A form of the molecule is also released into the pancreatic juice where it undergoes coversion into a stable protein aggregate (Rindler and Hoops 1990). Considering the fact that intra-ductal plug formation is one of the early events in the pathophysiology of CP and GP2 is a major constituent of these plugs (Freedman et al. 1993), it was speculated that variations in GP2 may possibly influence the risk of duct obstruction and hence chronic pancreatitis. To address this question we screened exons 3 and 9 of the *GP2* gene in TCP patients and identified two variants of which the variant c.1275A>G showed a disease predisposing effect that was in contrast to the observations made in French white patients (Masson et al. 2010). A recent study has shown that c.1275A>G variant significantly reduces the rate of exon 9 inclusion and hence the last 116 amino acids are substituted by 15 new amino acids. Consequently there is a decrease in the ratio of full-length transcript: total transcript compared with that derived from the wild type (Boulling et al. 2010). These changes may lead to structural alterations and hence compromise the function of the protein.

Transcription Factor 7-Like 2 (*TCF7L2*)

TCP patients often progress to developing secondary diabetes also known as FCPD. Interestingly, FCPD patients present characteristics of both, type 1 (T1D) and type 2 (T2D) diabetes. An early study from our group proposed that the nature and mechanism of diabetes in these patients can be inferred by investigating a known genetic risk factor for T1D or T2D (Mahurkar et al. 2008). Therefore, two polymorphisms (rs7903146 and rs12255372) in transcription factor 7 like protein 2 (TCF7L2, MIM602228) that were reported to be strongly associated with T2D were genotyped in TCP and FCPD patients. Although neither polymorphism showed an independent association with FCPD, the data indicated that these polymorphisms might interact with *SPINK1* and *CTSB* mutations and result in FCPD (Mahurkar et al. 2008).

Claudin 2 (*CLDN2*)

The CP GWAS, in addition to rs10273639 in *PRSS1*, also reported the association of two other common variants namely rs12688220 and rs7057398 (Whitcomb et al. 2012). These variants lie in the *CLDN2-MORC4* loci on X chromosome. Similar to *PRSS1* rs10273639, the European replication study could not establish the association of these two SNPs with NACP (Derikx et al. 2015). We addressed this inconsistency by genotyping a large case-control cohort (Paliwal et al. 2016). We observed a strong association of both, rs12688220 [OR (95% CI) = 1.54 (1.35–1.75); $P = 1.22 \times 10^{-10}$] and rs7057398 [OR (95% CI) = 1.50 (1.29–1.75); $P = 1.44 \times 10^{-7}$] with TCP. Noticeably, although the major alleles for these variants are same in different populations, their frequencies vary considerably. For instance, the frequency of the proposed risk (T) allele at rs12688220 in Indians ($AF_T = 0.48$) is nearly double compared with other Asian ($AF_T = 0.24$–0.28; $P < 1 \times 10^{-4}$) or European ($AF_T = 35$; $P = 7 \times 10^{-4}$) populations (Fig. 11.5). Similarly, for rs7057398, the risk allele (C) frequency is highest in Indians (AFc = 0.52) compared with other Asian or European population (AFc = 0.28–0.35; $P = 6 \times 10^{-3}$) (Fig. 11.5). Although the GWAS reported altered localisation of CLDN2 to the baso-lateral membrane of acinar cells in patients carrying high-risk genotype at rs12688220, the exact mechanism is still unclear. A recent report attributed half of pancreatic injury during pancreatitis to NFkB-mediated inflammatory pathways (Dawra et al. 2011). *CLDN2* promoter harbors binding site for NFkB (Sakaguchi et al. 2002). CLDN2 expression is shown to correlate with inflammation and

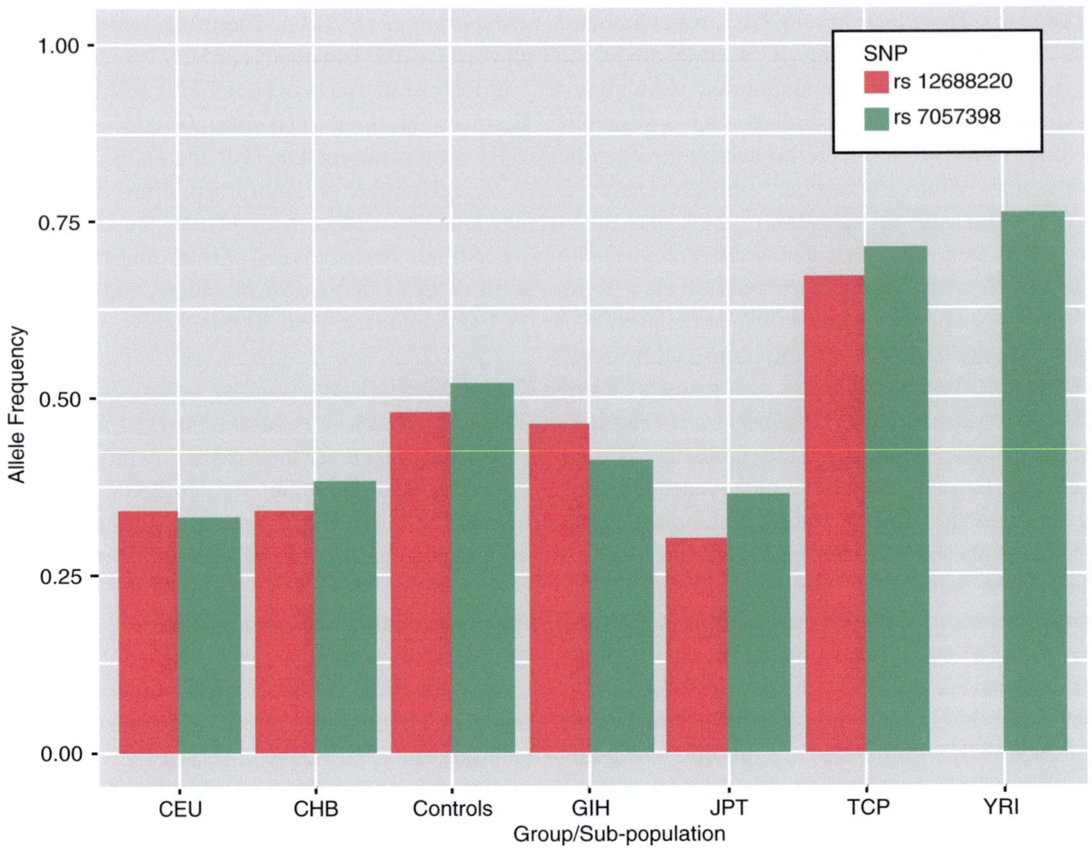

Fig. 11.5 Risk allele frequency of *CLDN2-MORC4* loci variants (rs12688220 and rs7057398) in various groups/sub-populations including TCP patients and controls. *TCP* Tropical calcific pancreatitis, *GIH* Gujarati Indians in Houston, *CEU* Utah residents with ancestry from northern and western Europe, *CHB* Han Chinese in Beijing, China, *JPT* Japanese in Tokyo, Japan, *YRI* Yoruba in Ibadan, Nigeria

increases under conditions of stress and injury by regulation through different cytokines (Suzuki et al. 2011). Thus, it is likely that these variants might be involved in the altered inflammatory response. However, further investigation is needed to confirm its role in the etiopathogenesis of chronic pancreatitis.

Carboxyl-Ester Lipase (*CEL*)

CEL is a non-specific lipolytic enzyme capable of hydrolyzing a variety of lipid substrates and aids in their digestion and absorption. It is a major constituent of pancreatic juice. Mutation in *CEL* lead to maturity-onset diabetes of the young and pancreatic exocrine dysfunction (Raeder et al. 2006). CEL-HYB is a fusion gene between carboxyl ester lipase (*CEL*) and its identical pseudo gene (*CELP*) arranged in tandem. *CEL-CELP* genic constellation is one of the good examples for possible occurrence of non-allelic homologous recombination (NAHR). The product of NAHR event at this region named CEL-HYB is indeed reported to be associated with chronic pancreatitis in European populations (Fjeld et al. 2014). Expression of CEL-HYB in cellular models showed reduced lipolytic activity, impaired secretion, prominent intra acinar accumulation and induced autophagy. Our recent study from three Asian populations including Indians

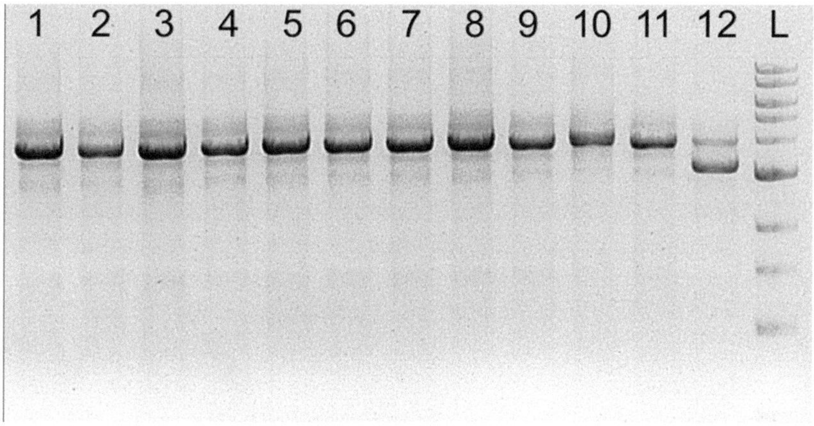

Fig. 11.6 A representative gel image showing presence of *CEL-HYB2b* allele in an individual (lane 12). L, 1Kb ladder

failed to detect this recombination allele and replicate the association (Zou et al. 2016). We, instead found an alternative NAHR allele CEL-HYB2 (Fig. 11.6) with the breakpoint region spanning 239bp between intron9-exon10. The CEL-HYB2 that we observed in the Indian cohort corresponds to the minor allele of CEL-HYB2 (CEL-HYB2b) and is also not associated with TCP. The non-association of CEL-HYB2a/b could be because of the fact that its transcribed mRNA significantly undergoes non-sense mediated decay owing to the absence of truncated protein and its toxic effects.

2.4 Concluding Remarks

The phenotype of TCP has undergone a remarkable change over the last few decades. There is more heterogeneity in the clinical profile which has prompted the researchers to investigate newer aspects of the disease pathophysiology. In addition to the role of (micro) nutrient deficiencies and other environmental factors, involvement of genetics is being emphasized. Genetic studies have provided some insights about the mechanistic of the disease pathophysiology. Several studies including ours have indicated that akin to phenotypic heterogeneity, genetic heterogeneity also exists between TCP and CP in the West. Further, our recent report demonstrates that rs10273639/rs4726576 variants that regulate PRSS1 expression, and *CLDN2-MORC4* loci variants (rs7057398 and rs12688220) predict risk for non-alcoholic chronic pancreatitis entities like TCP as well. These results bear significance on several aspects. Firstly, it is one of the first reports suggesting a direct role for PRSS1 in the pathogenesis of TCP. Secondly, co-inheritance of p.N34S SPINK1 with *PRSS1* or *CLDN2-MORC4* risk allele is predicted to have an influence on the age of onset/presentation. These observations suggest potential utility of risk screening for these variants. Thirdly, risk allele frequency at these two loci vary significantly between different ethnic groups: the significantly lower frequency of rs10273639 risk allele in Asian populations including Indians compared with Europeans undermine a central role for *PRSS1* in CP in Asians; contrastingly, higher frequency of the inflammation related SNPs in *CLDN2-MORC4* loci suggest a more prominent role for inflammatory pathway in TCP pathophysiology. Above observations clearly indicate that that genetic predisposition likely plays a significant role in pathogenesis of TCP. These risk factors work via both 'trypsin-central' and 'trypsin-independent' pathways (Fig. 11.7). These genetic differences along with the environmental factors (nutrition, alcohol abuse) might be responsible for the observed phenotypic differences.

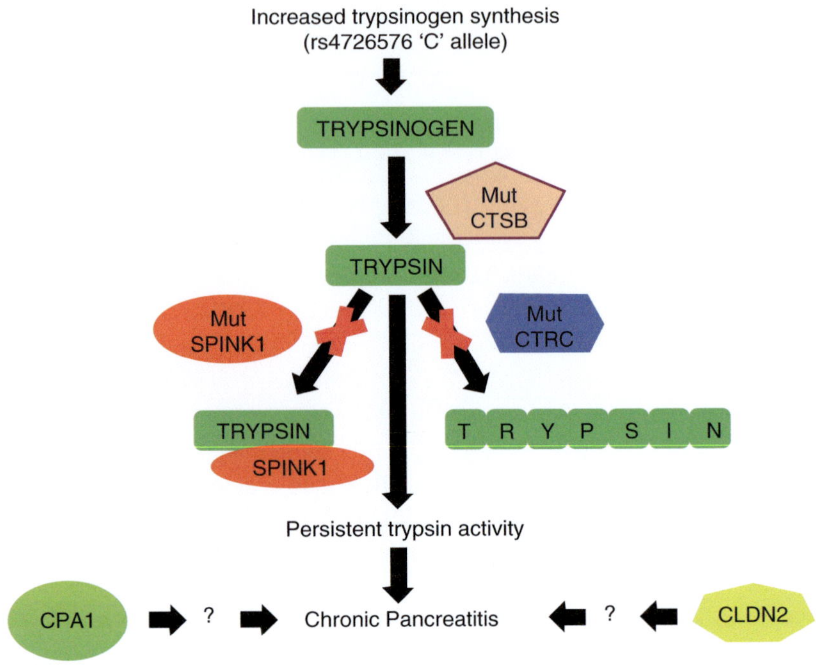

Fig. 11.7 Advanced model for chronic pancreatitis in Indians: The presence of *PRSS1* rs4726576 risk allele results in increased expression of trypsinogen within the pancreatic acinar cells. Compounding presence of mutated CTSB, mutated SPINK1 and defective CTRC leads to increased and persistent intracellular trypsin activity. Functionally defective CPA1 along with the presence of CLDN2 variants work via an alternative 'trypsin-independent' pathway

2.5 Future Directions

Aforementioned observations suggest that there are multiple factors that can alter the phenotype of a complex disease as exemplified by TCP. However, we have not been able to translate these understandings to individual patient care. It is thus emphasized that genotype-phenotype correlation needs to be investigated thoroughly further to track the changes in disease presentation with underlying genetic susceptibility when exposed to certain environmental risk factors.

Acknowledgements We express our sincere gratitude to the patients and normal subjects who agreed to participate in our study. The support of Dr. D Nageshwar Reddy and Dr. G V Rao from Asian Institute of Gastroenterology, Hyderabad, India in generating a case-control cohort is greatly acknowledged. We also appreciate the efforts of our other collaborators Dr. S P Singh, Cuttack Medical College, Cuttack, India and Dr. Varghese Thomas, Calicut Medical College, Calicut, India in recruiting individuals and providing biological samples. We also thank Council of Scientific and Industrial Research, Indian Council of Medical Research, and Department of Biotechnology, Ministry of Science and technology, Government of India, India for financial assistance.

3 Pediatric Pancreatitis

Maisam Abu-El-Haija and Aliye Uc

3.1 Introduction

Pancreatitis results from an insult to the pancreas that may lead to trypsin activation, inflammatory cell infiltration, edema, cell death, fibrosis and organ damage (Sarles 1991). In the majority of children, the inflammation is self-limited and reversible with only one acute pancreatitis (AP) episode over their lifetime (~1:10,000) (Morinville et al. 2010; Nydegger et al. 2007). In a subset of patients (~10–34%), AP may progress to acute recurrent pancreatitis (ARP) (Bai et al. 2011; Beger et al. 1997) and a subset (~0.5–2.7/100,000 cases) may develop chronic pancreatitis (CP) (Pant and Sferra 2015; Spanier et al. 2013; Yadav et al. 2011).

The incidence, characteristics, of CP in children are poorly defined and mostly based on retrospective cohorts. A recent pediatric multi-center collaboration, INternational Study Group of Pediatric Pancreatitis: In Search for a CuRE (INSPPIRE) has assumed the task of studying the disease characteristics of ARP and CP in pediatrics (Morinville et al. 2012, 2014; Schwarzenberg et al. 2015; Ting et al. 2015). Diagnostic criteria for pediatric AP, ARP and CP are listed on Table 11.6 (Conwell and Banks 2008; Deng et al. 2005; Morinville et al. 2012; Muddana et al. 2010; Whitcomb 2004).

Recurrent inflammation and subsequent fibrosis may further lead to organ dysfunction with pancreatic exocrine and/or endocrine insufficiency (Conwell and Banks 2008; Deng et al. 2005; Muddana et al. 2010; Whitcomb 2004). Current diagnostic criteria is reflective of the injury sustained by the pancreas and can include changes in duct morphology, gland atrophy, calcifications or pancreatic insufficiency. An evidence-based algorithm to confirm the diagnosis of CP proposed by the American Pancreatic Association utilizes criteria that can be sequentially assessed starting with imaging findings as well as pancreatic functional studies (Conwell et al. 2014). There are no established criteria to diagnose early or minimal change CP.

Table 11.6 Definitions of pancreatitis in children (Conwell and Banks 2008; Deng et al. 2005; Morinville et al. 2012; Muddana et al. 2010; Whitcomb 2004)

Acute Pancreatitis (AP)
Requires at least two out of three criteria:
1. Abdominal pain suggestive of, or compatible with AP (ie, abdominal pain of acute onset, especially in the epigastric region)
2. Serum levels of pancreatic amylase and/or lipase equal to or greater than three times the upper limit of normal
3. Radiographic findings consistent with AP on ultrasound (US), computed tomography (CT), endoscopic ultrasonography (EUS) or magnetic resonance imaging/magnetic resonance cholangiopancreatography (MRI/MRCP)
Acute Recurrent Pancreatitis (ARP)
Requires at least two distinct episodes of AP (each as defined above), along with:
1. Complete resolution of pain (≥1 month pain-free interval between the diagnoses of AP)
OR
2. Complete normalization of serum pancreatic enzyme levels (amylase and lipase), before the subsequent episode of AP is diagnosed, along with complete resolution of pain symptoms, irrespective of a specific time interval between AP episodes
Chronic Pancreatitis (CP)
Requires at least one of the following three:
1. Abdominal pain consistent with pancreatic origin *and* imaging findings suggestive of chronic pancreatic damage[a]
2. Evidence of exocrine pancreatic insufficiency *and* suggestive pancreatic imaging findings[a]
3. Evidence of endocrine pancreatic insufficiency *and* suggestive pancreatic imaging findings[a]

[a]Suggestive imaging findings of CP include:
- *Ductal changes:* irregular contour of the main pancreatic duct or its radicles; intraductal filling defects; calculi, stricture or dilation
- *Parenchymal changes:* generalized or focal enlargement, irregular contour (accentuated lobular architecture), cavities, calcifications, heterogeneous echotexture

3.2 Risk Factors

The risk factors associated with pediatric CP are listed in Table 11.7. While ARP and CP in adults are most often secondary to gallstones or excessive alcohol usage, (Cote et al. 2011; Muniraj

Table 11.7 Risk factors of chronic pancreatitis in children

Idiopathic
Genetic
• *PRSS1*
• *CFTR*
• *SPINK1*
• *CTRC*
• *CPA1*
• *CEL*
Medications (L-asparaginase, valproate, metronidazole, azathioprine, tetracycline, pentamidine, etc.)
Metabolic disease
• Hyperlipidemia
• Hypercalcemia
• Glycogen storage disease
• Organic acidemias
Autoimmune
Anatomic
• Pancreas divisum
• Anomalous junction of the biliary and pancreatic ducts
• Annular pancreas
• Ampullary obstruction
• Crohn disease

et al. 2014; Yadav et al. 2009) the risk factors involved in disease progression in children are poorly delineated (Lucidi et al. 2011; Morinville et al. 2012). In contrast to the adult population, alcohol use, smoking and other environmental factors are uncommon in children with CP (Schwarzenberg et al. 2015). Since the identification of *PRSS1* as a cause of hereditary pancreatitis, single center-studies with small cohorts reported that children with ARP or CP often have mutations in the *cationic trypsinogen (PRSS1), cystic fibrosis transmembrane generator (CFTR), serine protease inhibitor Kazal type I (SPINK1), chymotrypsin-C (CTRC)* and *carboxypeptidase 1 (CPA1)* genes (Lucidi et al. 2011; Sanchez-Ramirez et al. 2007; Schnur et al. 2014; Sobczynska-Tomaszewska et al. 2006; van Geenen et al. 2011; Werlin et al. 2015; Witt 2001; Witt et al. 2013). Indeed, in the largest pediatric CP population reported by INSPPIRE, two third of children had at least one mutation identified in *PRSS1*, *SPINK1*, *CFTR*, or *CTRC* (Schwarzenberg et al. 2015). In the last decade, more genetic associations have been reported with CP including *claudin 2 (CLDN2), carboxylesterlipase (CEL) and CEL-Hybrid (CEL-HYB)* (Derikx et al. 2015; Fjeld et al. 2015; Ragvin et al. 2013; Witt et al. 2013). A strong association with the *CPA1* gene and early childhood pancreatitis (less than ten years of age) highlights the importance of genetic influences at an early age (Witt et al. 2013). While additional pediatric studies have reported varying proportions of genetic associations with ARP or CP, the impact of genetic mutations on natural history and disease outcome should be studied on well-defined and prospectively followed cohorts.

Environmental risk factors (i.e. medications, alcohol, smoking, chronic renal failure, hypercalcemia) are uncommon in pediatric CP (0–4%) (Oracz et al. 2015; Schwarzenberg et al. 2015). It is not known whether obstructive factors and specifically pancreas divisum are sufficient to cause CP in children. In the INSPPIRE cohort, pancreas divisum was present in ~20% of children with CP (Schwarzenberg et al. 2015), which is higher than what has been reported in subjects without pancreatic disease (7%) (Rebours et al. 2009). Future studies are needed whether pancreas divisum has an impact on pediatric pancreatic disease progression and development of CP. Autoimmune pancreatitis (AIP) is scarce in the pediatric population with only a few centers publishing cases or case series (Friedlander et al. 2012; Fujii et al. 2013; Zen et al. 2014). Most cases are type 2 AIP and the response to steroids in general is good.

3.3 Pathophysiology

While the pathophysiology of CP is not fully defined, a number of factors have been proposed. These pathophysiological models, mostly originated from animal studies, will be briefly discussed below.

3.3.1 Trypsin Pathways

In this model, the balance between proteolytic enzymes and anti-protease defense mechanisms is disturbed, leading to premature activation of zymogens within pancreas and autodigestion of the organ. The supportive models of this theory are gene mutations and specifically, the breakthrough discovery of the *PRSS1* gene in 1996 (Le Bodic et al. 1996; Pandya et al. 1996; Whitcomb et al. 1996a, b). This discovery substantiated the decades-old observation of familial clustering of chronic pancreatitis (Comfort and Steinberg 1952). The most common mutations in *PRSS1* linked to hereditary pancreatitis are R122H and N29I, leading to autoactivation of trypsinogen (Whitcomb et al. 1996b). *SPINK1* encodes a protein that is involved in preventing trypsin-catalyzed premature activation of zymogens within pancreas. Because 1–4% of the general population carry one *SPINK1* mutation (most commonly N34S), this gene is regarded as a modifier of the inflammatory process possibly tilting the balance in favor of ARP/CP (Aoun et al. 2010; Pfutzer et al. 2000; Threadgold et al. 2002; Witt et al. 2000). Of note, children with *PRSS1* or *SPINK1* mutations were more likely to present with CP compared with ARP in the INSPPIRE cohort, suggesting that these genes may influence the development of CP (Kumar et al. 2016). Another candidate gene is *CFTR*. If CFTR function is completely or almost completely lost, children are born with cystic fibrosis (CF), severe pancreatic damage and exocrine pancreatic insufficiency (EPI). A subset of pancreatic-sufficient CF patients develop recurrent attacks of AP and patients with compound heterozygous *CFTR* mutations have higher likelihood for CP (Cohn et al. 1998; Sharer et al. 1998). The pathogenesis of *CFTR*-associated pancreatic damage is not clear, but thickened and acidic secretions in pancreas causing zymogen activation have been proposed (Whitcomb 2013). The risk of pancreatitis increases up to 900-fold in the presence of both *CFTR* and *SPINK1* mutations (Noone et al. 2001). Other candidate gene variants and their association with pancreatitis in the trypsin pathway have been described, including *chymotrypsin C (CTRC)* and *calcium sensing receptor (CASR)* (Baudry et al. 2010; Felderbauer et al. 2006; Masson et al. 2008b; Muddana et al. 2008; Rosendahl et al. 2008).

3.3.2 Inflammatory Pathways

This theory is supported by animal models lacking trypsinogen that still develop inflammation in their pancreas following an insult (Dawra et al. 2011). Sustained activation of inflammatory pathways by various stimuli may lead to of CP in animal models. Different mechanisms have been postulated to play a role, including regulatory T cells, CD28, TNF, NFκB, IL-6 and IL-8, complement pathways and TGF- β (Abu-El-Haija et al. 2011; Huang et al. 2013; Meagher et al. 2008). In Autoimmune pancreatitis (AIP), T helper cells, IgG4 (+) cells may also be involved (Okazaki et al. 2000; Zen et al. 2007).

Other pathogenic cellular events such as abnormal calcium signaling, mitochondrial dysfunction, endoplasmic reticulum stress, autophagy and impaired trafficking, lysosomal and secretory responses also synergize with inflammatory pathways (Sah et al. 2012).

3.3.3 Fibrosis

The hallmark of CP is fibrosis and acinar cell loss of. Stellate cell activation has been proposed to have a role in progression to CP (Masamune and Shimosegawa 2013). Smoking have a role in activating pancreatic stellate cells through the nicotinic acetylcholine receptors, as an agent on its own, or that effect might be enhanced with alcohol exposure (Lee et al. 2015). Stellate cells may induce fibrogenesis by activating Transforming Growth factor β1 (TGF β1) and inhibition of Matrix metalloproteinases (Shek et al. 2002). Understanding the pathways involved in stellate cell activation may lead to designing effective therapies that could halt the progression to CP (Apte et al. 2015).

3.4 Clinical Manifestations

The main clinical symptom from CP in children is pain that ranges from mild to severe, episodic to constant (Schwarzenberg et al. 2015). In the INSPPIRE population, 36% of children with ARP and 72% with CP received pain medications. Acetaminophen and ibuprofen were the leading pain medications for ARP while patients with CP utilized acetaminophen and hydrocodone for pain (Kumar et al. 2016). The disease burden was higher in CP compared with ARP (more emergency department visits, hospitalizations, missed school days, medical, endoscopic and surgical interventions).

Children with CP also report other gastrointestinal symptoms including indigestion, nausea, vomiting, weight loss, diarrhea, steatorrhea, symptoms related to diabetes. In general, GI symptoms are attributed to impaired pancreatic duct drainage caused by duct strictures, fibrosis, calcification, etc. (Troendle and Barth 2016). In a subset of patients, pancreatic duct is of normal caliber and symptoms are attributed to small duct or “minimal change” disease (Wilson et al. 2015). The management is based on the underlying etiology, disease course and whether CP is manifesting as small or large duct disease (Troendle and Barth 2016).

3.5 Diagnostic Testing

3.5.1 Biochemistry

There are no specific laboratory tests for CP. In most cases, serum amylase and lipase are normal or only mildly elevated (Steer et al. 1995). Patients with CP may continue to have acute exacerbations and elevations in their amylase and lipase.

3.5.2 Radiology

Imaging studies play an important role in the diagnosis of CP but they are not sensitive enough to detect early or minimal changes in the pancreas. In the INSPPIRE cohort, pancreatic calcifications were present in only nine (12%) on initial imaging, while ductal dilatation (61%), irregularity (47%), and stricture (21%), and pancreatic atrophy (21%) were more common (Schwarzenberg et al. 2015). Calcifications were rare in the pediatric age group.

Ultrasonography. Ultrasonography (US) is the first imaging of choice as it has high likelihood to delineate pancreas anatomy in children without the risk of radiation exposure (Darge and Anupindi 2009). Although US performs well in pediatric AP (Abu-El-Haija et al. 2014), the diagnostic accuracy in CP has not been studied (Nydegger et al. 2006). US is helpful in assessing the pancreatic duct diameter in children with CP (normals are: ≤1.5 mm in children 1–6 years; ≤1.9 mm at ages 7–12 years; ≤2.2 mm at ages 13–18 years). Calcifications and intraductal stones can also be detected with US in CP (Darge and Anupindi 2009).

Endoscopic US (EUS). EUS is technically feasible in children as young as 5 years of age (Varadarajulu et al. 2005), but the experience is limited only to few studies (Stevens 2013). There are no pediatric-specific EUS criteria for CP.

Magnetic resonance cholangiopancreatography (MRCP). Due to its non-invasive nature and lack of radiation, MRCP has become the diagnostic imaging test of choice in children with CP (Delaney et al. 2008; Tipnis and Werlin 2007). MRCP can reliably detect pancreas atrophy, ductal dilatations, small filling defects, strictures, irregularities of the main pancreatic duct, and irregularity of side branches (Hansen et al. 2013) (Fig. 11.8). Unlike ERCP that images ducts under pressure, MRCP visualizes the ducts in their normal physiologic state (Darge and Anupindi 2009). Therefore MRCP may not reveal the details of small ducts, which may be important in diagnosing early CP. Secretin may be more important in children than in adults as it increases the detectability of the normally smaller pancreatic ducts on MRCP (Manfredi et al. 2002). More studies are needed whether secretin-MRCP (s-MRCP) is superior to MRCP in children for the diagnosis of CP (Manfredi et al. 2002; Trout et al. 2013).

Endoscopic Retrograde Cholangiopancreatography (ERCP). ERCP should mainly be reserved for therapeutic interventions (pancreatic duct stenting, sphincterotomy, stone extraction) in children. Although relatively safe and widely available, ERCP carries an overall morbidity of ~7%, which includes acute pancreatitis (4%), hemorrhage (1%), cholangitis (1%), perforation (0.5%), and death (0.1%) (Lee and Conwell 2012). In pediatric CP, ERCP findings include main pancreatic duct dilatation, ductal

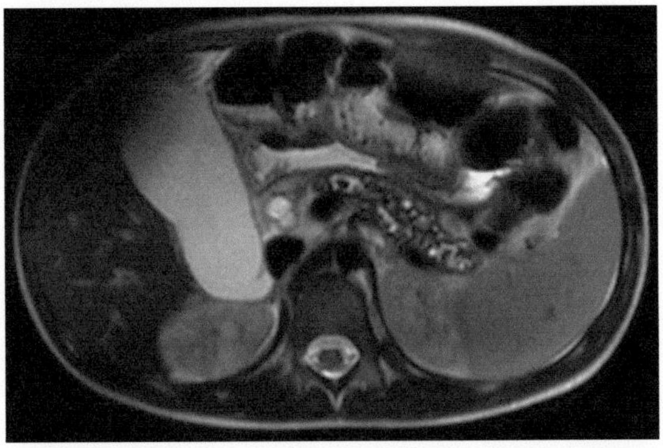

Fig. 11.8 MRCP findings in chronic pancreatitis. Magnetic resonance imaging (MRI/ MRCP) in in a 9-year-old male with CP showing diffuse parenchymal atrophy, duct dilatations in the head and neck of the pancreas with several dilated side branches elsewhere. There are several foci of low signal intensity consistent with extensive pancreatic calcifications, including intraductal stones. (Image is courtesy of Dr. Andrew Trout, Cincinnati Children's Hospital, Cincinnati, Ohio, USA)

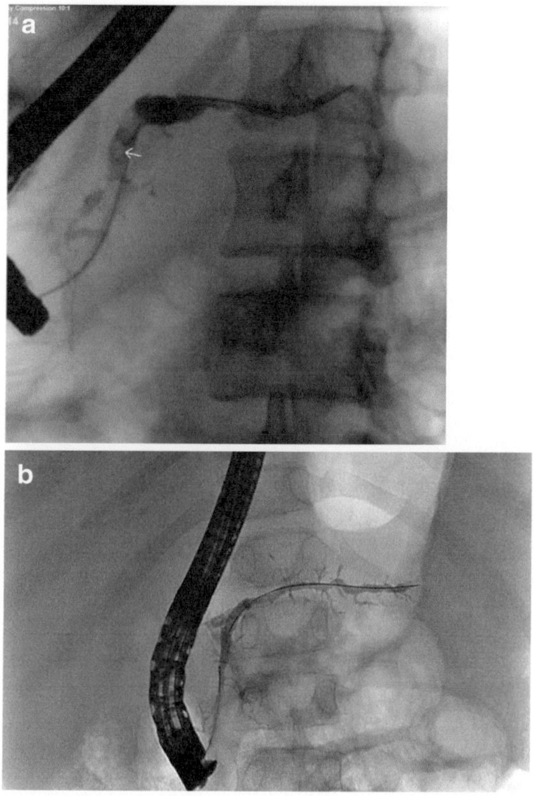

Fig. 11.9 ERCP changes in chronic pancreatitis. (**a**) ERCP fluoroscopy image from a child with idiopathic CP showing intraductal stone (*arrow*) with dilated main pancreatic duct; (**b**) dilated main pancreatic duct with dilated main side branches in a child with CP. (Image is courtesy of Dr. Tom K. Lin, Cincinnati Children's Hospital, Cincinnati, Ohio, USA)

stones, and changes in the main duct branches and small ducts (Fig. 11.9). The ERCP-based grading system of CP severity has been developed in adults (Cambridge classification), but it has not been validated in children (Axon et al. 1984).

Computerized tomography (CT) with contrast. CT can detect advanced changes in CP, including calcifications, pancreas atrophy, fat replacement, and ductal dilatation (Fig. 11.10). CT has poor sensitivity to identify ductal abnormalities and subtle parenchymal changes and the radiation exposure is not preferred in the pediatric age range (Kinney and Freeman 2008; Nydegger et al. 2006).

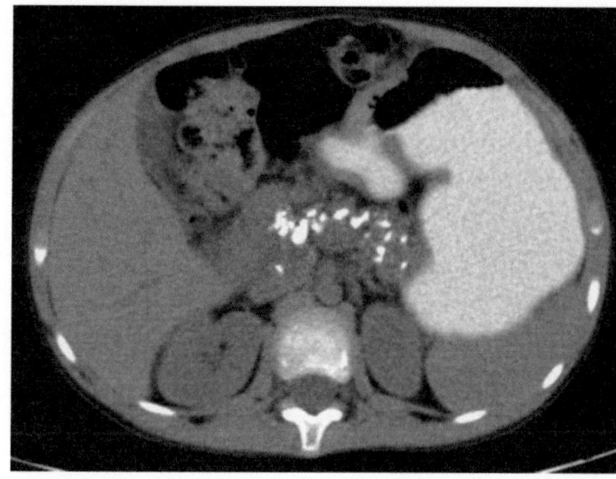

Fig. 11.10 CT changes in chronic pancreatitis. Computed tomography with intravenous and oral contrast, in a 9-year-old male with CP showing findings consistent with chronic pancreatitis including diffuse parenchymal atrophy and calcifications. (Image is courtesy of Dr. Andrew Trout, Cincinnati Children's Hospital, Cincinnati, Ohio, USA)

3.6 Complications of CP in Children

3.6.1 Exocrine Pancreatic Insufficiency (EPI)

In children with long-standing CP, EPI may develop when a large portion of pancreatic acini are permanently damaged (>95%). In adults, exocrine pancreatic insufficiency occurs in 50–80% of patients in a median time of 5.6–13.1 years (Ammann et al. 1984; Layer et al. 1994). In the INSPPIRE cohort, 34% of children were exocrine pancreatic insufficient at the time of diagnosis (Schwarzenberg et al. 2015). It should be noted that EPI may develop in other forms of exocrine pancreatic disease in children (CF, Shwachman-Diamond syndrome, etc). There is not a perfect exocrine pancreatic function test that could accurately measure acinar and/or ductal functions of the pancreas. Below is a brief review of currently available tests.

Pancreatic stimulation test (PFT). In this test, pancreatic fluid is collected as it is secreted into the duodenum and measured for volume, pancreatic enzymes and electrolytes before and after stimulation with cholecystokinin and/or secretin (Schibli et al. 2006). Although it is considered "gold standard" to quantify the exocrine pancreatic function, PFTs are not widely performed due to their invasive nature. The collection of the duodenal fluid via the endoscope (endoscopic pancreatic function test or ePFT) has been proposed as an alternative and is currently performed by few pediatric centers using various protocols. This approach has the potential to underestimate the pancreatic secretory capacity and classify patients as pancreatic insufficient erroneously (Schibli et al. 2006).

72-hour fecal fat collection. This test relies on the exocrine pancreas losing greater than 95% of its enzyme secretory output and development of steatorrhea (DiMagno et al. 1973). Steatorrhea can be measured by a 72-h stool collection and calculation of coefficient of fat absorption [CFA: (grams of fat ingested-grams of fat excreted)/(grams of fat ingested) × 100]. In children younger than 6 months of age, a fecal fat greater than 15% of fat intake is considered abnormal; this value is 7% for children over 6 months of age. It is not a specific test for EPI as it can be abnormal in other diseases causing fat malabsorption.

Fecal elastase-1 (FE1). This widely available ELISA-based stool test is the preferred method to diagnose EPI. A value of less than100 μg/g is considered diagnostic. Intermediate values of fecal elastase (100–200 μg/g) may be due to loss of pancreatic function, but not severe enough to cause clinical EPI. The sensitivity of FE1 to diagnose moderate and severe EPI is approximately 100%. In patients with mild loss of pancreatic function, the test sensitivity is ~25% with a specificity of 96% (Daftary et al. 2006). Therefore, FE1 is not reliable to determine mild or borderline loss of exocrine pancreatic function. FE1 may be falsely low when the stool is diluted in cases of diarrhea (i.e. infectious diarrhea, severe enteropathies, short gut, collected from an ileostomy).

Secretin-MRCP. s-MRCP findings (changes in pancreatic duct caliber, anteroposterior diameter of the pancreas, signal intensity ratio between pancreas and spleen on T1-weighted and arterial-venous enhancement ratios and duodenal filling) show correlation with other exocrine pancreatic tests including ePFT (Balci et al. 2010) and fecal elastase (Manfredi et al. 2012). This test has not been validated in children.

Treatment of EPI. Pancreatic enzymes are only recommended for the treatment of CP and EPI in children, as their role in controlling pain in CP has not been established. Pancreatic enzyme replacement therapy (PERT) is based on number of lipase units administered per meal. Children <4 years of age require 1000 lipase units/kg per meal; 500 lipase units/kg per meal are used for those >4 years of age and 25,000–40,000 units/meal are used for adults. For snacks half the dose is recommended. The daily dose for most patients is less than 10,000 units of lipase/kg per day or 6000 units of lipase/kg per meal to prevent fibrosing colonopathy. For children who cannot swallow capsules, delayed release capsules containing enteric coated microspheres or microtablets may be opened and the contents sprinkled on soft food that does not require chewing and has a low pH (applesauce, gelatins, pureed apricot, banana or sweet potatoes). Foods having a pH greater than 7.3, such as milk, custard or ice cream should be avoided as a vehicle for the sprinkled enzymes because the protective enteric coating can dissolve in these foods, leaving the enzymes vulnerable to inactivation by gastric acid. Pancrealipase tablets or capsules should not be crushed or chewed. Concurrent administration with H_2 antagonists or proton pump inhibitors may enhance enzyme efficacy.

3.6.2 Pancreatogenic Diabetes Mellitus (T3cDM)

Diabetes mellitus can also occur in 40–70% of adults with CP with a median time to onset of 11.9–26.3 years (Ammann et al. 1984; Layer et al. 1994). The diabetes occurs in ~5% of patients with hereditary pancreatitis by 10 years after the onset of symptoms, and 18% by 20 years (Howes et al. 2004). This form of diabetes is called type 3c or pancreatogenic diabetes and is the result of partial or complete loss of insulin secretion. In the INSPPIRE cohort, 1% of children already had diabetes at the time of enrollment (Schwarzenberg et al. 2015). Although there are no consensus definition and diagnostic criteria for T3DM, a deficient pancreatic polypeptide response to nutrients in the setting of CP and EPI and no evidence for type 1 or 2 diabetes mellitus have been proposed as discriminating factors. The exact mechanism of pancreatic diabetes is unknown, but patients have evidence of islet dysfunction and altered glucose metabolism (Lundberg et al. 2016). Endocrine pancreatic insufficiency can be diagnosed via 2006 WHO criteria for the diagnosis of diabetes mellitus (fasting glucose ≥7.0 mmol/L (126 mg/dL) or plasma glucose ≥11.1 mmol/L (200 mg/dL) 2 h after glucose load 1.75 g/kg children (to maximum 75 g glucose load) (Report of the Expert Committee on the Diagnosis and Classification of Diabetes Mellitus 1997). Children should routinely be followed and monitored for the development of EPI and diabetes. Screening tests for early diagnosis of T3cDM are not established but may involve fasting blood glucose, oral glucose tolerance test and mixed meal glucose tolerance test. It is also not known how frequently children with CP should be monitored for EPI and T3cDM. The experience with the treatment of pancreatogenic diabetes comes mostly from total pancreatectomy with islet cell autotransplantation (TPIAT) studies and involves insulin therapy (Bellin et al. 2008, 2012, 2013).

3.6.3 Pain and Impaired Quality of Life

In the INSPPIRE cohort, substantial disease burden was associated with pediatric CP: ~80% reported abdominal pain within the previous year and one-third were taking narcotic analgesics (Schwarzenberg et al. 2015). Hospitalizations, emergency department visits and school absences were common. Overall, burden of pain is significant in children with ARP to CP contributing significantly to impaired quality of life, as well as higher level of fatigue (Pohl et al. 2012).

Medical therapies. The experience with the medical therapy of pain in pediatric CP is limited. Nonsteroidal anti-inflammatory drugs and acetaminophen should be the first-line agents for pain control. The addictive profile of narcotics and their gastrointestinal side effects should be considered when initiating the therapy. Tramadol and Gabapentin have shown efficacy in controlling pain in adults with CP, but there are no pediatric studies (Olesen et al. 2011).

Endoscopic Interventions. In adults with uncomplicated CP, endoscopic therapy may be useful in treating chronic pain (Cahen et al. 2005, 2007). The main goal is to alleviate a pancreatic duct obstruction in the presence of ductal stone or stricture, placement of a stent in the main pancreatic duct or pancreatic portion of the bile duct (Cremer et al. 1991; Ponchon et al. 1995). In adults with CP, endoscopic stenting of bile duct strictures may result in high response rates (Costamagna et al. 2001; Draganov et al. 2002).

ERCP can be done successfully in over 90% of children (Issa et al. 2007) and therapeutic ERCP is frequently utilized in children with ARP or CP. In a small pediatric study, children were evaluated with ERCP for recurrent acute and chronic pancreatitis; in 52% of patients ERCP altered the therapy (Graham et al. 1998). In another pediatric study, the majority of children with pancreas divisum and CP had resolution of symptoms and did not require surgery following placement of a pancreatic duct stent (Bhasin et al. 2013). In the INSPPIRE cohort, ~40% of children undergo therapeutic ERCP during the course of their illness and their response to therapy is currently being evaluated.

Surgical Therapies. Surgical techniques include drainage operations that aim to decompress dilated ducts or resections of strictures and removal of pancreatic stones (Andersen and Frey 2010). In the majority of cases, a Puestow-type procedure (longitudinal pancreatojejunostomy that involves opening the pancreatic duct throughout the body and tail of the gland) is used. The timing and choice of interventions are not well-defined for pediatric CP, but a recent study recommended a step-wise approach for children with hereditary pancreatitis with early endoscopic interventions; surgical drainage procedures reserved in case therapeutic ERCP was unsuccessful (Kargl et al. 2015). In general, drainage procedures are not encouraged if the patient will undergo TPIAT in the future, because this procedure has been reported to decrease the islet yield from the pancreas (Bellin et al. 2011; Kobayashi et al. 2010). TPIAT is increasingly being proposed as a treatment for pediatric CP. Currently, there are no consensus guidelines for TPIAT eligibility. Children with intractable abdominal pain due to CP who have failed other therapies are proposed as candidates for this operation. The decision for TPIAT requires a multidisciplinary team including pediatric gastroenterologists, pediatric surgeons, pediatric endocrinologists, psychologists, and anesthesiologists. The child's physical and emotional status in coping with and managing diabetes must be assessed. Within a year of this operation, 50–80% of patients from a single center have become narcotic independent on follow-up (Bellin et al. 2008, 2011; Chinnakotla et al. 2014a, b; Sutherland et al. 2012; Wilson et al. 2013). The pain improvement was largely sustained at 10-year follow-up, whereby 10–20% of patients continued to take narcotics (Chinnakotla et al. 2014a, b). Similar to the narcotic independence, insulin independence was also generally sustained over the 10-year follow-up in the majority of children (~40%) (Chinnakotla et al. 2014a). Both children and adults demonstrate significant improvement in physical and mental health after TPIAT (Bellin et al. 2011; Chinnakotla et al. 2014b; Walsh et al. 2012; Wilson et al. 2013).

Conclusion

Pediatric chronic pancreatitis continues to be a challenging disease. It is relatively uncommon and poorly characterized. Although there have been pediatric focused reports recently, little is known about its epidemiology, natural history, prognostic factors and response to therapies. Current studies suggest that pediatric CP has unique features with a high prevalence of genetic risk factors and few confounding environmental factors, thus distinguishing it from adult pancreatitis populations. Future studies should focus on early identification of pediatric CP, better understanding of its natural history and prognostic factors and better therapeutic strategies to improve pain and quality of life.

References

Abu-El-Haija M, et al. An activated immune and inflammatory response targets the pancreas of newborn pigs with cystic fibrosis. Pancreatology. 2011;11(5):506–15.

Abu-El-Haija M, Lin TK, Palermo J. Update to the management of pediatric acute pancreatitis: highlighting areas in need of research. J Pediatr Gastroenterol Nutr. 2014;58(6):689–93.

Ammann RW, et al. Course and outcome of chronic pancreatitis. Longitudinal study of a mixed medical-surgical series of 245 patients. Gastroenterology. 1984;86(5 Pt 1):820–8.

Andersen DK, Frey CF. The evolution of the surgical treatment of chronic pancreatitis. Ann Surg. 2010;251(1):18–32.

Aoun E, et al. SPINK1 N34S is strongly associated with recurrent acute pancreatitis but is not a risk factor for the first or sentinel acute pancreatitis event. Am J Gastroenterol. 2010;105(2):446–51.

Apte M, Pirola RC, Wilson JS. Pancreatic stellate cell: physiologic role, role in fibrosis and cancer. Curr Opin Gastroenterol. 2015;31(5):416–23.

Axon AT, et al. Pancreatography in chronic pancreatitis: international definitions. Gut. 1984;25(10):1107–12.

Azad Khan A, Banik N, Mahatab H. Malnutrition related diabetes mellitus in Bangladesh. In: ICS; 1991. p. 944–9.

Bai HX, Lowe ME, Husain SZ. What have we learned about acute pancreatitis in children? J Pediatr Gastroenterol Nutr. 2011;52(3):262–70.

Balakrishnan V. Pancreatic tropicale. In: Progress en hepatogastroenterologie: maladies du pancreas exocrine Paris. Doin Editeurs; 1987. p. 207–27.

Balakrishnan V. Tropical chronic pancreatitis: a historical perspective. Gut. 2011;60(10):1441; author reply 1441–2. doi:10.1136/gut.2010.223321.

Balakrishnan V, Hariharan M, Rao VR, Anand BS. Endoscopic pancreatography in chronic pancreatitis of the tropics. Digestion. 1985;32(2):128–31.

Balakrishnan V, Sauniere JF, Hariharan M, Sarles H. Diet, pancreatic function, and chronic pancreatitis in south India and France. Pancreas. 1988;3(1):30–5.

Balakrishnan V, Nair P, Radhakrishnan L, Narayanan VA. Tropical pancreatitis—a distinct entity, or merely a type of chronic pancreatitis? Indian J Gastroenterol. 2006;25(2):74–81.

Balakrishnan V, Unnikrishnan AG, Thomas V, Choudhuri G, Veeraraju P, Singh SP, Garg P, Pai CG, Devi RNS, Bhasin D, Jayanthi V, Premalatha N, Chacko A, Kar P, Rai RR, Rajan R, Subhalal N, Mehta R, Mishra SP, Dwivedi M, Vinayakumar KRN, Jain AK, Biswas K, Mathai S, Varghese J, Ramesh H, Alexander T, Philip J, Raj VV, Vinodkumar A, Mukevar S, Sawant P, Nair P, Kumar H, Sudhindran S, Dhar P, Sudheer OV, Sundaram KR, Tantri BV, Singh D, Nath TR. Chronic pancreatitis. A prospective nationwide study of 1,086 subjects from India. JOP. 2008;9(5):593–600.

Balakrishnan V, Lakshmi R, Nandakumar R. Tropical pancreatitis—what is happening to it? In: Chronic pancreatitis and pancreatic diabetes in India. The Indian Pancreatitis Study Group, Cochin; n.d. p. 23–54.

Balci NC, et al. MRI and S-MRCP findings in patients with suspected chronic pancreatitis: correlation with endoscopic pancreatic function testing (ePFT). J Magn Reson Imaging. 2010;31(3):601–6.

Baudry C, et al. Recurrent acute pancreatitis caused by association of a novel mutation of the calcium-sensing receptor gene and a heterozygous mutation of the SPINK1 gene. Pancreas. 2010;39(3):420–1.

Beer S, Zhou J, Szabó A, Keiles S, Chandak GR, Witt H, Sahin-Tóth M. Comprehensive functional analysis of chymotrypsin C (CTRC) variants reveals distinct loss-of-function mechanisms associated with pancreatitis risk. Gut. 2013;62(11):1616–24. doi:10.1136/gutjnl-2012-303090.

Beger HG, et al. Natural course of acute pancreatitis. World J Surg. 1997;21(2):130–5.

Bellin MD, et al. Outcome after pancreatectomy and islet autotransplantation in a pediatric population. J Pediatr Gastroenterol Nutr. 2008;47(1):37–44.

Bellin MD, et al. Quality of life improves for pediatric patients after total pancreatectomy and islet autotransplant for chronic pancreatitis. Clin Gastroenterol Hepatol. 2011;9(9):793–9.

Bellin MD, Sutherland DE, Robertson RP. Pancreatectomy and autologous islet transplantation for painful chronic pancreatitis: indications and outcomes. Hosp Pract (1995). 2012;40(3):80–7.

Bellin MD, et al. Islet autotransplantation to preserve beta cell mass in selected patients with chronic pancreatitis and diabetes mellitus undergoing total pancreatectomy. Pancreas. 2013;42(2):317–21.

Bhasin DK, Singh G, Rana SS, Chowdry SM, Shafiq N, Malhotra S, Sinha SK, Nagi B. Clinical profile of idiopathic chronic pancreatitis in North India. Clinical Gastroenterol Hepatol. 2009;7(5):594–9. doi:10.1016/j.cgh.2009.01.009.

Bhasin DK, et al. Clinical presentation and outcome of endoscopic therapy in patients with symptomatic chronic pancreatitis associated with pancreas divisum. JOP. 2013;14(1):50–6.

Bhatia E. Fibrocalculous pancreatic diabetes as currently seen in Lucknow, Uttar Pradesh. In: Chronic pancreatitis and pancreatic diabetes in India. The Indian Pancreatitis Study Group, Cochin, n.d. p. 197–210.

Bhatia E, Choudhuri G, Sikora SS, Landt O, Kage A, Becker M, Witt H. Tropical calcific pancreatitis: strong association with SPINK1 trypsin inhibitor mutations. Gastroenterology. 2002;123(4):1020–5.

Boonyasrisawat W, Pulsawat P, Yenchitsomanus P-T, Vannasaeng S, Pramukkul P, Deerochanawong C, Sriussadaporn S, Ploybutr S, Pasurakul T, Banchuin N. Analysis of the reg1alpha and reg1beta gene transcripts in patients with fibrocalculous pancreatopathy. Southeast Asian J Trop Med Public Health. 2002;33(2):365–72.

Boulling A, Le Gac G, Dujardin G, Chen J-M, Férec C. The c.1275A>G putative chronic pancreatitis-associated synonymous polymorphism in the glycoprotein 2 (GP2) gene decreases exon 9 inclusion. Mol Genet Metab. 2010;99(3):319–24. doi:10.1016/j.ymgme.2009.10.176.

Boulling A, Witt H, Chandak GR, Masson E, Paliwal S, Bhaskar S, Reddy DN, Cooper DN, Chen J-M, Férec C. Assessing the pathological relevance of SPINK1 promoter variants. Eur J Hum Genet. 2011;19(10):1066–73. doi:10.1038/ejhg.2011.79.

Boulling A, Sato M, Masson E, Génin E, Chen J-M, Férec C. Identification of a functional PRSS1 promoter variant in linkage disequilibrium with the chronic pancreatitis-protecting rs10273639. Gut. 2015;64(11):1837–8. doi:10.1136/gutjnl-2015-310254.

Braganza JM, Schofield D, Snehalatha C, Mohan V. Micronutrient antioxidant status in tropical compared with temperate-zone chronic pancreatitis. Scand J Gastroenterol. 1993;28(12):1098–104.

Cahen DL, et al. Long-term results of endoscopic drainage of common bile duct strictures in chronic pancreatitis. Eur J Gastroenterol Hepatol. 2005;17(1):103–8.

Cahen DL, et al. Endoscopic versus surgical drainage of the pancreatic duct in chronic pancreatitis. N Engl J Med. 2007;356(7):676–84.

Cerini C, Peyrot V, Garnier C, Duplan L, Veesler S, Le Caer JP, Bernard JP, Bouteille H, Michel R, Vazi A, Dupuy P, Michel B, Berland Y, Verdier JM. Biophysical characterization of lithostathine. Evidences for a polymeric structure at physiological pH and a proteolysis mechanism leading to the formation of fibrils. J Biol Chem. 1999;274(32):22266–74.

Chandak GR, Idris MM, Reddy DN, Bhaskar S, Sriram PVJ, Singh L. Mutations in the pancreatic secretory trypsin inhibitor gene (PSTI/SPINK1) rather than the cationic trypsinogen gene (PRSS1) are significantly associated with tropical calcific pancreatitis. J Med Genet. 2002;39(5):347–51.

Chandak GR, Idris MM, Reddy DN, Mani KR, Bhaskar S, Rao GV, Singh L. Absence of PRSS1 mutations and association of SPINK1 trypsin inhibitor mutations in hereditary and non-hereditary chronic pancreatitis. Gut. 2004;53(5):723–8.

Chari ST, Smyrk TC, Levy MJ, et al. Diagnosis of autoimmune pancreatitis: the Mayo Clinic experience. Clin Gastroenterol Hepatol. 2006;4:1010–6.

Chari ST, Takahashi N, Levy MJ, et al. A diagnostic strategy to distinguish autoimmune pancreatitis from pancreatic cancer. Clin Gastroenterol Hepatol. 2009;10:1097–103.

Chari ST, Klöppel G, Zhang L, et al. Histologic and clinical subtypes of autoimmune pancreatitis: the Honolulu consensus document. Pancreas. 2010;39:549–54.

Chen JM, Audrezet MP, Mercier B, Quere I, Ferec C. Exclusion of anionic trypsinogen and mesotrypsinogen involvement in hereditary pancreatitis without cationic trypsinogen gene mutations. Scand J Gastroenterol. 1999;34(8):831–2.

Chiari H. Über die selbstverdaung des menschlichen panckreas. Z Helik. 1896;17:69–96.
Chinnakotla S, et al. Total pancreatectomy and islet autotransplantation in children for chronic pancreatitis: indication, surgical techniques, postoperative management, and long-term outcomes. Ann Surg. 2014a;260(1):56–64.
Chinnakotla S, et al. Long-term outcomes of total pancreatectomy and islet auto transplantation for hereditary/genetic pancreatitis. J Am Coll Surg. 2014b;218(4):530–43.
Chowdhury ZM, McDermott MF, Davey S, Hassan Z, Sinnott PJ, Hemmatpour SK, Sherwin S, Ali L, Aganna E, Allotey RA, North BV, Cassell PG, Azad Khan AK, Hitman GA. Genetic susceptibility to fibrocalculous pancreatic diabetes in Bangladeshi subjects: a family study. Genes Immun. 2002;3(1):5–8. doi:10.1038/sj.gene.6363814.
Ciesla M, Skrzypek K, Kozakowska M, et al. MiRNAs as biomarkers of disease onset. Anal Bioanal Chem. 2011;401:2051–61.
Cohn JA, et al. Relation between mutations of the cystic fibrosis gene and idiopathic pancreatitis. N Engl J Med. 1998;339(10):653–8.
Comfort MW, Steinberg AG. Pedigree of a family with hereditary chronic relapsing pancreatitis. Gastroenterology. 1952;21(1):54–63.
Conwell DL, Banks PA. Chronic pancreatitis. Curr Opin Gastroenterol. 2008;24(5):586–90.
Conwell DL, et al. American Pancreatic Association Practice Guidelines in Chronic Pancreatitis: evidence-based report on diagnostic guidelines. Pancreas. 2014;43(8):1143–62.
Costamagna G, et al. Long-term results of endoscopic management of postoperative bile duct strictures with increasing numbers of stents. Gastrointest Endosc. 2001;54(2):162–8.
Cote GA, et al. Alcohol and smoking as risk factors in an epidemiology study of patients with chronic pancreatitis. Clin Gastroenterol Hepatol. 2011;9(3):266–73; quiz e27.
Cremer M, et al. Stenting in severe chronic pancreatitis: results of medium-term follow-up in seventy-six patients. Endoscopy. 1991;23(3):171–6.
Daftary A, et al. Fecal elastase-1: utility in pancreatic function in cystic fibrosis. J Cyst Fibros. 2006;5(2):71–6.
Dani R, Penna FJ, Nogueira CE. Etiology of chronic calcifying pancreatitis in Brazil: a report of 329 consecutive cases. Int J Pancreatol. 1986;1(5–6):399–406. doi:10.1007/BF02801872.
Darge K, Anupindi S. Pancreatitis and the role of US, MRCP and ERCP. Pediatr Radiol. 2009;39(Suppl 2):S153–7.
Dawra R, Sah RP, Dudeja V, Rishi L, Talukdar R, Garg P, Saluja AK. Intra-acinar trypsinogen activation mediates early stages of pancreatic injury but not inflammation in mice with acute pancreatitis. Gastroenterology. 2011;141(6):2210–2217.e2. doi:10.1053/j.gastro.2011.08.033.
De Caro A, Lohse J, Sarles H. Characterization of a protein isolated from pancreatic calculi of men suffering from chronic calcifying pancreatitis. Biochem Biophys Res Commun. 1979;87(4):1176–82.
De Reggi M, Gharib B, Patard L, Stoven V. Lithostathine, the presumed pancreatic stone inhibitor, does not interact specifically with calcium carbonate crystals. J Biol Chem. 1998;273(9):4967–71.
Delaney L, et al. MR cholangiopancreatography in children: feasibility, safety, and initial experience. Pediatr Radiol. 2008;38(1):64–75.
Deng X, et al. Chronic alcohol consumption accelerates fibrosis in response to cerulein-induced pancreatitis in rats. Am J Pathol. 2005;166(1):93–106.
Derikx MHM, Szmola R, te Morsche RHM, Sunderasan S, Chacko A, Drenth JPH. Tropical calcific pancreatitis and its association with CTRC and SPINK1 (p.N34S) variants. Eur J Gastroenterol Hepatol. 2009;21(8):889–94. doi:10.1097/MEG.0b013e32832183cf.
Derikx MH, Kovacs P, Scholz M, Masson E, Chen J-M, Ruffert C, Lichtner P, Te Morsche RHM, Cavestro GM, Férec C, JPH D, Witt H, Rosendahl J, PanEuropean Working group on Alcoholic Chronic Pancreatitis Members and Collaborators. Polymorphisms at PRSS1-PRSS2 and CLDN2-MORC4 loci associate with alcoholic and non-alcoholic chronic pancreatitis in a European replication study. Gut. 2015;64(9):1426–33. doi:10.1136/gutjnl-2014-307453.
Report of the Expert Committee on the Diagnosis and Classification of Diabetes Mellitus. Diabetes Care. 1997;20(7):1183–97.
DiMagno EP, Go VL, Summerskill WH. Relations between pancreatic enzyme outputs and malabsorption in severe pancreatic insufficiency. N Engl J Med. 1973;288(16):813–5.
Draganov P, et al. Long-term outcome in patients with benign biliary strictures treated endoscopically with multiple stents. Gastrointest Endosc. 2002;55(6):680–6.
Farazi TA, Spitzer JI, Morozov P, et al. miRNAs in human cancer. J Pathol. 2011;223:102–15.
Felderbauer P, et al. Mutations in the calcium-sensing receptor: a new genetic risk factor for chronic pancreatitis? Scand J Gastroenterol. 2006;41(3):343–8.
Fjeld K, Johansson S, Rosendahl J, Chen J-M, Lasher D, Cnop M, Johansson BB, Masson E, Mayerle J, Mössner J. A recombination allele of the lipase gene CEL and its pseudogene CELP encodes a hybrid protein and is a genetic risk factor for chronic pancreatitis. Pancreatology. 2014;14(3):S16.
Fjeld K, et al. A recombined allele of the lipase gene CEL and its pseudogene CELP confers susceptibility to chronic pancreatitis. Nat Genet. 2015;47(5):518–22.
Freedman SD, Sakamoto K, Venu RP. GP2, the homologue to the renal cast protein uromodulin, is a major component of intraductal plugs in chronic pancreatitis. J Clin Invest. 1993;92(1):83–90. doi:10.1172/JCI116602.

Friedlander J, et al. Diagnosis of autoimmune pancreatitis vs neoplasms in children with pancreatic mass and biliary obstruction. Clin Gastroenterol Hepatol. 2012;10(9):1051–5.e1.

Fujii LL, et al. Pediatric pancreatic EUS-guided trucut biopsy for evaluation of autoimmune pancreatitis. Gastrointest Endosc. 2013;77(5):824–8.

Garg PK, Tandon RK. Survey on chronic pancreatitis in the Asia-Pacific region. J Gastroenterol Hepatol. 2004;19(9):998–1004. doi:10.1111/j.1440-1746.2004.03426.x.

Geevarghese PJ. Pancreatic diabetes: a clinico-pathologic study of growth onset diabetes with pancreatic calculi. Popular Prakashan; 1968.

Ghazale A, Chari ST, Zhang L, et al. Immunoglobulin G4-associated cholangitis: clinical profile and response to therapy. Gastroenterology. 2008;134:706–15.

Giorgi D, Bernard JP, Rouquier S, Iovanna J, Sarles H, Dagorn JC. Secretory pancreatic stone protein messenger RNA. Nucleotide sequence and expression in chronic calcifying pancreatitis. J Clin Invest. 1989;84(1):100–6. doi:10.1172/JCI114128.

Girish BN, Rajesh G, Vaidyanathan K, Balakrishnan V. Zinc status in chronic pancreatitis and its relationship with exocrine and endocrine insufficiency. JOP. 2009;10(6):651–6.

Girish BN, Rajesh G, Vaidyanathan K, Balakrishnan V. Assessment of cassava toxicity in patients with tropical chronic pancreatitis. Trop Gastroenterol. 2011a;32(2):112–6.

Girish BN, Rajesh G, Vaidyanathan K, Balakrishnan V. Assessment of oxidative status in chronic pancreatitis and its relation with zinc status. Indian J Gastroenterol. 2011b;30(2):84–8. doi:10.1007/s12664-011-0094-8.

Girish BN, Vaidyanathan K, Rajesh G, Balakrishnan V. Effects of micronutrient status on oxidative stress and exocrine pancreatic function in patients with chronic pancreatitis. Indian J Biochem Biophys. 2012;49(5):386–91.

Govindarajan M, Mohan V, Deepa R, Ashok S, Pitchumoni CS. Histopathology and immunohistochemistry of pancreatic islets in fibrocalculous pancreatic diabetes. Diabetes Res Clin Pract. 2001;51(1):29–38.

Graham KS, et al. ERCP in the management of pediatric pancreatitis. Gastrointest Endosc. 1998;47(6):492–5.

Greenbaum LM, Hirshkowitz A. Endogenous cathepsin activation of trypsinogen in extracts of dog pancreas. Proc Soc Exp Biol Med. 1961;107:74–6.

Hamada S, Masamune A, Kanno A, et al. Comprehensive analysis of serum microRNAs in autoimmune pancreatitis. Digestion. 2015;91:263–71.

Hamano H, Kawa S, Horiuchi A, et al. High serum IgG4 concentrations in patients with sclerosing pancreatitis. N Engl J Med. 2001;344:732–8.

Hansen TM, et al. Morphological and functional evaluation of chronic pancreatitis with magnetic resonance imaging. World J Gastroenterol. 2013;19(42):7241–6.

Hart PA, Kamisawa T, Brugge WR, et al. Long-term outcomes of autoimmune pancreatitis: a multicentre, international analysis. Gut. 2013a;62:1771–6.

Hart PA, Topazian MD, Witzig TE, et al. Treatment of relapsing autoimmune pancreatitis with immunomodulators and rituximab: the Mayo Clinic experience. Gut. 2013b;62:1607–15.

Hart PA, Law RJ, Dierkhising RA, et al. Risk of cancer in autoimmune pancreatitis: a case-control study and review of the literature. Pancreas. 2014;43:417–21.

Hart PA, Levy MJ, Smyrk TC, et al. Clinical profiles and outcomes in idiopathic duct-centric chronic pancreatitis (type 2 autoimmune pancreatitis): the Mayo Clinic experience. Gut. 2015a. pii:gutjnl-2015-309275. doi:10.1136/gutjnl-2015-309275. [Epub ahead of print].

Hart PA, Zen Y, Chari ST. Recent advances in autoimmune pancreatitis. Gastroenterology. 2015b;149:39–51.

Hassan Z, Mohan V, Ali L, Allotey R, Barakat K, Faruque MO, Deepa R, McDermott MF, Jackson AE, Cassell P, Curtis D, Gelding SV, Vijayaravaghan S, Gyr N, Whitcomb DC, Khan AKA, Hitman GA. SPINK1 is a susceptibility gene for fibrocalculous pancreatic diabetes in subjects from the Indian subcontinent. Am J Hum Genet. 2002;71(4):964–8. doi:10.1086/342731.

Havinga JR, Slot JW, Strous GJ. Membrane detachment and release of the major membrane glycoprotein of secretory granules in rat pancreatic exocrine cells. Eur J Cell Biol. 1985;39(1):70–6.

Hawrami K, Mohan V, Bone A, Hitman GA. Analysis of islet regenerating (reg) gene polymorphisms in fibrocalculous pancreatic diabetes. Pancreas. 1997;14(2):122–5.

Hirano K, Isayama H, Tada M, et al. Association between autoimmune pancreatitis and malignancy. Clin J Gastroenterol. 2014;7:200–4.

Hofbauer B, Saluja AK, Lerch MM, Bhagat L, Bhatia M, Lee HS, Frossard JL, Adler G, Steer ML. Intra-acinar cell activation of trypsinogen during caerulein-induced pancreatitis in rats. Am J Physiol. 1998;275(2 Pt 1):G352–62.

Howes N, et al. Clinical and genetic characteristics of hereditary pancreatitis in Europe. Clin Gastroenterol Hepatol. 2004;2(3):252–61.

Huang H, et al. Activation of nuclear factor-kappaB in acinar cells increases the severity of pancreatitis in mice. Gastroenterology. 2013;144(1):202–10.

Idris MM, Bhaskar S, Reddy DN, Mani KR, Rao GV, Singh L, Chandak GR. Mutations in anionic trypsinogen gene are not associated with tropical calcific pancreatitis. Gut. 2005;54(5):728–9. doi:10.1136/gut.2004.055335.

Illangovekara V. Malnutritiion related diabetes in Sri Lanka fact or fiction. J Ceylon Coll Phys. 1995;28:16–25.

Issa H, Al-Haddad A, Al-Salem AH. Diagnostic and therapeutic ERCP in the pediatric age group. Pediatr Surg Int. 2007;23(2):111–6.

Kambo PK, Hitman GA, Mohan V, Ramachandran A, Snehalatha C, Suresh S, Metcalfe K, Ryait BK,

Viswanathan M. The genetic predisposition to fibrocalculous pancreatic diabetes. Diabetologia. 1989;32(1):45–51.
Kamisawa T, Shimosegawa T, Okazaki K, et al. Standard steroid treatment for autoimmune pancreatitis. Gut. 2009;58:1504–7.
Kamisawa T, Okazaki K, Kawa S, et al. Japanese consensus guidelines for management of autoimmune pancreatitis: III. Treatment and prognosis of AIP. J Gastroenterol. 2010;45:471–7.
Kamisawa T, Chari ST, Lerch MM, et al. Recent advances in autoimmune pancreatitis: type 1 and type 2. Gut. 2013;62:1373–80.
Kamisawa T, Okazaki K, Kawa S, et al. Amendment of the Japanese consensus guidelines for autoimmune pancreatitis, 2013 III. Treatment and prognosis of autoimmune pancreatitis. J Gastroenterol. 2014;49:961–70.
Kamisawa T, Zen Y, Pillai S, et al. IgG4-related disease. Lancet. 2015;385:1460–71.
Kanno A, Masamune A, Okazaki K, et al. Nationwide epidemiological survey of autoimmune pancreatitis in Japan in 2011. Pancreas. 2015a;44:535–9.
Kanno A, Masamune A, Shimosegawa T. Endoscopic approaches for the diagnosis of autoimmune pancreatitis. Dig Endosc. 2015b;27:250–8.
Kanno A, Masamune A, Fujishima F, et al. Diagnosis of autoimmune pancreatitis by EUS-guided FNA using a 22-gauge needle: a prospective multicenter study. Gastrointest Endosc. 2016;84:797–804.e1.
Kargl S, et al. Therapeutic step-up strategy for management of hereditary pancreatitis in children. J Pediatr Surg. 2015;50(4):511–4.
Kim KP, Kim MH, Kim JC, et al. Diagnostic criteria for autoimmune chronic pancreatitis revisited. World J Gastroenterol. 2006;12:2487–96.
Kini M. Multiple pancreatic calculi with chronic pancreatitis. Br J Surg. 1938;25(99):705–6.
Kinnear TW. The pattern of diabetes mellitus in a Nigerian teaching hospital. East Afr Med J. 1963;40:288–94.
Kinney TP, Freeman ML. Recent advances and novel methods in pancreatic imaging. Minerva Gastroenterol Dietol. 2008;54(1):85–95.
Ko SB, Mizuno N, Yatabe Y, et al. Corticosteroids correct aberrant CFTR localization in the duct and regenerate acinar cells in autoimmune pancreatitis. Gastroenterology. 2010;138:1988–96.
Kobayashi T, et al. Correlation of pancreatic histopathologic findings and islet yield in children with chronic pancreatitis undergoing total pancreatectomy and islet autotransplantation. Pancreas. 2010;39(1):57–63.
Kosaka N, Iguchi H, Ochiya T. Circulating miRNA in body fluid: a new potential biomarker for cancer diagnosis and prognosis. Cancer Sci. 2010;101:2087–92.
Kubota K, Watanabe S, Uchiyama T, et al. Factors predictive of relapse and spontaneous remission of autoimmune pancreatitis patients treated/not treated with corticosteroids. J Gastroenterol. 2011;46:834–42.
Kukor Z, Mayerle J, Krüger B, Tóth M, Steed PM, Halangk W, Lerch MM, Sahin-Tóth M. Presence of cathepsin B in the human pancreatic secretory pathway and its role in trypsinogen activation during hereditary pancreatitis. J Biol Chem. 2002;277(24):21389–96. doi:10.1074/jbc.M200878200.
Kumar S, et al. Risk factors associated with pediatric acute recurrent and chronic pancreatitis: lessons from INSPPIRE. JAMA Pediatr. 2016;170(6):562–9.
Layer P, et al. The different courses of early- and late-onset idiopathic and alcoholic chronic pancreatitis. Gastroenterology. 1994;107(5):1481–7.
Le Bodic L, et al. The hereditary pancreatitis gene maps to long arm of chromosome 7. Hum Mol Genet. 1996;5(4):549–54.
LeBel D, Beattie M. Identification of the proteins exposed on the cytoplasmic surface of the pancreatic zymogen granule. Biochim Biophys Acta. 1984a;769(3):622–4.
LeBel D, Beattie M. The integral and peripheral proteins of the zymogen granule membrane. Biochim Biophys Acta. 1984b;769(3):611–21.
Lee LS, Conwell DL. Update on advanced endoscopic techniques for the pancreas: endoscopic retrograde cholangiopancreatography, drainage and biopsy, and endoscopic ultrasound. Radiol Clin N Am. 2012;50(3):547–61.
Lee AT, et al. Alcohol and cigarette smoke components activate human pancreatic stellate cells: implications for the progression of chronic pancreatitis. Alcohol Clin Exp Res. 2015;39(11):2123–33.
Lerch MM, Gorelick FS. Early trypsinogen activation in acute pancreatitis. Med Clin North Am. 2000;84(3):549–63. viii
Lucidi V, et al. The etiology of acute recurrent pancreatitis in children: a challenge for pediatricians. Pancreas. 2011;40(4):517–21.
Lundberg R, et al. Early alterations in glycemic control and pancreatic endocrine function in nondiabetic patients with chronic pancreatitis. Pancreas. 2016;45(4):565–71.
MacDonald RJ, Ronzio RA. Comparative analysis of zymogen granule membrane polypeptides. Biochem Biophys Res Commun. 1972;49(2):377–82.
Mahurkar S, Idris MM, Reddy DN, Bhaskar S, Rao GV, Thomas V, Singh L, Chandak GR. Association of cathepsin B gene polymorphisms with tropical calcific pancreatitis. Gut. 2006;55(9):1270–5. doi:10.1136/gut.2005.087403.
Mahurkar S, Bhaskar S, Reddy DN, Rao GV, Chandak GR. Comprehensive screening for reg1alpha gene rules out association with tropical calcific pancreatitis. World J Gastroenterol. 2007;13(44):5938–43.
Mahurkar S, Bhaskar S, Reddy DN, Prakash S, Rao GV, Singh SP, Thomas V, Chandak GR. TCF7L2 gene polymorphisms do not predict susceptibility to diabetes in tropical calcific pancreatitis but may interact with SPINK1 and CTSB mutations in predicting diabetes. BMC Med Genet. 2008;9:80. doi:10.1186/1471-2350-9-80.
Mahurkar S, Bhaskar S, Reddy DN, Rao GV, Singh SP, Thomas V, Chandak GR. The G191R variant in the

PRSS2 gene does not play a role in protection against tropical calcific pancreatitis. Gut. 2009;58(6):881–2. doi:10.1136/gut.2008.170753.

Manfredi R, et al. Idiopathic chronic pancreatitis in children: MR cholangiopancreatography after secretin administration. Radiology. 2002;224(3):675–82.

Manfredi R, et al. Quantitative MRCP assessment of pancreatic exocrine reserve and its correlation with faecal elastase-1 in patients with chronic pancreatitis. Radiol Med. 2012;117(2):282–92.

Maruyama M, Arakura N, Ozaki Y, et al. Type 1 autoimmune pancreatitis can transform into chronic pancreatitis: a long-term follow-up study of 73 Japanese patients. Int J Rheumatol. 2013;2013:272595.

Masamune A, Shimosegawa T. Pancreatic stellate cells—multi-functional cells in the pancreas. Pancreatology. 2013;13(2):102–5.

Masamune A, Nishimori I, Kikuta K, et al. Randomised controlled trial of long-term maintenance corticosteroid therapy in patients with autoimmune pancreatitis. Gut. 2016. pii:gutjnl-2016-312049. doi:10.1136/gutjnl-2016-312049. [Epub ahead of print].

Masson E, Le Maréchal C, Chandak GR, Lamoril J, Bezieau S, Mahurkar S, Bhaskar S, Reddy DN, Chen J-M, Férec C. Trypsinogen copy number mutations in patients with idiopathic chronic pancreatitis. Clin Gastroenterol Hepatol. 2008a;6(1):82–8. doi:10.1016/j.cgh.2007.10.004.

Masson E, et al. Association of rare chymotrypsinogen C (CTRC) gene variations in patients with idiopathic chronic pancreatitis. Hum Genet. 2008b;123(1):83–91.

Masson E, Paliwal S, Bhaskar S, Prakash S, Scotet V, Reddy DN, Le Maréchal C, Ratan Chandak G, Chen J-M, Férec C. Genetic analysis of the glycoprotein 2 gene in patients with chronic pancreatitis. Pancreas. 2010;39(3):353–8. doi:10.1097/MPA.0b013e3181bb9620.

Mathangi DC, Deepa R, Mohan V, Govindarajan M, Namasivayam A. Long-term ingestion of cassava (tapioca) does not produce diabetes or pancreatitis in the rat model. International J Pancreatol. 2000;27(3):203–8. doi:10.1385/IJGC:27:3:203.

Meagher C, et al. Spontaneous development of a pancreatic exocrine disease in CD28-deficient NOD mice. J Immunol. 2008;180(12):7793–803.

Members of the Criteria Committee for Autoimmune Pancreatitis of the Japan Pancreas Society. Diagnostic criteria for autoimmune pancreatitis by the Japan Pancreas Society. J Jpn Pancreas (Suizou). 2002;17:587.

Midha S, Singh N, Sachdev V, Tandon RK, Joshi YK, Garg PK. Cause and effect relationship of malnutrition with idiopathic chronic pancreatitis: prospective case-control study. J Gastroenterol Hepatol. 2008;23(9):1378–83. doi:10.1111/j.1440-1746.2008.05459.x.

Midha S, Khajuria R, Shastri S, Kabra M, Garg PK. Idiopathic chronic pancreatitis in India: phenotypic characterisation and strong genetic susceptibility due to SPINK1 and CFTR gene mutations. Gut. 2010;59(6):800–7. doi:10.1136/gut.2009.191239.

Mngola EN. Diabetes mellitus in the African enviornment—the dilemma. In: Mngola EN, ed. Diabetes 1982. Proceedings of the II Congress of the IDF. Amsterdam: Excerpta Medica, 1983:309–13.

Mohan V, Chari ST, Hitman GA, Suresh S, Madanagopalan N, Ramachandran A, Viswanathan M. Familial aggregation in tropical fibrocalculous pancreatic diabetes. Pancreas. 1989;4(6):690–3.

Mohan V, Nagalotimath SJ, Yajnik CS, Tripathy BB. Fibrocalculous pancreatic diabetes. Diabetes Metab Rev. 1998;14(2):153–70.

Moorthy TR, Nalini N, Narendranathan M. Ultrasound imaging in tropical pancreatitis. J Clin Ultrasound. 1992;20(6):389–93.

Morinville VD, Barmada MM, Lowe ME. Increasing incidence of acute pancreatitis at an American pediatric tertiary care center: is greater awareness among physicians responsible? Pancreas. 2010;39(1):5–8.

Morinville VD, et al. Definitions of pediatric pancreatitis and survey of present clinical practices. J Pediatr Gastroenterol Nutr. 2012;55(3):261–5.

Morinville VD, et al. Design and Implementation of INSPPIRE (International Study Group of Pediatric Pancreatitis: in Search for a Cure). J Pediatr Gastroenterol Nutr. 2014;59(3):360–4.

Muddana V, et al. Association between calcium sensing receptor gene polymorphisms and chronic pancreatitis in a US population: role of serine protease inhibitor Kazal 1type and alcohol. World J Gastroenterol. 2008;14(28):4486–91.

Muddana V, et al. Are genetic variants in the platelet-derived growth factor [beta] gene associated with chronic pancreatitis? Pancreas. 2010;39(8):1215–9.

Multigner L, De Caro A, Lombardo D, Campese D, Sarles H. Pancreatic stone protein, a phosphoprotein which inhibits calcium carbonate precipitation from human pancreatic juice. Biochem Biophys Res Commun. 1983;110(1):69–74.

Muniraj T, et al. Chronic pancreatitis, a comprehensive review and update. Part I: epidemiology, etiology, risk factors, genetics, pathophysiology, and clinical features. Dis Mon. 2014;60(12):530–50.

Nemoda Z, Sahin-Tóth M. Chymotrypsin C (caldecrin) stimulates autoactivation of human cationic trypsinogen. J Biol Chem. 2006;281(17):11879–86. doi:10.1074/jbc.M600124200.

Nishimori I, Tamakoshi A, Kawa S, et al. Influence of steroid therapy on the course of diabetes mellitus in patients with autoimmune pancreatitis: findings from a nationwide survey in Japan. Pancreas. 2006;32:244–8.

Noone PG, et al. Cystic fibrosis gene mutations and pancreatitis risk: relation to epithelial ion transport and trypsin inhibitor gene mutations. Gastroenterology. 2001;121(6):1310–9.

Notohara K, Burgart LJ, Yadav D, et al. Idiopathic chronic pancreatitis with periductal lymphoplasmacytic infiltration: clinicopathologic features of 35 cases. Am J Surg Pathol. 2003;27:1119–27.

Notohara K, Nishimori I, Mizuno N, et al. Clinicopathological features of type 2 autoimmune pancreatitis in Japan: results of a multicenter survey. Pancreas. 2015;44:1072–7.

Nydegger A, Couper RT, Oliver MR. Childhood pancreatitis. J Gastroenterol Hepatol. 2006;21(3):499–509.

Nydegger A, et al. Changing incidence of acute pancreatitis: 10-year experience at the Royal Children's Hospital, Melbourne. J Gastroenterol Hepatol. 2007;22(8):1313–6.

Okazaki K, Uchida K. Autoimmune pancreatitis: the past, present, and future. Pancreas. 2015;44:1006–16.

Okazaki K, et al. Autoimmune-related pancreatitis is associated with autoantibodies and a Th1/Th2-type cellular immune response. Gastroenterology. 2000;118(3):573–81.

Okazaki K, Kawa S, Kamisawa T, et al. Clinical diagnostic criteria of autoimmune pancreatitis: revised proposal. J Gastroenterol. 2006;41:626–31.

Olesen SS, et al. Pregabalin reduces pain in patients with chronic pancreatitis in a randomized, controlled trial. Gastroenterology. 2011;141(2):536–43.

Oracz G, et al. Toxic-metabolic risk factors in pediatric chronic pancreatitis—single center experience. J Pediatr Gastroenterol Nutr. 2015;62(6):e66.

Paliwal S, Bhaskar S, Rao GV, Reddy DN, Chandak GR. What's there in a name: tropical calcific pancreatitis and idiopathic chronic pancreatitis in India. Gut. 2011;60(10):1440–1; author reply 1441–2. doi:10.1136/gut.2010.228452.

Paliwal S, Bhaskar S, Mani KR, Reddy DN, Rao GV, Singh SP, Thomas V, Chandak GR. Comprehensive screening of chymotrypsin C (CTRC) gene in tropical calcific pancreatitis identifies novel variants. Gut. 2013;62(11):1602–6. doi:10.1136/gutjnl-2012-302448.

Paliwal S, Bhaskar S, Reddy DN, Rao GV, Thomas V, Singh SP, Chandak GR. Association analysis of PRSS1-PRSS2 and CLDN2-MORC4 variants in nonalcoholic chronic pancreatitis using tropical calcific pancreatitis as model. Pancreas. 2016;45(8):1153–7. doi:10.1097/MPA.0000000000000608.

Pandya A, et al. Linkage studies in a large kindred with hereditary pancreatitis confirms mapping of the gene to a 16-cM region on 7q. Genomics. 1996;38(2):227–30.

Pannala R, Chari ST. Corticosteroid treatment for autoimmune pancreatitis. Gut. 2009;58:1438–9.

Pant C, Sferra TJ. Emergency department visits and hospitalizations in children with chronic pancreatitis in the United States. J Pediatr Gastroenterol Nutr. 2015;61(5):568–70.

Papita R, Nazir A, Anbalagan VP, Anjana RM, Pitchumoni C, Chari S, Mohan V. Secular trends of fibrocalculous pancreatic diabetes and diabetes secondary to alcoholic chronic pancreatitis at a tertiary care diabetes centre in South India. JOP. 2012;13(2):205–9.

Paquet MR, St-Jean P, Roberge M, Beaudoin AR. Isolation of zymogen granules from rat pancreas and characterization of their membrane proteins. Eur J Cell Biol. 1982;28(1):20–6.

Pfutzer RH, et al. SPINK1/PSTI polymorphisms act as disease modifiers in familial and idiopathic chronic pancreatitis. Gastroenterology. 2000;119(3):615–23.

Pitchumoni C. Familial pancreatitis. Pancreatic diabetes. Trivandrum: Geoprinters; 1970. p. 46–8.

Pohl JF, et al. Health-related quality of life in pediatric patients with long-standing pancreatitis. J Pediatr Gastroenterol Nutr. 2012;54(5):657–63.

Ponchon T, et al. Endoscopic stenting for pain relief in chronic pancreatitis: results of a standardized protocol. Gastrointest Endosc. 1995;42(5):452–6.

Raeder H, Johansson S, Holm PI, Haldorsen IS, Mas E, Sbarra V, Nermoen I, Eide SA, Grevle L, Bjorkhaug L, Sagen JV, Aksnes L, Sovik O, Lombardo D, Molven A, Njolstad PR. Mutations in the CEL VNTR cause a syndrome of diabetes and pancreatic exocrine dysfunction. Nat Genet. 2006;38(1):54–62. doi:10.1038/ng1708.

Ragvin A, et al. The number of tandem repeats in the carboxyl-ester lipase (CEL) gene as a risk factor in alcoholic and idiopathic chronic pancreatitis. Pancreatology. 2013;13(1):29–32.

Raina A, Yadav D, Krasinskas AM, et al. Evaluation and management of autoimmune pancreatitis: experience at a large US center. Am J Gastroenterol. 2009;104:2295–306.

Rajesh G, Girish BN, Vaidyanathan K, Saumya M, Balakrishnan V. Folate deficiency in chronic pancreatitis. JOP. 2010;11(4):409–10; author reply 413-404.

Rajesh G, Veena AB, Menon S, Balakrishnan V. Clinical profile of early-onset and late-onset idiopathic chronic pancreatitis in South India. Indian J Gastroenterol. 2014a;33(3):231–6. doi:10.1007/s12664-013-0421-3.

Rajesh G, Girish BN, Panicker S, Balakrishnan V. Time trends in the etiology of chronic pancreatitis in South India. Trop Gastroenterol. 2014b;35(3):164–7.

Rebours V, et al. The natural history of hereditary pancreatitis: a national series. Gut. 2009;58(1):97–103.

Rindler MJ, Hoops TC. The pancreatic membrane protein GP-2 localizes specifically to secretory granules and is shed into the pancreatic juice as a protein aggregate. Eur J Cell Biol. 1990;53(1):154–63.

Rosendahl J, Witt H, Szmola R, Bhatia E, Ozsvári B, Landt O, Schulz H-U, Gress TM, Pfützer R, Löhr M, Kovacs P, Blüher M, Stumvoll M, Choudhuri G, Hegyi P, te Morsche RHM, Drenth JPH, Truninger K, Macek M, Puhl G, Witt U, Schmidt H, Büning C, Ockenga J, Kage A, Groneberg DA, Nickel R, Berg T, Wiedenmann B, Bödeker H, Keim V, Mössner J, Teich N, Sahin-Tóth M. Chymotrypsin C (CTRC) variants that diminish activity or secretion are associated with chronic pancreatitis. Nat Genet. 2008;40(1):78–82. doi:10.1038/ng.2007.44.

Rosling H. Cassava toxicity and food security. A review of health effects of cyanide exposure from cassava and of ways to prevent these effects. Rosling MD; 1987.

Sah RP, Chari ST. Serologic issues in IgG4-related systemic disease and autoimmune pancreatitis. Curr Opin Rheumatol. 2011;23:108–13.

Sah RP, Chari ST, Pannala R, et al. Differences in clinical profile and relapse rate of type 1 versus type 2 autoimmune pancreatitis. Gastroenterology. 2010;139:140–8; quiz e12–3.

Sah RP, Garg P, Saluja AK. Pathogenic mechanisms of acute pancreatitis. Curr Opin Gastroenterol. 2012;28(5):507–15.

Sakaguchi T, Gu X, Golden HM, Suh E, Rhoads DB, Reinecker H-C. Cloning of the human claudin-2 5'-flanking region revealed a TATA-less promoter with conserved binding sites in mouse and human for caudal-related homeodomain proteins and hepatocyte nuclear factor-1alpha. J Biol Chem. 2002;277(24):21361–70. doi:10.1074/jbc.M110261200.

Saluja A, Hashimoto S, Saluja M, Powers RE, Meldolesi J, Steer ML. Subcellular redistribution of lysosomal enzymes during caerulein-induced pancreatitis. Am J Physiol. 1987;253(4 Pt 1):G508–16.

Sanchez-Ramirez CA, et al. Acute and recurrent pancreatitis in children: etiological factors. Acta Paediatr. 2007;96(4):534–7.

Sandhyamani S, Vijayakumari A, Balaraman Nair M. Bonnet monkey model for pancreatic changes in induced malnutrition. Pancreas. 1999;18(1):84–95.

Sarles H. Definitions and classifications of pancreatitis. Pancreas. 1991;6(4):470–4.

Sarles H, Sarles JC, Muratore R, et al. Chronic inflammatory sclerosis of the pancreas—an autonomous pancreatic disease? Am J Dig Dis. 1961;6:688–98.

Sathiaraj E, Gupta S, Chutke M, Mahurkar S, Mansard MJ, Rao GV, Reddy DN. Malnutrition is not an etiological factor in the development of tropical pancreatitis—a case-control study of southern Indian patients. Trop Gastroenterol. 2010;31(3):169–74.

Schibli S, et al. Towards the ideal quantitative pancreatic function test: analysis of test variables that influence validity. Clin Gastroenterol Hepatol. 2006;4(1):90–7.

Schneider A, Suman A, Rossi L, Barmada MM, Beglinger C, Parvin S, Sattar S, Ali L, Khan AKA, Gyr N, Whitcomb DC. SPINK1/PSTI mutations are associated with tropical pancreatitis and type II diabetes mellitus in Bangladesh. Gastroenterology. 2002;123(4):1026–30.

Schnur A, et al. Functional effects of 13 rare PRSS1 variants presumed to cause chronic pancreatitis. Gut. 2014;63(2):337–43.

Schwarzenberg SJ, et al. Pediatric chronic pancreatitis is associated with genetic risk factors and substantial disease burden. J Pediatr. 2015;166(4):890–6.e1.

Shaper AG. Chronic pancreatic disease and protein malnutrition. Lancet. 1960;1(7136):1223–4.

Sharer N, et al. Mutations of the cystic fibrosis gene in patients with chronic pancreatitis. N Engl J Med. 1998;339(10):645–52.

Shek FW, et al. Expression of transforming growth factor-beta 1 by pancreatic stellate cells and its implications for matrix secretion and turnover in chronic pancreatitis. Am J Pathol. 2002;160(5):1787–98.

Shimosegawa T, Chari ST, Frulloni L, et al. International consensus diagnostic criteria for autoimmune pancreatitis: guidelines of the International Association of Pancreatology. Pancreas. 2011;40:352–8.

Shiokawa M, Kodama Y, Yoshimura K, et al. Risk of cancer in patients with autoimmune pancreatitis. Am J Gastroenterol. 2013;108:610–7.

Singh S, Choudhuri G, Agarwal S. Frequency of CFTR, SPINK1, and cathepsin B gene mutation in North Indian population: connections between genetics and clinical data. ScientificWorldJournal. 2014;2014:763195. doi:10.1155/2014/763195.

Sobczynska-Tomaszewska A, et al. Analysis of CFTR, SPINK1, PRSS1 and AAT mutations in children with acute or chronic pancreatitis. J Pediatr Gastroenterol Nutr. 2006;43(3):299–306.

Spanier B, Bruno MJ, Dijkgraaf MG. Incidence and mortality of acute and chronic pancreatitis in the Netherlands: a nationwide record-linked cohort study for the years 1995-2005. World J Gastroenterol. 2013;19(20):3018–26.

Steer ML, Meldolesi J, Figarella C. Pancreatitis. The role of lysosomes. Dig Dis Sci. 1984;29(10):934–8.

Steer ML, Waxman I, Freedman S. Chronic pancreatitis. N Engl J Med. 1995;332(22):1482–90.

Stevens T. Role of endoscopic ultrasonography in the diagnosis of acute and chronic pancreatitis. Gastrointest Endosc Clin N Am. 2013;23(4):735–47.

Sutherland DE, et al. Total pancreatectomy and islet autotransplantation for chronic pancreatitis. J Am Coll Surg. 2012;214(4):409–24; discussion 424–6.

Suzuki T, Yoshinaga N, Tanabe S. Interleukin-6 (IL-6) regulates claudin-2 expression and tight junction permeability in intestinal epithelium. J Biol Chem. 2011;286(36):31263–71. doi:10.1074/jbc.M111.238147.

Szilágyi L, Kénesi E, Katona G, Kaslik G, Juhász G, Gráf L. Comparative in vitro studies on native and recombinant human cationic trypsins. Cathepsin B is a possible pathological activator of trypsinogen in pancreatitis. J Biol Chem. 2001;276(27):24574–80. doi:10.1074/jbc.M011374200.

Szmola R, Sahin-Tóth M. Chymotrypsin C (caldecrin) promotes degradation of human cationic trypsin: identity with Rinderknecht's enzyme Y. Proc Natl Acad Sci U S A. 2007;104(27):11227–32. doi:10.1073/pnas.0703714104.

Szmola R, Sahin-Tóth M. Pancreatitis-associated chymotrypsinogen C (CTRC) mutant elicits endoplasmic reticulum stress in pancreatic acinar cells. Gut. 2010;59(3):365–72. doi:10.1136/gut.2009.198903.

Szmola R, Bence M, Carpentieri A, Szabó A, Costello CE, Samuelson J, Sahin-Tóth M. Chymotrypsin C is a co-activator of human pancreatic procarboxypeptidases A1 and A2. J Biol Chem. 2011;286(3):1819–27. doi:10.1074/jbc.M110.187369.

Threadgold J, et al. The N34S mutation of SPINK1 (PSTI) is associated with a familial pattern of idiopathic chronic pancreatitis but does not cause the disease. Gut. 2002;50(5):675–81.

Ting J, et al. Direct costs of acute recurrent and chronic pancreatitis in children in the INSPPIRE registry. J Pediatr Gastroenterol Nutr. 2015;62(3):443–9.

Tipnis NA, Werlin SL. The use of magnetic resonance cholangiopancreatography in children. Curr Gastroenterol Rep. 2007;9(3):225–9.

Troendle DM, Barth BA. Pediatric considerations in endoscopic retrograde cholangiopancreatography. Gastrointest Endosc Clin N Am. 2016;26(1):119–36.

Trout AT, et al. Does secretin add value in pediatric magnetic resonance cholangiopancreatography? Pediatr Radiol. 2013;43(4):479–86.

Tsujii-Hayashi Y, Kitahara M, Yamagaki T, Kojima-Aikawa K, Matsumoto I. A potential endogenous ligand of annexin IV in the exocrine pancreas. Carbohydrate structure of GP-2, a glycosylphosphatidylinositol-anchored glycoprotein of zymogen granule membranes. J Biol Chem. 2002;277(49):47493–9. doi:10.1074/jbc.M206572200.

Umehara H, Okazaki K, Masaki Y, et al. Comprehensive diagnostic criteria for IgG4-related disease (IgG4-RD), 2012. Mod Rheumatol. 2012;22:21–30.

van Geenen EJ, et al. Smoking is related to pancreatic fibrosis in humans. Am J Gastroenterol. 2011;106(6):1161–6; quiz 1167.

Vannasaeng S, Nitiyanant W, Vachayanrat A, Ploybutr S. Characteristics of diabetes with onset under 30 years in Thailand. Childhood and juvenile diabetes mellitus. Amsterdam: Excerpta Medica; 1998. p. 75–9.

Varadarajulu S, Wilcox CM, Eloubeidi MA. Impact of EUS in the evaluation of pancreaticobiliary disorders in children. Gastrointest Endosc. 2005;62(2):239–44.

Walsh RM, et al. Improved quality of life following total pancreatectomy and auto-islet transplantation for chronic pancreatitis. J Gastrointest Surg. 2012;16(8):1469–77.

Watanabe T, Yonemura Y, Yonekura H, Suzuki Y, Miyashita H, Sugiyama K, Moriizumi S, Unno M, Tanaka O, Kondo H, et al. Pancreatic beta-cell replication and amelioration of surgical diabetes by Reg protein. Proc Natl Acad Sci U S A. 1994;91(9):3589–92.

Werlin S, et al. Genetic and electrophysiological characteristics of recurrent acute pancreatitis. J Pediatr Gastroenterol Nutr. 2015;60(5):675–9.

Whitcomb DC. Inflammation and Cancer V. Chronic pancreatitis and pancreatic cancer. Am J Physiol Gastrointest Liver Physiol. 2004;287(2):G315–9.

Whitcomb DC. Genetic risk factors for pancreatic disorders. Gastroenterology. 2013;144(6):1292–302.

Whitcomb DC, Gorry MC, Preston RA, Furey W, Sossenheimer MJ, Ulrich CD, Martin SP, Gates LK, Amann ST, Toskes PP, Liddle R, McGrath K, Uomo G, Post JC, Ehrlich GD. Hereditary pancreatitis is caused by a mutation in the cationic trypsinogen gene. Nat Genet. 1996a;14(2):141–5. doi:10.1038/ng1096-141.

Whitcomb DC, et al. A gene for hereditary pancreatitis maps to chromosome 7q35. Gastroenterology. 1996b;110(6):1975–80.

Whitcomb DC, LaRusch J, Krasinskas AM, Klei L, Smith JP, Brand RE, Neoptolemos JP, Lerch MM, Tector M, Sandhu BS, Guda NM, Orlichenko L, Alzheimer's Disease Genetics Consortium, Alkaade S, Amann ST, Anderson MA, Baillie J, Banks PA, Conwell D, Coté GA, Cotton PB, DiSario J, Farrer LA, Forsmark CE, Johnstone M, Gardner TB, Gelrud A, Greenhalf W, Haines JL, Hartman DJ, Hawes RA, Lawrence C, Lewis M, Mayerle J, Mayeux R, Melhem NM, Money ME, Muniraj T, Papachristou GI, Pericak-Vance MA, Romagnuolo J, Schellenberg GD, Sherman S, Simon P, Singh VP, Slivka A, Stolz D, Sutton R, Weiss FU, Wilcox CM, Zarnescu NO, Wisniewski SR, O'Connell MR, Kienholz ML, Roeder K, Barmada MM, Yadav D, Devlin B. Common genetic variants in the CLDN2 and PRSS1-PRSS2 loci alter risk for alcohol-related and sporadic pancreatitis. Nat Genet. 2012;44(12):1349–54. doi:10.1038/ng.2466.

Wilson GC, et al. Surgical outcomes after total pancreatectomy and islet cell autotransplantation in pediatric patients. Surgery. 2013;154(4):777–83; discussion 783–4.

Wilson GC, et al. Total pancreatectomy with islet cell autotransplantation as the initial treatment for minimal-change chronic pancreatitis. HPB (Oxford). 2015;17(3):232–8.

Witt H. Gene mutations in children with chronic pancreatitis. Pancreatology. 2001;1(5):432–8.

Witt H, Luck W, Hennies HC, Classen M, Kage A, Lass U, Landt O, Becker M. Mutations in the gene encoding the serine protease inhibitor, Kazal type 1 are associated with chronic pancreatitis. Nat Genet. 2000;25(2):213–6. doi:10.1038/76088.

Witt H, Sahin-Tóth M, Landt O, Chen J-M, Kähne T, Drenth JP, Kukor Z, Szepessy E, Halangk W, Dahm S, Rohde K, Schulz H-U, Le Maréchal C, Akar N, Ammann RW, Truninger K, Bargetzi M, Bhatia E, Castellani C, Cavestro GM, Cerny M, Destro-Bisol G, Spedini G, Eiberg H, Jansen JBMJ, Koudova M, Rausova E, Macek M, Malats N, Real FX, Menzel H-J, Moral P, Galavotti R, Pignatti PF, Rickards O, Spicak J, Zarnescu NO, Böck W, Gress TM, Friess H, Ockenga J, Schmidt H, Pfützer R, Löhr M, Simon P, Weiss FU, Lerch MM, Teich N, Keim V, Berg T, Wiedenmann B, Luck W, Groneberg DA, Becker M, Keil T, Kage A, Bernardova J, Braun M, Güldner C, Halangk J, Rosendahl J, Witt U, Treiber M, Nickel R, Férec C. A degradation-sensitive anionic trypsinogen (PRSS2) variant protects against chronic pancreatitis. Nat Genet. 2006;38(6):668–73. doi:10.1038/ng1797.

Witt H, Beer S, Rosendahl J, Chen J-M, Chandak GR, Masamune A, Bence M, Szmola R, Oracz G, Macek M, Bhatia E, Steigenberger S, Lasher D, Bühler F, Delaporte C, Tebbing J, Ludwig M, Pilsak C, Saum K, Bugert P, Masson E, Paliwal S, Bhaskar S, Sobczynska-

Tomaszewska A, Bak D, Balascak I, Choudhuri G, Nageshwar Reddy D, Rao GV, Thomas V, Kume K, Nakano E, Kakuta Y, Shimosegawa T, Durko L, Szabó A, Schnúr A, Hegyi P, Rakonczay Z, Pfützer R, Schneider A, Groneberg DA, Braun M, Schmidt H, Witt U, Friess H, Algül H, Landt O, Schuelke M, Krüger R, Wiedenmann B, Schmidt F, Zimmer K-P, Kovacs P, Stumvoll M, Blüher M, Müller T, Janecke A, Teich N, Grützmann R, Schulz H-U, Mössner J, Keim V, Löhr M, Férec C, Sahin-Tóth M. Variants in CPA1 are strongly associated with early onset chronic pancreatitis. Nat Genet. 2013;45(10):1216–20. doi:10.1038/ng.2730.

Yadav D, et al. Alcohol consumption, cigarette smoking, and the risk of recurrent acute and chronic pancreatitis. Arch Intern Med. 2009;169(11):1035–45.

Yadav D, et al. Incidence, prevalence, and survival of chronic pancreatitis: a population-based study. Am J Gastroenterol. 2011;106(12):2192–9.

Yajnik CS, Shelgikar KM, Sahasrabudhe RA, Naik SS, Pai VR, Alberti KG, Hockaday TD, Katrak A, Dandona P. The spectrum of pancreatic exocrine and endocrine (beta-cell) function in tropical calcific pancreatitis. Diabetologia. 1990;33(7):417–21.

Yoshida K, Toki F, Takeuchi T, et al. Chronic pancreatitis caused by an autoimmune abnormality. Proposal of the concept of autoimmune pancreatitis. Dig Dis Sci. 1995;40:1561–8.

Zen Y, et al. Th2 and regulatory immune reactions are increased in immunoglobin G4-related sclerosing pancreatitis and cholangitis. Hepatology. 2007;45(6):1538–46.

Zen Y, Grammatikopoulos T, Hadzic N. Autoimmune pancreatitis in children: insights into the diagnostic challenge. J Pediatr Gastroenterol Nutr. 2014;59(5):e42–5.

Zou WB, Boulling A, Masamune A, Issarapu P, Masson E, Wu H, Sun XT, Hu LH, Zhou DZ, He L, Fichou Y, Nakano E, Hamada S, Kakuta Y, Kume K, Isayama H, Paliwal S, Mani KR, Bhaskar S, Cooper DN, Ferec C, Shimosegawa T, Chandak GR, Chen JM, Li ZS, Liao Z. No association between CEL-HYB hybrid allele and chronic pancreatitis in Asian populations. Gastroenterology. 2016;150(7):1558–1560.e55. doi:10.1053/j.gastro.2016.02.071.

Zuidema PJ. Calcification and cirrhosis of the pancreas in patients with deficient nutrition. Doc Med Geogr Trop. 1955;7(3):229–51.

Zuidema PJ. Cirrhosis and disseminated calcification of the pancreas in patients with malnutrition. Trop Geogr Med. 1959;11(1):70–4.

Chronic Pancreatitis and Pancreatic Cancer

12

Xiang-Yu Kong and Ke-Ping Xie

1 Introduction

Pancreatic cancer is a fast progressive and highly aggressive malignancy. Clinically, pancreatic cancer exhibits profound resistance to existing treatment modalities and surgical resection remains the only chance for cure of pancreatic cancer patients (Vincent et al. 2011). Development of efficient early detection modality is of highest priority. Epidemiological studies have shown that chronic pancreatitis is one of the major risk factors for pancreatic cancer, and patients with chronic pancreatitis have 2.3 to 18.5-fold increased risk than normal controls (Malka et al. 2002). Delineating the progression from chronic pancreatitis to pancreatic cancer and identifying the genetic and epigenetic events in this process will help detect early-stage pancreatic cancer in chronic pancreatitis cases and improve prognosis of these patients.

Hereditary pancreatitis represents the best model to dissect the causal linkage between chronic pancreatitis and pancreatic cancer. Epidemiological analysis has shown that hereditary pancreatitis ranks the strongest known risk factor for pancreatic cancer (Schneider and Whitcomb 2002). With the advent of molecular techniques, several germ-line mutations within certain genes, *e.g.*, PRSS1 and CFTR, are identified as the major cause for hereditary pancreatitis (Keiles and Kammesheidt 2006). However, these mutations are rarely detected in common chronic pancreatitis cases, indicating that these genes are not directly associated with development of pancreatic cancer (Hengstler et al. 2000; Malats et al. 2001). It is widely believed that inflammation itself, but not those hereditary genes, promotes pancreatic cancer development and progression (Lu et al. 2006).

Once inflammation is initiated, inflammatory cells, especially macrophages, are recruited to the inflicted sites and release cytokines, growth factors, matrix-degrading enzymes and others (Jackson and Evers 2006). All those inflammatory factors, in combination with macrophages, constitute the extrinsic signals, which reprogram the microenvironment to facilitate pancreatic cancer development and progression (Jackson and Evers 2006). Evidently, the inflammatory milieu may disable surveillance mechanisms and destabilize the genome in normal pancreatic cells, which will enhance the generation and accumulation of genetic events within these cells

X.-Yu. Kong
Department of Gastroenterology, Shanghai Changhai Hospital, Shanghai, China

K.-P. Xie (✉)
Departments of Gastroenterology, Hepatology and Nutrition, Unit 1644, The University of Texas MD Anderson Cancer Center, 1515 Holcombe Boulevard, Houston, TX 77030, USA
e-mail: kepxie@mdanderson.org

Z.-S. Li et al. (eds.), *Chronic Pancreatitis*, DOI 10.1007/978-981-10-4515-8_12

and accelerate the process of pancreatic tumor formation. Mechanistically, a number of dysregulated signaling pathways are commonly identified in both chronic pancreatitis and pancreatic cancer tissues. Of clinical significance, most of those altered pathways, including cytokines, NF-κB, reactive oxygen species, PPARγ, and so on, have potential value in pancreatic cancer treatment (Uomo et al. 2010).

However, chronic pancreatitis and pancreatic cancer are two entirely different diseases with distinct prognosis. Under certain circumstances, it is clinically difficult to distinguish from each other (Sakorafas and Tsiotou 1999). Given that numerous signaling pathways are similarly altered in both chronic pancreatitis and pancreatic cancer; it is a daunting challenge to identify potential biomarkers for the differential diagnosis of the two diseases. Currently, all the global proteomic studies have failed to identify pancreatic cancer specific biomarkers, which may arguably be due to the low abundance of those biomarkers in human tissues. Nonetheless, recent studies have discovered a list of protein markers, a combination of which may enhance the diagnostic efficacy for pancreatic cancer (Chan et al. 2014). Moreover, the stability and abundance of DNA and microRNAs in human tissues have also been explored for their clinical utility as pancreatic cancer biomarkers (Schultz et al. 2014).

2 Pancreatic Cancer Is Inflammatory Malignancy

Extensive histopathological studies have identified different precursor lesions as having the potential to evolve into highly malignant and invasive pancreatic cancer, including chronic pancreatitis, pancreatic intraepithelial neoplasia (PanIN), mucinous cystic neoplasms, and intraductal papillary mucinous neoplasms (Brugge et al. 2004; Maitra et al. 2005). PanINs are the most common precancerous lesions in pancreas, constituting the development course of pancreatic cancer (Costello et al. 2012), which is somewhat similar to that of adenoma-carcinoma sequence in the development of colon cancer (Vogelstein et al. 1988).

It have now well documented concerning the genetic and epigenetic alterations accompanying the sequential course of cellular transformation from normal pancreas to pancreatic cancer (Bardeesy and DePinho 2002). Multi-modality analyses with clinic-pathological parameters have further characterized the clinical significance of those alterations in detection and diagnosis, prognostic prediction, treatment selection, and etc. *K-ras* is the most notable and prevalent oncogene identified in pancreatic cancer cells. Although occasionally occurring in normal pancreatic tissue and only 30% of pancreatic lesions at the earliest stage of histopathological disturbance (Klimstra and Longnecker 1994), the frequency of K-ras activation increases as the disease progresses and is found in almost all PDAC cases, making this mutational activation virtually essential for PDAC pathogenesis (Rozenblum et al. 1997). Identification of K-ras mutation as the first notable genetic alteration led to much better understanding of pancreatic cancer genetics, which are including inactivation of tumor-suppressive genes, *e.g.*, p16/CDKN2A, TP53, and SMAD4 (Bardeesy and DePinho 2002). A recent landmark study of sequencing of 23,219 transcripts reveals 20,661 protein-coding genes in 24 PDAC cases. This detailed global genomic study has identified a large number of genetic alterations, among which a core set of 12 signaling pathways and processes are shown to have an altered gene expression in 67–100% of pancreatic cancer cases (Jones et al. 2008).

Apparently, pancreatic cancer takes 20 years to grow into a detectable tumor, and during this time course, an average of 63 genetic alterations happen in each case (Jones et al. 2008). Two prerequisites for pancreatic cancer are proposed: first, there must be immortal pancreatic cells to accumulate these genetic events; second, there must be harsh milieu to efficiently induce the genetic events to happen. Existence of cancer stem cells meets the first prerequisite, whereas the second prerequisite may largely be attributed to chronic inflammation surrounding pancreatic cells (Cooks et al. 2014). Lessons from ulcerative colitis show that the inflammation process will lead to repeated cycles of epithelial cell damage and regeneration, which presumably increase the possibility of somatic mutations and favor cellular transformation and tumorigenesis (Itzkowitz and Yio 2004). Chronic pancreatitis may follow a similar path to pancreatic cancer.

On the other hand, the entire process of pancreatic cancer development and progression is full of inflammation. The inflammatory response is observed at the early stages of pancreatic cancer initiation. For example, we have recently found that active infiltration of inflammatory cells and immune cells is observed during acinar-to-ductal metaplasia phase and KLF4 plays a critical role in inflammatory response, which appears to be important for PanIN formation and progression to late-stage invasive pancreatic cancer. The inflammation is also important to pancreatic desmoplasia. Therefore, pancreatic inflammation could be a cause of pancreatic cellular transformation and cancer initiation, and also could be a driver force of pancreatic cancer promotion and progression.

3 Chronic Pancreatitis Is Malignant Driver

Chronic pancreatitis is a progressive inflammatory disease with irreversibly functional and morphological changes caused by various etiological factors (Liao et al. 2013). Recent investigation on 2008 patients with chronic pancreatitis shows that its incidence in China is increasing (13/100,000) (Wang et al. 2009). Given that inflammation is one of the major risk factor for carcinogenesis, chronic pancreatitis patients would be more susceptible to pancreatic cancer. However, it was Lowenfels and colleagues, who published an international cohort study on clarification of the nature of the risk in 1993 (Lowenfels et al. 1993). In their multicenter cohort study, 2015 chronic pancreatitis cases were enrolled and 56 cancers were identified during a mean follow-up of 7.4 years. The standardized incidence ratio was 14.4 and the risk of developing pancreatic cancer, 20 years after diagnosis, was as high as 4%. Similar studies further confirmed the increased cancer risk in chronic pancreatitis patients, which underlines the significance of differential diagnosis between chronic pancreatitis and pancreatic cancer (Bansal and Sonnenberg 1995).

Hereditary pancreatitis represents the best model to dissect the causal link between chronic pancreatitis and pancreatic cancer. Epidemiological and experimental analyses show that hereditary pancreatitis ranks the strongest known risk factor for pancreatic cancer (Schneider and Whitcomb 2002). By the age of 70 years old, 40% of patients with hereditary pancreatitis will develop pancreatic tumors (Lowenfels et al. 1997). Genetic studies identified germ-line mutations in the PRSS1 gene and CFTR gene as leading causes to hereditary pancreatitis. One important question was whether these genes actually oncogenes for development of sporadic pancreatic carcinomas. To address this question, Hengstler et al. analyzed genomic DNA in pancreatic tissue for R122H mutations in the trypsinogen gene from 34 patients and corresponding normal tissue from 28 of these individuals. No mutations were found (Hengstler et al. 2000). Malats et al. have also shown that the incidence of mutations of CFTR gene in sporadic pancreatic cancers were similar to that in healthy controls (Malats et al. 2001). These studies suggest that PRSS1 and CFTR gene mutations are not directly associated with the development of pancreatic cancer. Interestingly, hereditary pancreatitis arises mainly during or soon after childhood, which means that those patients with hereditary pancreatitis will endure chronic inflammation with onset of an early age (Raimondi et al. 2009). Though mutations in PRSS1 and CFTR genes do not directly contribute to pancreatic cancer development and progression, the high-risk inflammation milieu caused by them may play important roles in this regard.

Histopathologically, pancreatic cancer contains two compartments as major components of pancreatic cancer, the malignant ductal cells and the surrounding stromal cells, with the latter accounts for 90% of total tumor mass (Neesse et al. 2011). Previous studies establish that the stroma formation was initiated and sustained by the out-of-control inflammation, and recent studies from genetic mouse models indicate that inflammation induced by pancreatitis will significantly promote pancreatic tumor formation (Carriere et al. 2009; Gidekel Friedlander et al. 2009; Guerra et al. 2007; Morris et al. 2010). Though it is evident that chronic pancreatitis is a significant risk factor in inducing cellular transformation and pancreatic carcinogenesis, detailed mechanisms underlying the progression from chronic pancreatitis to pancreatic cancer remain to be explored (Kong et al. 2012).

4 Pathways Linking Chronic Pancreatitis to Pancreatic Cancer

The concept of the strong link between inflammation and cancer was first proposed in the nineteenth century by Virchow, who observed the presence of inflammation cells within neoplastic tissues (Balkwill and Mantovani 2001). Epidemiological and clinical researches support his hypothesis and reveal the causal link between chronic inflammation and cancer. For example, the ulcerative colitis, which is a common chronic inflammatory disease affecting the large bowel mucosa, may provide the strongest evidence to whether and how inflammation affect carcinogenesis progress. Patients with ulcerative colitis are more predisposed to colorectal cancer, which is in the order of tenfold greater than that in the general Western population (Itzkowitz and Yio 2004). Inflammation-cancer connection is not unique to a subset of tumors, but universally identified within different cancer types, including lung, bladder, gastrointestinal tract, skin and vulva. Use of anti-inflammatory medications, *e.g.*, aspirin, is usually associated with protection against various tumors, which to some extent substantiate that inflammation is a risk factor for many types of cancer (McKay et al. 2008). While the link between inflammation and cancer is clearly strong, detailed mechanisms underlying this connection warrant more studies.

The chronic pancreatitis-pancreatic cancer link has also been established in different ethnic cohorts independently by different groups. Nonetheless, "chronic pancreatitis-pancreatic cancer" connection holds certain traits different from other cancer types. For example, COX-2 levels were significantly elevated in chronic pancreatitis patients, and targeted therapy against COX-2 appears be a good therapeutic strategy to treat chronic pancreatitis (Reding et al. 2006). However, aspirin, the most commonly used COX-2 inhibitor, exhibits controversial effects to pancreatic cancer (Jacobs et al. 2004). Extended periods of regular aspirin use may likely increase risk of pancreatic cancer among women (Schernhammer et al. 2004). These inconsistent results suggested that there exist a complex network among pancreatic cells and inflammatory milieu, and a list of comprehensive studies is needed to explore or validate current knowledge framework concerning "inflammation-cancer" connection in pancreatic cancer. To this end, multiple animal models have been established for dissecting the effects of inflammatory mediators and anti-inflammatory drugs on "chronic pancreatitis-pancreatic cancer" progression (Mazur et al. 2015). Currently used animal models are primarily developed based on the genetic activation of resident *K-ras* oncogenes knocked-in within the endogenous *K-ras* locus (Olive et al. 2009). These models faithfully recapitulate the histological lesions that characterize many aspects of human pancreatic tumors, including a desmoplastic stroma and inflammatory responses that closely resemble those observed in human patients. Of particular interest, these animals will not develop into pancreatic cancer, unless undergo pancreatic damage in the form of pancreatitis (Hingorani et al. 2003). These results further confirm the indispensable functions of inflammation in pancreatic carcinogenesis. Many insightful mechanisms have been identified linking pancreatitis and pancreatic cancer by using the genetic animal models and can be arguably grouped into intrinsic pathway and extrinsic pathway.

4.1 Extrinsic Pathways Linking Chronic Pancreatitis and Pancreatic Cancer

Besides neoplastic cells, the pancreatic cancer mass is composed of a stroma constituting of fibroblasts, vessels and leukocytes. Inflammation is the primary insult causing the robust stroma reaction surrounding pancreatic cancer cells (Elinav et al. 2013). Significantly, inflammatory cells, especially those leukocytes, are the major players in initiating and sustaining the inflammation reaction. The leukocytes within tumor stroma, as well as those cytokines and growth factors derived from leukocytes, constitute the complex extrinsic pathways, which play a critical role in cellular transformation and tumorigenesis process (Hidalgo 2010).

Tumor associated macrophages (TAMs) are the principal leukocytes driving an amplification of the inflammatory response in the tumor milieu. TAMs belong to the myeloid cell lineage and derive from myeloid progenitor cells. These precursor cells are located in the bone marrow; upon maturation, monocytes are released into the bloodstream. At the recruitment by certain chemokines, *e.g.*, CCL2 and CCL5, TAMs accumulate in tumor stroma, where TAMs are educated to facilitate cancer progression. TAMs assists tumor cell malignant behavior in many ways by releasing cytokines, growth factors and matrix-degrading enzymes and many angiogenic factors (Colotta et al. 2009). Numerous molecular alterations are involved in "TAM-pancreatic cancer" connection. For examples, administration of agonist CD40 antibody will activate macrophages, which help macrophages infiltrate tumors, became tumoricidal, and facilitated the depletion of tumor stroma (Beatty et al. 2011). TAMs secrete MIP3α to increase migration ability of pancreatic cancer cells by binding to the transmembrane receptor CCR6 (Campbell et al. 2005). TAMs could convey proangiogenetic effects to pancreatic cancer cells. Blocking angiopoietin-2 (ANG2), a TIE2 ligand and angiogenic factor, could impede the upregulation of Tie2 in TAMs, and decrease tumor angiogenesis of pancreatic cancer (Mazzieri et al. 2011). Furthermore, TAMs could help maintain the cancer stem cells, which have been linked to chemoresistance, metastatic dissemination, and the induction of immune suppression (Mitchem et al. 2013). Blockage the connection between TAMs and cancer stem cells could eliminate the cancer stem cells, improve chemotherapeutic response, and generate promising therapeutic efficacy. Therefore, TAMs and the complex cytokines network greatly enhance the tumorigenesis of pancreatic cancer. Targeted treatment against TAM may be promising in future pancreatic cancer therapeutics.

4.2 Intrinsic Pathways Within Pancreatic Cancer Cells Modulated by Chronic Pancreatitis

Previous studies have reported that each pancreatic cancer case contain an average of 63 genetic alterations, most of which are point mutations. These alterations define a core set of 12 cellular signaling pathways (Jones et al. 2008). However, the rates of spontaneous mutations within normal pancreatic cells are very low. Compared with normal pancreatic cells, the widespread destabilization of gene copy number and nucleotide sequence assure us that instability of the genome is universally inherent within pancreatic cancer cells (Hanahan and Weinberg 2011). In normal cells, there is extraordinary ability of genome maintenance systems to detect and resolve defects in the DNA, whereas in cancer cells, the protection mechanisms are defected and enable these cells to accumulate more genetic alterations and advantageously develop into a tumor (Hanahan and Weinberg 2011).

Evidently, inflammatory microenvironment participates in genome instability of pancreatic cancer cells. For example, Bielas et al. have reported that the mutation rate in the inflamed microenvironment is higher than in normal tissues, with a mutation frequency of 4×10^{-8} and $<1 \times 10^{8}$ per base pair, respectively (Bielas et al. 2006). The hallmark suppressor p53, critical in protecting genomes from instability, shows high frequency of mutations in chronic pancreatitis (Gansauge et al. 1998). Higher incidence of mutations within pancreatic cancer cells is largely attributed to the deregulate DNA repair systems and altered cell cycle checkpoints, whereas derivatives generated by inflammatory cells are also responsible for the destruction against these genome maintainers. For example, inflammatory cytokines, *e.g.*, TNF and IL-1β, could induce HIF-α in pancreatic cancer cells, which may destruct the mismatch repair mechanisms and leads to instability of genomes (Akakura et al. 2001). Nitrogen oxide (NO), another important mediator derived from inflammation microenvironment, could induce upregulation of DNA methyltransferase and result in promoter silencing and loss of gene expression of the mismatch repair member hMLH1 (Fleisher et al. 2000). NO and its derivatives could also inhibit the function of p53 and are associated with p53 mutations (Jaiswal et al. 2001), which will significantly attenuate its detection and repair ability against genome instability. Other inflammatory elements, including COX-2, reactive oxygen species, and MMPs can also tamper the genome surveillance machinery (Hanahan and Weinberg 2011). Through these different mechanisms, inflammatory elements render the cancer genomes instable, which leads to a genomically heterogeneous population of expanding cells naturally selected for their ability to proliferate, invade and metastasize to distant tissues, and evading host defenses (Hanahan and Weinberg 2011).

5 Common Alterations Involved in Pancreatic Cancer and Chronic Pancreatitis

Epidemiologic data identified inflammation as a significant risk factor for solid tumors. Both hereditary and sporadic forms of chronic pancreatitis are associated with increased risk of pancreatic cancer. In such context, the focus of cancer research have recently shifted from pancreatic cancer cells to the inflammatory milieu surrounding them, and identified a list of notable targets involved in inflammation-associated carcinogenesis. Targeted therapy against certain molecules generates promising effects in clinic. Novel therapeutics targeting the extrinsic and intrinsic pathways linking chronic pancreatitis and pancreatic cancer would decrease the levels of tumor-promoting properties of the inflammatory cells, and ultimately balance the inflammatory network to regain a normal homeostasis.

Cytokines The progressive and irreversible desmoplasia within chronic pancreatitis are largely attributed to the cytokines existing in stroma (Cavestro et al. 2003). Many cytokines have been identified within chronic pancreatitis, including TNF-α, IL-1, IL-6, IL-8, PDGF, TGF-β, and etc. A similar expression pattern of chemokines is found in pancreatic cancer (Farrow and Evers 2002). As pancreatic inflammation represents an early step in the development of pancreatic cancer (McKay et al. 2008), it is logical to believe that these cytokines are engaged in pancreatic carcinogenesis. Numerous studies have demonstrated the tumor-promoting roles of these cytokines in pancreatic carcinogenesis (Yu and Kim 2014). For example, TNF-α is normally expressed under the context of pancreatic acinar cell injury, whereas in chronic pancreatitis, TNF-α could upregulate PDGF expression, which is known to strongly stimulate fibrogenesis (Friess et al. 1999). PDGF, as well as other TNF-α downstream targets, *e.g.*, EGFR and TGF-α, are all well-known oncogenes in pancreatic carcinogenesis (Kalthoff et al. 1993). Through NF-κB activation, TNF-α may also inhibit apoptosis of pancreatic cancer cells (McDade et al. 1999). These data suggest that abnormal cytokine expressions in chronic pancreatitis are significantly associated with pancreatic carcinogenesis. A new generation of vaccines directed against cytokine activity could be beneficial in future treatment of cancer (Zagury et al. 2001).

Nuclear factor kappa B Nuclear factor kappa B (NF-κB) is an important transcription factor proved to be involved in multiple cellular activities (Suzuki et al. 2011). The functional NF-κB in pancreas is a p65/p50 heterodimer. Under normal conditions, NF-κB dimers are bound to inhibitory proteins, IκBs, which block nuclear localization sequences and thus trap the dimers within the cytoplasm where they were inactive (DiDonato et al. 1997). However, in inflammatory response, *e.g.*, pancreatitis, IκBs are degraded and NF-κB subsequently translocate into the nucleus, where it interacts with other transcription factors and binds to its consensus sequence on promoters of target genes (Huang et al. 2013). Enhanced NF-κB activity is associated with increased severity of acute and chronic pancreatitis (Huang et al. 2013). NF-κB activity is ubiquitously unregulated in many cancer types. It has been suggested that NF-κB plays its role in carcinogenesis through its inhibition of apoptosis of preneoplastic cells and the maintenance of a pro-neoplastic microenvironment rich in proinflammatory mediators (McKay et al. 2008). Targeted therapy against NF-κB could induce apoptosis and increase gemcitabine effectiveness in a subset of pancreatic cancer cells (Pan et al. 2008). Due to the critical role that NF-κB plays in linking chronic pancreatitis and pancreatic cancer, restoration of its expression and function may decrease the tumor-promoting effects of inflammatory cells, with hope to orchestrate the homeostatic relationship between inflammation and pancreatic cells.

Peroxisome proliferator-activated receptor-γ Peroxisome proliferator-activated receptor-γ (PPARγ) is a nuclear receptor and transcription factor, which can repress inflammatory genes and orchestrate inflammation homeostasis (Glass and Saijo 2010). Ligands of PPARγ play important roles in preventing the out-of-control inflammation in various tissues. For examples, different PPARγ agonists could reduce the severity of cerulein-induced acute pancreatitis (Hashimoto et al. 2003; Cuzzocrea et al. 2004). PPARγ agonists could inhibit the proinflammatory cytokine gene expression within macrophages to prevent the development of chronic pancreatitis (Shimizu et al. 2002). Also, PPARγ overexpression could inhibit pro-fibrogenic activities of immortalized rat pancreatic stellate cells to suppress chronic inflammation process (Jaster et al. 2005). Furthermore, the impact of PPARγ on pancreatic cancer development and progression has support the notion that chronic pancreatitis is strongly associated pancreatic cancer. For examples, PPARγ ligand could suppress cancer growth (Elnemr et al. 2000). A list of targets, including cyclin D1, p27KiP1, and PTEN are implicated in its anti-tumor effects (Diao and Chen 2007). Troglitazone is a well-known PPARγ ligand, and clinical studies have shown that troglitazone could significantly lower PSA levels in prostate cancer patients (Mueller et al. 2000). However, its therapeutic efficacy against pancreatic cancer have not been evaluated in clinics.

Reactive oxygen species Reactive oxygen species are generated by activated neutrophils and macrophages during inflammation. Reactive oxygen species has been implicated in the pathogenesis of acute and chronic pancreatitis, and antioxidants could be potentially effective against the development of pancreatic fibrosis in patients with chronic pancreatitis (Asaumi et al. 2007). Furthermore, highly reactive oxygen species could promote repeated tissue damage and regeneration during chronic pancreatitis. In this process, reactive oxygen species can induce genotoxic effects, including DNA strand breaks, sister chromatid exchanges, and formation of adducts with DNA (Jackson and Loeb 2001). Repeated damage-regeneration stimuli could impose permanent genomic alterations into pancreatic cells, which further accelerate the mutation accumulation, and subsequently the carcinogenesis process (Campisi and d'Adda di Fagagna 2007). Though the anti-tumor effects of those compounds with anti-oxidant activity have not been validated in clinic, epidemiologic studies show that intake of fresh fruit and vegetables appears to be inversely correlated with pancreatic cancer (Wiseman and Halliwell 1996). Eradication of reactive oxygen species from chronic inflammatory milieu will protect pancreatic cells DNA from genotoxic damage, and could perhaps lower the incident of transformation of these cells.

6 Differential Diagnosis Between Pancreatic Cancer and Chronic Pancreatitis

Chronic pancreatitis and pancreatic cancer are two distinct diseases with entirely different prognosis. However, it is a great challenge to discriminate them from each other in many cases. Several reasons contribute to this challenge. First, just like chronic pancreatitis tissues which are mostly made of fibrosis, more than 90% of pancreatic tumor mass is also made of the stroma element. Fine needle aspiration, the most commonly used technique to sample a pancreatic mass, usually could not obtain the tissue containing pancreatic cells. Second, there are too many common pathways dysregulated among chronic pancreatitis and pancreatic cancer tissues, such as reactive oxygen species, Hedgehog, NF-κB, and etc. At the present time, none of the global proteomic studies have identified cancer-specific proteins (Goggins 2005). Third, as chronic pancreatitis patients are more susceptible to develop into pancreatic cancer, the chronic pancreatitis patients are frequently followed up. However, even using the most advanced techniques, one cannot exclude the existence of malignant cells hidden within a chronic inflammatory mass (Cote et al. 2013).

It is generally accepted that stroma formation is a critical hallmark characteristic for pancreatic cancer, and the transformation of pancreatic cells usually occur in inflamed tissues (Xie and Xie 2015). Most previous cancer biomarker studies using modern technologies are methodologically flawed as they compare samples from cancer patients with those of healthy, inflammation-free people (Morcos et al. 2013). An accurate and non-invasive test to differentiate pancreatic cancer from chronic pancreatitis would be extremely helpful to detect pancreatic cancer at an early stage and help physicians to make the right treatment decisions and prolong patients' survival.

Protein Biomarkers CA19-9 is the most widely used tumor maker for pancreatic cancer, and its sensitivity is ~80%, while only about 55% for small and resectable cancers (<3 cm) (Ballehaninna and Chamberlain 2011). Disappointingly, in high-risk, asymptomatic individuals harboring IPMNs or high-grade PanINs, serum CA19-9 is often normal (Maitra and Hruban 2008). Furthermore, chronic pancreatitis tissues also exhibit high positive rates of CA19-9 expression (Shi et al. 2014). These data showed that CA19-9 is not an optimal biomarker to detect those non-malignant pancreatic tumors, nor is suitable to distinguish pancreatic cancer from chronic pancreatitis and other nonneoplastic pancreatic diseases. Recent efforts have been devoted to those markers with capacity to distinguish pancreatic cancer from chronic pancreatitis cases, and have identified a list of markers with potential clinical application (Crnogorac-Jurcevic et al. 2005). For example, using quantitative RT-PCR and immunohistochemistry to analyze the expression of UHRF1, ATP7A and aldehyde oxidase 1 in combination could potentially provide an additional useful diagnostic tool for fine-needle aspirated or cytological specimens obtained during endoscopic procedures (Crnogorac-Jurcevic et al. 2005). PAM4 is a monoclonal antibody expressed by 90% of PDAC, as well as the precursor lesions PanIN and intraductal papillary mucinous neoplasm, and shows high specificity for PDAC and precursor lesions versus benign, nonneoplastic pancreatic tissues. Interestingly, approximately 80% of chronic pancreatitis patients are negative for circulating PAM4 antigen, which highlights PAM4's potential use in differential diagnosis between chronic pancreatitis and pancreatic cancer (Shi et al. 2014).

DNA and RNA biomarkers Early studies indicate that human plasma are rich in nuclease, so that DNA and RNA fragments could not be stably detected as markers for cancer detection and diagnosis (Kong et al. 2011). However, recent studies show that DNA and RNA molecules could also serve as markers with potential clinical applications. For example, KRAS2 mutations in codon 12 could stably be detected in circulating deoxyribo nucleic acid, and its positive rate is significantly higher in pancreatic cancer than in chronic pancreatitis patients (47% *vs.* 13%). A combined normal serum CA19-9 and absence of circulating KRAS2 mutations may significantly increase the differential diagnosis efficacy between chronic pancreatitis and pancreatic cancer (Maire et al. 2002).

microRNAs microRNAs (miRNAs) are endogenous, small, non-coding RNAs that repress the expression of target mRNAs. More than 1500 mature human miRNA sequences are listed in the miRNA database (Kozomara and Griffiths-Jones 2014). These sequences play important roles in virtually all biological pathways in mammals and other multicellular organisms (Berezikov 2011). Despite their subtle effects on individual targets, miRNAs are responsible for the modulation of multiple signaling pathways involved in cell growth, proliferation, differentiation, motility, and apoptosis (Kang et al. 2016). In fact, a number of miRNAs are located in fragile regions of the human genome that are associated with cancer development, and dysregulated miRNAs play crucial roles in tumor initiation, progression, and metastasis and are often associated with diagnosis, prognosis, and response to therapy (Rachagani et al. 2015).

There are many miRNAs that play important roles in pancreatic cancer development and progression, including miR-494 (Li et al. 2014). Our recent study has suggested that miRNAs could be stably detected in plasma and may serve as good markers for pancreatic cancer diagnosis (Kong et al. 2011). Among seven miRNAs evaluated in our study, miR-21 is able to distinguish pancreatic cancer from chronic pancreatitis and healthy patients; whereas miR-155 and miR-196a are able to differentiate sera with diseased pancreas (pancreatic cancer/chronic pancreatitis) from normal pancreas. Further quantitation of miRNAs in whole blood from pancreatic cancer, chronic pancreatitis and healthy controls has identified two panels of microRNAs with potential to distinguish pancreatic cancer patients from chronic pancreatitis and healthy controls (Schultz et al. 2014).

7 Summary

Pancreatic cancer is a lethal disease with unknown etiology. Chronic pancreatitis is a common chronic inflammatory disease, which affects the structural integrity and functions of pancreas. Clinical and experimental studies have suggested that chronic pancreatitis is a major risk factor for pancreatic cancer, whereas numerous extrinsic and intrinsic pathways have been linked to chronic pancreatitis to pancreatic cancer pathogenesis. Intriguingly, many genetic and epigenetic alterations are commonly detected in both chronic pancreatitis and pancreatic cancer tissues, while therapy targeting some alterations produces certain efficacy in pancreatic cancer treatment. However, chronic pancreatitis and pancreatic cancer patients have entirely distinct prognosis and require different management, differential diagnosis between them in clinic is extremely important. Most cancer biomarker studies using modern technologies are methodologically flawed as they compare samples from cancer patients with those from healthy, inflammation-free people. Future studies regarding pancreatic cancer biomarker discovery should exclude those molecules that are dysregulated in chronic pancreatitis tissues, thus uncovering pancreatic cancer specific biomarkers for diagnosis and treatment.

Acknowledgment *Funding*: Supported in part by grants R01-CA129956, R01-CA148954, R01CA152309 and R01CA172233, and R01CA195651; and grant No.81402017 from NSFC of China.

Conflicts of Interest: The authors disclose no conflicts.

References

Akakura N, et al. Constitutive expression of hypoxia-inducible factor-1alpha renders pancreatic cancer cells resistant to apoptosis induced by hypoxia and nutrient deprivation. Cancer Res. 2001;61:6548–54.

Asaumi H, Watanabe S, Taguchi M, Tashiro M, Otsuki M. Externally applied pressure activates pancreatic stellate cells through the generation of intracellular reactive oxygen species. Am J Physiol Gastrointest Liver Physiol. 2007;293:G972–8.

Balkwill F, Mantovani A. Inflammation and cancer: back to Virchow? Lancet. 2001;357:539–45.
Ballehaninna UK, Chamberlain RS. Serum CA 19-9 as a biomarker for pancreatic cancer—a comprehensive review. Indian J Surg Oncol. 2011;2:88–100.
Bansal P, Sonnenberg A. Pancreatitis is a risk factor for pancreatic cancer. Gastroenterology. 1995;109:247–51.
Bardeesy N, DePinho RA. Pancreatic cancer biology and genetics. Nat Rev Cancer. 2002;2:897–909.
Beatty GL, et al. CD40 agonists alter tumor stroma and show efficacy against pancreatic carcinoma in mice and humans. Science. 2011;331:1612–6.
Berezikov E. Evolution of microRNA diversity and regulation in animals. Nat Rev Genet. 2011;12:846–60.
Bielas JH, Loeb KR, Rubin BP, True LD, Loeb LA. Human cancers express a mutator phenotype. Proc Natl Acad Sci U S A. 2006;103:18238–42.
Brugge WR, Lauwers GY, Sahani D, Fernandez-del Castillo C, Warshaw AL. Cystic neoplasms of the pancreas. N Engl J Med. 2004;351:1218–26.
Campbell AS, Albo D, Kimsey TF, White SL, Wang TN. Macrophage inflammatory protein-3alpha promotes pancreatic cancer cell invasion. J Surg Res. 2005;123:96–101.
Campisi J, d'Adda di Fagagna F. Cellular senescence: when bad things happen to good cells. Nat Rev Mol Cell Biol. 2007;8:729–40.
Carriere C, Young AL, Gunn JR, Longnecker DS, Korc M. Acute pancreatitis markedly accelerates pancreatic cancer progression in mice expressing oncogenic Kras. Biochem Biophys Res Commun. 2009;382:561–5.
Cavestro GM, Comparato G, Nouvenne A, Sianesi M, Di Mario F. The race from chronic pancreatitis to pancreatic cancer. JOP. 2003;4:165–8.
Chan A, et al. Validation of biomarkers that complement CA19.9 in detecting early pancreatic cancer. Clin Cancer Res. 2014;20:5787–95.
Colotta F, Allavena P, Sica A, Garlanda C, Mantovani A. Cancer-related inflammation, the seventh hallmark of cancer: links to genetic instability. Carcinogenesis. 2009;30:1073–81.
Cooks T, Harris CC, Oren M. Caught in the cross fire: p53 in inflammation. Carcinogenesis. 2014;35:1680–90.
Costello E, Greenhalf W, Neoptolemos JP. New biomarkers and targets in pancreatic cancer and their application to treatment. Nat Rev Gastroenterol Hepatol. 2012;9:435–44.
Cote GA, Smith J, Sherman S, Kelly K. Technologies for imaging the normal and diseased pancreas. Gastroenterology. 2013;144:1262–71.e1.
Crnogorac-Jurcevic T, et al. Proteomic analysis of chronic pancreatitis and pancreatic adenocarcinoma. Gastroenterology. 2005;129:1454–63.
Cuzzocrea S, et al. Rosiglitazone, a ligand of the peroxisome proliferator-activated receptor-gamma, reduces acute pancreatitis induced by cerulein. Intensive Care Med. 2004;30:951–6.
Diao L, Chen YG. PTEN, a general negative regulator of cyclin D expression. Cell Res. 2007;17:291–2.
DiDonato JA, Hayakawa M, Rothwarf DM, Zandi E, Karin M. A cytokine-responsive IkappaB kinase that activates the transcription factor NF-kappaB. Nature. 1997;388:548–54.
Elinav E, et al. Inflammation-induced cancer: crosstalk between tumours, immune cells and microorganisms. Nat Rev Cancer. 2013;13:759–71.
Elnemr A, et al. PPARgamma ligand (thiazolidinedione) induces growth arrest and differentiation markers of human pancreatic cancer cells. Int J Oncol. 2000;17:1157–64.
Farrow B, Evers BM. Inflammation and the development of pancreatic cancer. Surg Oncol. 2002;10:153–69.
Fleisher AS, et al. Microsatellite instability in inflammatory bowel disease-associated neoplastic lesions is associated with hypermethylation and diminished expression of the DNA mismatch repair gene, hMLH1. Cancer Res. 2000;60:4864–8.
Friess H, Guo XZ, Nan BC, Kleeff J, Buchler MW. Growth factors and cytokines in pancreatic carcinogenesis. Ann N Y Acad Sci. 1999;880:110–21.
Gansauge S, et al. Genetic alterations in chronic pancreatitis: evidence for early occurrence of p53 but not K-ras mutations. Br J Surg. 1998;85:337–40.
Gidekel Friedlander SY, et al. Context-dependent transformation of adult pancreatic cells by oncogenic K-Ras. Cancer Cell. 2009;16:379–89.
Glass CK, Saijo K. Nuclear receptor transrepression pathways that regulate inflammation in macrophages and T cells. Nat Rev Immunol. 2010;10:365–76.
Goggins M. Molecular markers of early pancreatic cancer. J Clin Oncol. 2005;23:4524–31.
Guerra C, et al. Chronic pancreatitis is essential for induction of pancreatic ductal adenocarcinoma by K-Ras oncogenes in adult mice. Cancer Cell. 2007;11:291–302.
Hanahan D, Weinberg RA. Hallmarks of cancer: the next generation. Cell. 2011;144:646–74.
Hashimoto K, Ethridge RT, Saito H, Rajaraman S, Evers BM. The PPARgamma ligand, 15d-PGJ2, attenuates the severity of cerulein-induced acute pancreatitis. Pancreas. 2003;27:58–66.
Hengstler JG, et al. Mutation analysis of the cationic trypsinogen gene in patients with pancreatic cancer. Anticancer Res. 2000;20:2967–74.
Hidalgo M. Pancreatic cancer. N Engl J Med. 2010;362:1605–17.
Hingorani SR, et al. Preinvasive and invasive ductal pancreatic cancer and its early detection in the mouse. Cancer Cell. 2003;4:437–50.
Huang H, et al. Activation of nuclear factor-kappaB in acinar cells increases the severity of pancreatitis in mice. Gastroenterology. 2013;144:202–10.
Itzkowitz SH, Yio X. Inflammation and cancer IV. Colorectal cancer in inflammatory bowel disease: the role of inflammation. Am J Physiol Gastrointest Liver Physiol. 2004;287:G7–17.
Jackson L, Evers BM. Chronic inflammation and pathogenesis of GI and pancreatic cancers. Cancer Treat Res. 2006;130:39–65.
Jackson AL, Loeb LA. The contribution of endogenous sources of DNA damage to the multiple mutations in cancer. Mutat Res. 2001;477:7–21.

Jacobs EJ, et al. Aspirin use and pancreatic cancer mortality in a large United States cohort. J Natl Cancer Inst. 2004;96:524–8.
Jaiswal M, LaRusso NF, Gores GJ. Nitric oxide in gastrointestinal epithelial cell carcinogenesis: linking inflammation to oncogenesis. Am J Physiol Gastrointest Liver Physiol. 2001;281:G626–34.
Jaster R, et al. Peroxisome proliferator-activated receptor gamma overexpression inhibits pro-fibrogenic activities of immortalised rat pancreatic stellate cells. J Cell Mol Med. 2005;9:670–82.
Jones S, et al. Core signaling pathways in human pancreatic cancers revealed by global genomic analyses. Science. 2008;321:1801–6.
Kalthoff H, Roeder C, Brockhaus M, Thiele HG, Schmiegel W. Tumor necrosis factor (TNF) up-regulates the expression of p75 but not p55 TNF receptors, and both receptors mediate, independently of each other, up-regulation of transforming growth factor alpha and epidermal growth factor receptor mRNA. J Biol Chem. 1993;268:2762–6.
Kang H, et al. Downregulation of microRNA-362-3p and microRNA-329 promotes tumor progression in human breast cancer. Cell Death Differ. 2016;23(3):484–95.
Keiles S, Kammesheidt A. Identification of CFTR, PRSS1, and SPINK1 mutations in 381 patients with pancreatitis. Pancreas. 2006;33:221–7.
Klimstra DS, Longnecker DS. K-ras mutations in pancreatic ductal proliferative lesions. Am J Pathol. 1994;145:1547–50.
Kong X, et al. Detection of differentially expressed microRNAs in serum of pancreatic ductal adenocarcinoma patients: miR-196a could be a potential marker for poor prognosis. Dig Dis Sci. 2011;56:602–9.
Kong X, Li L, Li Z, Xie K. Targeted destruction of the orchestration of the pancreatic stroma and tumor cells in pancreatic cancer cases: molecular basis for therapeutic implications. Cytokine Growth Factor Rev. 2012;23:343–56.
Kozomara A, Griffiths-Jones S. miRBase: annotating high confidence microRNAs using deep sequencing data. Nucleic Acids Res. 2014;42:D68–73.
Li L, et al. Down-regulation of microRNA-494 via loss of SMAD4 increases FOXM1 and beta-catenin signaling in pancreatic ductal adenocarcinoma cells. Gastroenterology. 2014;147:485–97.e18.
Liao Z, et al. Guidelines: diagnosis and therapy for chronic pancreatitis. J Interv Gastroenterol. 2013;3:133–6.
Lowenfels AB, et al. Pancreatitis and the risk of pancreatic cancer. International Pancreatitis Study Group. N Engl J Med. 1993;328:1433–7.
Lowenfels AB, et al. Hereditary pancreatitis and the risk of pancreatic cancer. International Hereditary Pancreatitis Study Group. J Natl Cancer Inst. 1997;89:442–6.
Lu H, Ouyang W, Huang C. Inflammation, a key event in cancer development. Mol Cancer Res. 2006;4:221–33.
Maire F, et al. Differential diagnosis between chronic pancreatitis and pancreatic cancer: value of the detection of KRAS2 mutations in circulating DNA. Br J Cancer. 2002;87:551–4.
Maitra A, Hruban RH. Pancreatic cancer. Annu Rev Pathol. 2008;3:157–88.
Maitra A, Fukushima N, Takaori K, Hruban RH. Precursors to invasive pancreatic cancer. Adv Anat Pathol. 2005;12:81–91.
Malats N, et al. Cystic fibrosis transmembrane regulator (CFTR) DeltaF508 mutation and 5T allele in patients with chronic pancreatitis and exocrine pancreatic cancer. PANKRAS II Study Group. Gut. 2001;48:70–4.
Malka D, et al. Risk of pancreatic adenocarcinoma in chronic pancreatitis. Gut. 2002;51:849–52.
Mazur PK, Herner A, Neff F, Siveke JT. Current methods in mouse models of pancreatic cancer. Methods Mol Biol. 2015;1267:185–215.
Mazzieri R, et al. Targeting the ANG2/TIE2 axis inhibits tumor growth and metastasis by impairing angiogenesis and disabling rebounds of proangiogenic myeloid cells. Cancer Cell. 2011;19:512–26.
McDade TP, Perugini RA, Vittimberga FJ Jr, Carrigan RC, Callery MP. Salicylates inhibit NF-kappaB activation and enhance TNF-alpha-induced apoptosis in human pancreatic cancer cells. J Surg Res. 1999;83:56–61.
McKay CJ, Glen P, McMillan DC. Chronic inflammation and pancreatic cancer. Best Pract Res Clin Gastroenterol. 2008;22:65–73.
Mitchem JB, et al. Targeting tumor-infiltrating macrophages decreases tumor-initiating cells, relieves immunosuppression, and improves chemotherapeutic responses. Cancer Res. 2013;73:1128–41.
Morcos NY, Zakhary NI, Said MM, Tadros MM. Postoperative simple biochemical markers for prediction of bone metastases in Egyptian breast cancer patients. Ecancermedicalscience. 2013;7:305.
Morris JP, Cano DA, Sekine S, Wang SC, Hebrok M. Beta-catenin blocks Kras-dependent reprogramming of acini into pancreatic cancer precursor lesions in mice. J Clin Invest. 2010;120:508–20.
Mueller E, et al. Effects of ligand activation of peroxisome proliferator-activated receptor gamma in human prostate cancer. Proc Natl Acad Sci U S A. 2000;97:10990–5.
Neesse A, et al. Stromal biology and therapy in pancreatic cancer. Gut. 2011;60:861–8.
Olive KP, et al. Inhibition of Hedgehog signaling enhances delivery of chemotherapy in a mouse model of pancreatic cancer. Science. 2009;324:1457–61.
Pan X, et al. Nuclear factor-kappaB p65/relA silencing induces apoptosis and increases gemcitabine effectiveness in a subset of pancreatic cancer cells. Clin Cancer Res. 2008;14:8143–51.
Rachagani S, et al. Clinical implications of miRNAs in the pathogenesis, diagnosis and therapy of pancreatic cancer. Adv Drug Deliv Rev. 2015;81:16–33.
Raimondi S, Maisonneuve P, Lowenfels AB. Epidemiology of pancreatic cancer: an overview. Nat Rev Gastroenterol Hepatol. 2009;6:699–708.
Reding T, et al. A selective COX-2 inhibitor suppresses chronic pancreatitis in an animal model (WBN/Kob

rats): significant reduction of macrophage infiltration and fibrosis. Gut. 2006;55:1165–73.

Rozenblum E, et al. Tumor-suppressive pathways in pancreatic carcinoma. Cancer Res. 1997;57:1731–4.

Sakorafas GH, Tsiotou AG. Pancreatic cancer in patients with chronic pancreatitis: a challenge from a surgical perspective. Cancer Treat Rev. 1999;25:207–17.

Schernhammer ES, et al. A prospective study of aspirin use and the risk of pancreatic cancer in women. J Natl Cancer Inst. 2004;96:22–8.

Schneider A, Whitcomb DC. Hereditary pancreatitis: a model for inflammatory diseases of the pancreas. Best Pract Res Clin Gastroenterol. 2002;16:347–63.

Schultz NA, et al. MicroRNA biomarkers in whole blood for detection of pancreatic cancer. JAMA. 2014;311:392–404.

Shi C, Merchant N, Newsome G, Goldenberg DM, Gold DV. Differentiation of pancreatic ductal adenocarcinoma from chronic pancreatitis by PAM4 immunohistochemistry. Arch Pathol Lab Med. 2014;138:220–8.

Shimizu K, et al. Thiazolidinedione derivatives as novel therapeutic agents to prevent the development of chronic pancreatitis. Pancreas. 2002;24:184–90.

Suzuki J, et al. Novel IkB kinase inhibitors for treatment of nuclear factor-kB-related diseases. Expert Opin Investig Drugs. 2011;20:395–405.

Uomo I, Miraglia S, Pastorello M. Inflammation and pancreatic ductal adenocarcinoma: a potential scenario for novel drug targets. JOP. 2010;11:199–202.

Vincent A, Herman J, Schulick R, Hruban RH, Goggins M. Pancreatic cancer. Lancet. 2011;378:607–20.

Vogelstein B, et al. Genetic alterations during colorectal-tumor development. N Engl J Med. 1988;319:525–32.

Wang LW, et al. Prevalence and clinical features of chronic pancreatitis in China: a retrospective multicenter analysis over 10 years. Pancreas. 2009;38:248–54.

Wiseman H, Halliwell B. Damage to DNA by reactive oxygen and nitrogen species: role in inflammatory disease and progression to cancer. Biochem J. 1996;313(Pt 1):17–29.

Xie D, Xie K. Pancreatic cancer stromal biology and therapy. Genes Dis. 2015;2:133–43.

Yu JH, Kim H. Oxidative stress and cytokines in the pathogenesis of pancreatic cancer. J Cancer Prev. 2014;19:97–102.

Zagury D, Burny A, Gallo RC. Toward a new generation of vaccines: the anti-cytokine therapeutic vaccines. Proc Natl Acad Sci U S A. 2001;98:8024–9.

Typical Cases of Chronic Pancreatitis

13

Jin-Huan Lin, Liang-Hao Hu, Jia-Yun Chen, Wen-Bin Zou, Zhuan Liao, and Zhao-Shen Li

1 Typical Case 1: Alcoholic Chronic Pancreatitis

Brief history: a 43-year-old man complained of steatorrhea for 3 years and upper abdominal pain for the last 15 days. Three years ago, he presented with yellowish-brown, loose and fatty feces 4–5 times daily after eating greasy food, which was alleviated by dietary management and oral digestive enzyme replacement. However, steatorrhea has been aggravated for the last 2 months. In the local hospital, CT showed chronic pancreatitis, pancreatic duct stones, biliary duct stones, and the main pancreatic duct dilatation. No treatment was given then. Half a month ago, the patient presented with severe upper abdominal pain radiating to the back, and was treated according to the diagnosis of an acute episode of chronic pancreatitis in the local hospital. After the pain was relieved partially, he had his admission to our department for further management.

Past history: type 2 diabetes with a normal blood glucose level controlled by insulin regimens for 12 years, regular consumption of 50 g alcohol daily for 20 years as well as of 150 cigarettes annually for 15 years.

Physical examination: no significant signs.

Laboratory parameters: normal blood lipid level, negative results of CEA, CA19-9, IgG4 and autoimmune antibodies.

CT and contrast-enhanced CT: pancreatic atrophy, marked dilatation of the pancreatic duct with irregular changes in caliber, multiple high-density shadows in the pancreatic head, and a patchy high-density shadow in the pancreatic tail (Fig. 13.1).

Diagnosis: chronic pancreatitis with pancreatic duct stones, type 2 diabetes, exocrine pancreatic insufficiency.

Treatment process: ESWL was performed on June 28, 2012 and July 2 respectively, and ERCP + EPT + stone extraction was carried out on July 4 (Figs. 13.2 and 13.3). The patient recovered well shortly afterwards.

J.-H. Lin, M.D. • L.-H. Hu, M.D. • W.-B. Zou, M.D.
Z. Liao, M.D. (✉) • Z.-S. Li, M.D. (✉)
Department of Gastroenterology, Changhai Hospital, The Second Military Medical University, Shanghai, China

Shanghai Institute of Pancreatic Diseases, Shanghai, China
e-mail: liaozhuan@smmu.edu.cn; zhaoshenli@hotmail.com

J.-Y. Chen
Department of Gastroenterology, Changhai Hospital, The Second Military Medical University, Shanghai, China

Z.-S. Li et al. (eds.), *Chronic Pancreatitis*, DOI 10.1007/978-981-10-4515-8_13

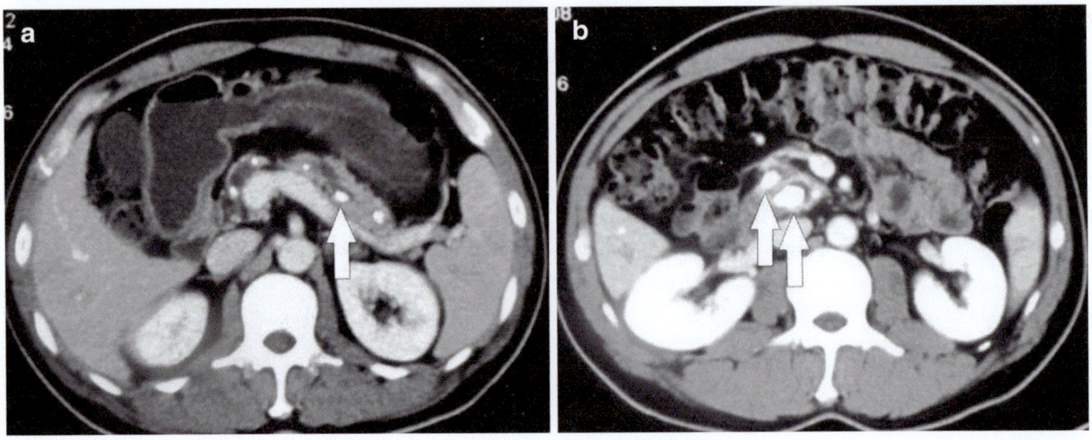

Fig. 13.1 (**a**) CT revealed marked dilatation of the pancreatic duct with irregular changes in caliber, and a patchy high-density shadow in the pancreatic tail (*arrow*). (**b**) Contrast-enhanced CT revealed pancreatic atrophy, and multiple high-density shadows in the pancreatic head (*arrows*)

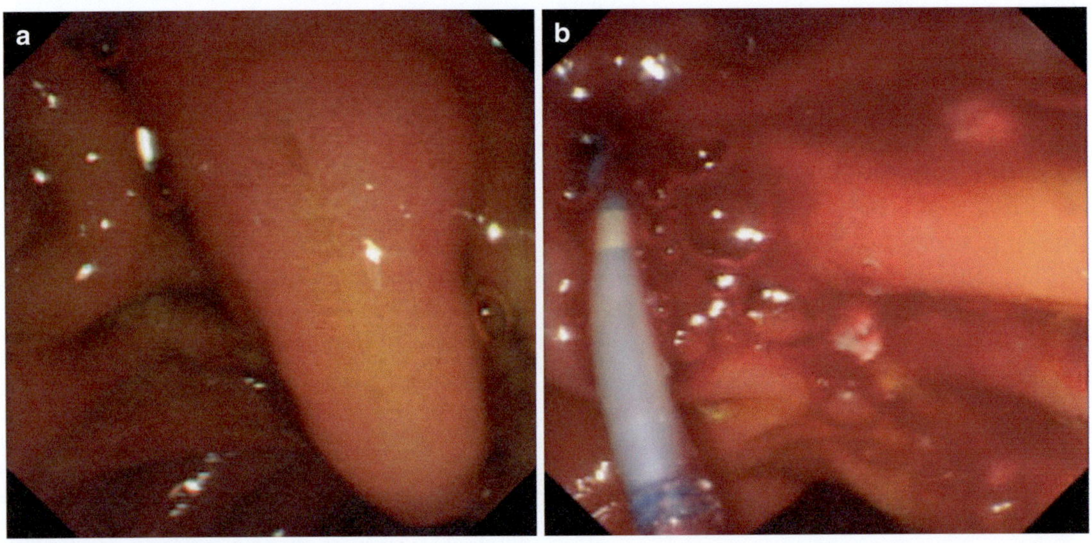

Fig. 13.2 (**a**) Endoscopy showed the major papilla on the descending duodenum before ERCP. (**b**) Endoscopy showed stone extraction from the papilla via retraction of the catheter with an inflated balloon after EPT

2 Typical Case 2: Chronic Pancreatitis with Main Pancreatic Duct Stricture and Upstream Dilatation

Brief history: a 47-year-old man complained of recurrent upper abdominal pain for 14 years with a recent bout for the last 4 days. In 1997, he presented with severe upper abdominal pain which radiated to the back right after drinking and was treated according to the diagnosis of acute pancreatitis in the local hospital. Since then, the similar symptom had recurred 3–4 times annually because of drinking or high-fat diets, requiring hospitalization each time. The patient could be free from any symptoms at the remission stage. In 2007, he was diagnosed as chronic pancreatitis since MRCP in our hospital demonstrated pancreatic atrophy and main pancreatic duct dilatation. Therefore, ERCP + pancreatic duct stent placement was performed and the symptom

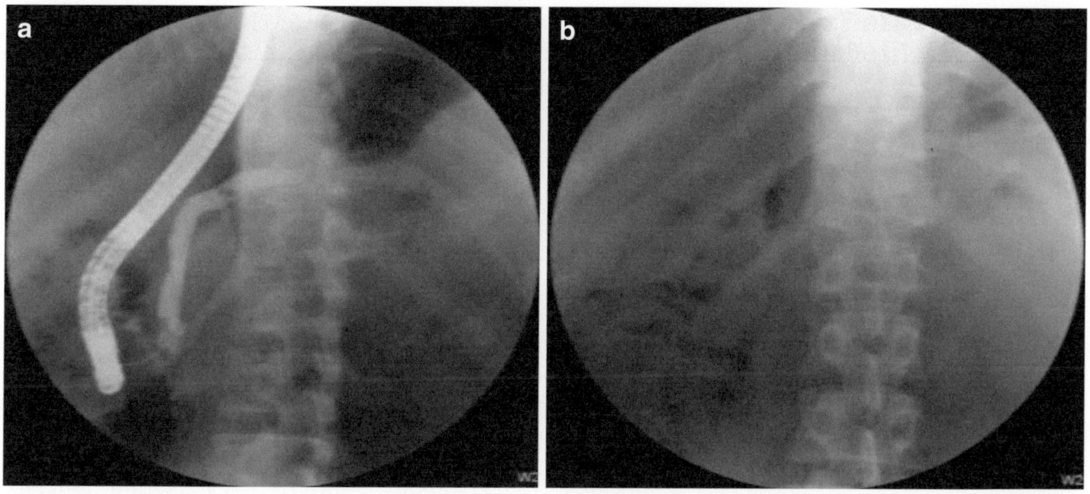

Fig. 13.3 (**a**) ERCP demonstrated irregular dilation of the entire pancreatic duct and multiple filling defects in the head and body of the pancreatic duct. (**b**) X-ray demonstrated the disappearance of filling defects after stone extraction

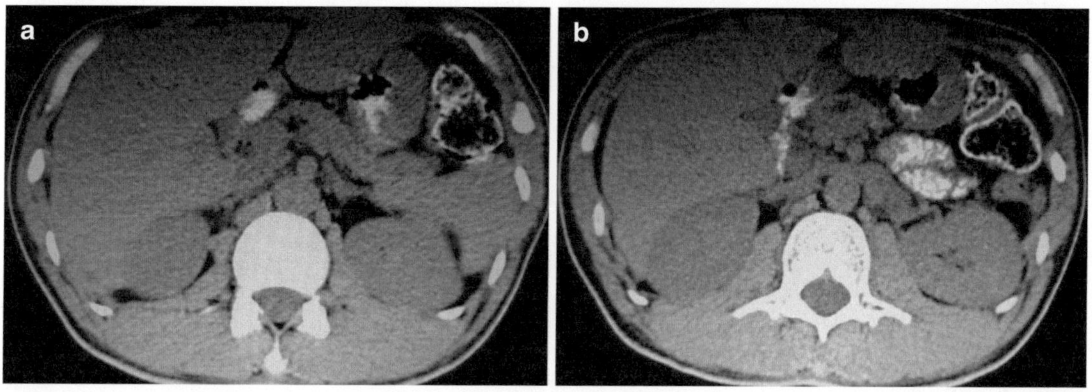

Fig. 13.4 CT revealed mild pancreatic atrophy, relatively low density in the body and tail of the pancreatic parenchyma with poorly defined organ margins, and segmental dilatation of the main pancreatic duct without stones

was improved significantly. Then he had periodical check-ups every year, underwent stent exchanges for several times, and took Creon, Nexium and Tylox intermittently. Due to a recent bout of abdominal pain, this man was admitted to our department for further management on June 13, 2011.

Physical examination: soft abdomen with epigastric tenderness, no rebound tenderness or guarding.

Laboratory parameters: CEA 5.63 ng/mL, triglyceride 3.72 mmol/L, total cholesterol 6.09 mmol/L, blood glucose 10.8 mmol/L, HbA1c 11.4%, and serum amylase 315 U/L.

CT: mild pancreatic atrophy, relatively low density in the body and tail of the pancreatic parenchyma with poorly defined organ margins, and segmental dilatation of the main pancreatic duct without stones (Fig. 13.4).

MRCP: segmental dilatation of the main pancreatic duct, mild peripancreatic fluid collections with the pancreas poorly demarcated (Fig. 13.5).

Diagnosis: an acute episode of chronic pancreatitis, secondary diabetes.

Treatment process: antacids, trypsin inhibitors and fluid replenishment were administered immediately. ERCP + pancreatic duct stent placement was performed on June 20, 2011 (Figs. 13.6 and 13.7).

3 Typical Case 3: Chronic Pancreatitis with Pancreatic Pseudocyst

Brief history: a 52-year-old man complained of recurrent upper abdominal pain for 1 year and aggravated for 1 month. In 2010, he presented with persistent upper abdominal pain concurrently with fever and nausea under no obvious precipitating causes. Blood tests in the local hospital showed a high serum amylase level and CT suggested pancreatic duct stones and an acute episode of chronic pancreatitis. Therefore, antacids, trypsin inhibitors and anti-inflammatory agents were administered to improve the symptoms. Since then, the pain had recurred for several times, relieved by fasting each time. Due to much more frequent bouts in the past month, the patient was admitted to our department for further management. Weight had been reduced by 8 kg since the onset of the pain.

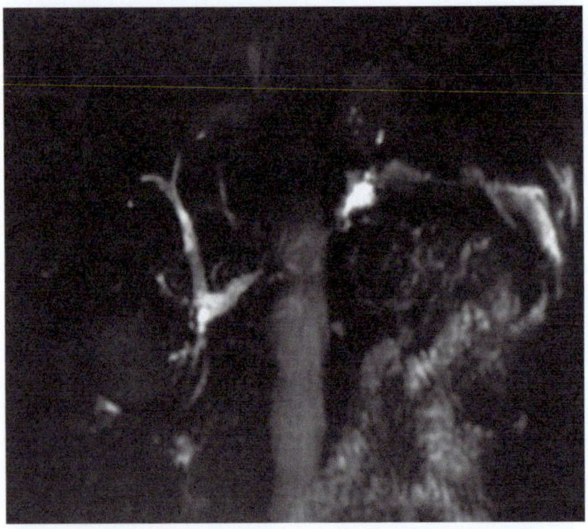

Fig. 13.5 MRCP revealed segmental dilatation of the main pancreatic duct, mild peripancreatic fluid collections with the pancreas poorly demarcated

Physical examination: soft abdomen with epigastric tenderness, no rebound tenderness or guarding.

Laboratory parameters: triglyceride 1.93 mmol/L, HbA1c 6.4%, serum amylase 293 U/L, and negative results of IgG4.

CT: atrophy in the pancreatic body and tail, bead-like dilatation of the main pancreatic duct, a cystic density lesion with clearly defined margins measuring 5.6 * 4.7 cm in the pancreatic neck, nodular and punctuate high-density shadows in the pancreatic head and body, and peripancreatic fluid collections (Fig. 13.8).

MRI and MRCP: significant atrophy in the pancreatic body and tail, bead-like dilatation of the main pancreatic duct, and a cystic density lesion with clearly defined margins measuring 5.6 * 4.7 cm in the pancreatic neck (Fig. 13.9).

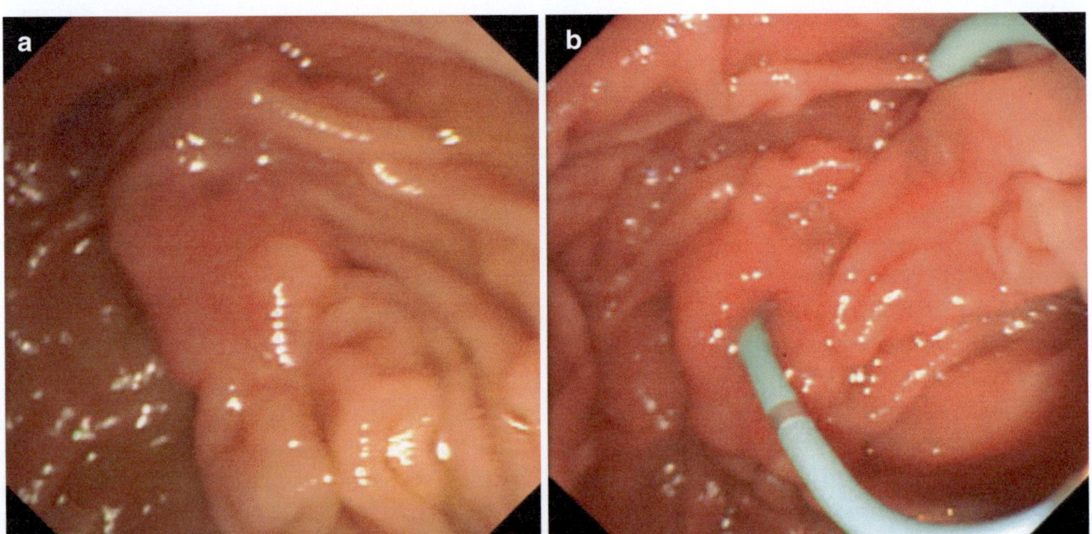

Fig. 13.6 (**a**) Endoscopy showed the major papilla on the descending duodenum after EPT. (**b**) Endoscopy showed pancreatic duct stent placement (5 Fr, 7 cm)

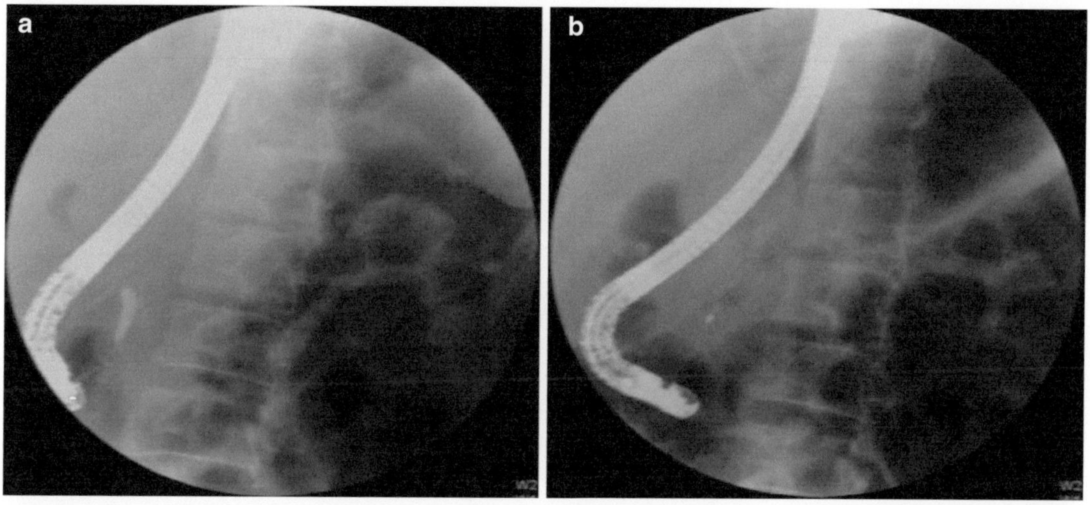

Fig. 13.7 (**a**) ERCP demonstrated the main pancreatic duct stricture at the junction of the head and body with upstream dilatation. (**b**) ERCP demonstrated that pancreatic duct stent had passed through the stricture

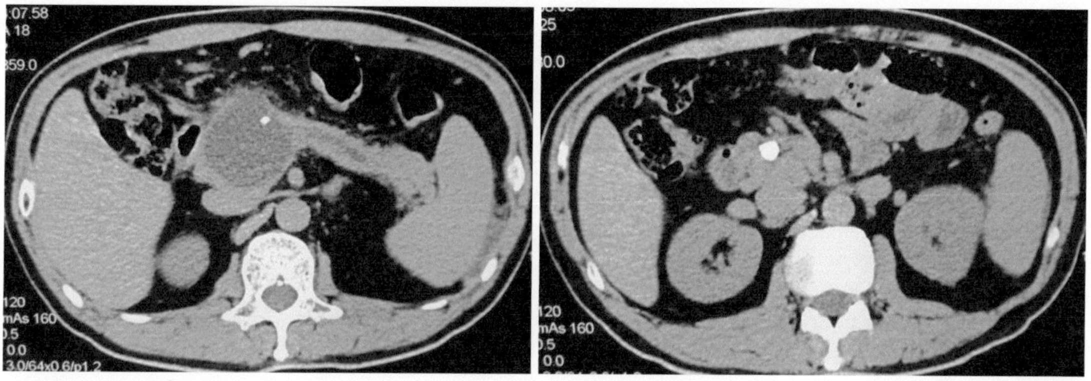

Fig. 13.8 CT revealed atrophy in the pancreatic body and tail, bead-like dilatation of the main pancreatic duct, a cystic density lesion with clearly defined margins measuring 5.6 * 4.7 cm in the pancreatic neck, nodular and punctuate high-density shadows in the pancreatic head and body, and peripancreatic fluid collections

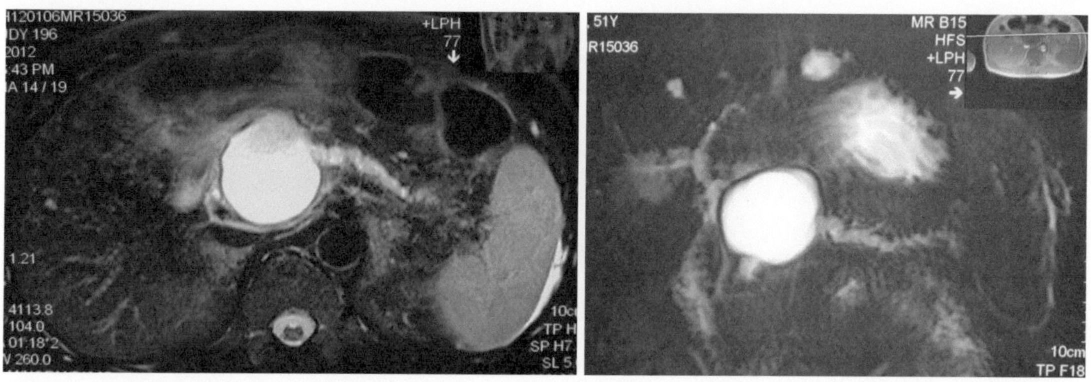

Fig. 13.9 MRI and MRCP revealed significant atrophy in the pancreatic body and tail, bead-like dilatation of the main pancreatic duct, and a cystic density lesion with clearly defined margins measuring 5.6 * 4.7 cm in the pancreatic neck

Diagnosis: an acute episode of chronic pancreatitis, pancreatic pseudocyst.

Treatment process: after conservative treatment, ERCP + EST was carried out on 17 January 2011, followed by ESWL on 31 January, 6 February and 7 February respectively. Then, ERCP + EPT + bougienage + stent placement across the connection between the pseudocyst and accessory pancreatic duct was performed on 8 February (Figs. 13.10 and 13.11). Three months later, CT showed a decrease in the volume of the pseudocyst (Fig. 13.12).

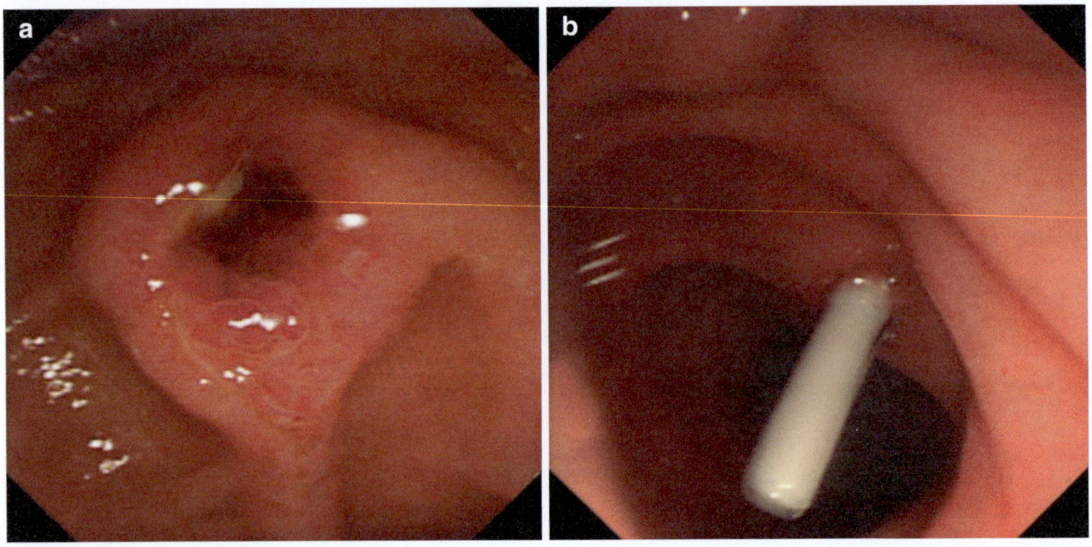

Fig. 13.10 (**a**) Endoscopy showed the major papilla on the descending duodenum after EPT and the repeated insertion of a guidewire into the accessory pancreatic duct. (**b**) Endoscopy showed stent insertion into the accessory pancreatic duct (8.5 Fr, 7 cm)

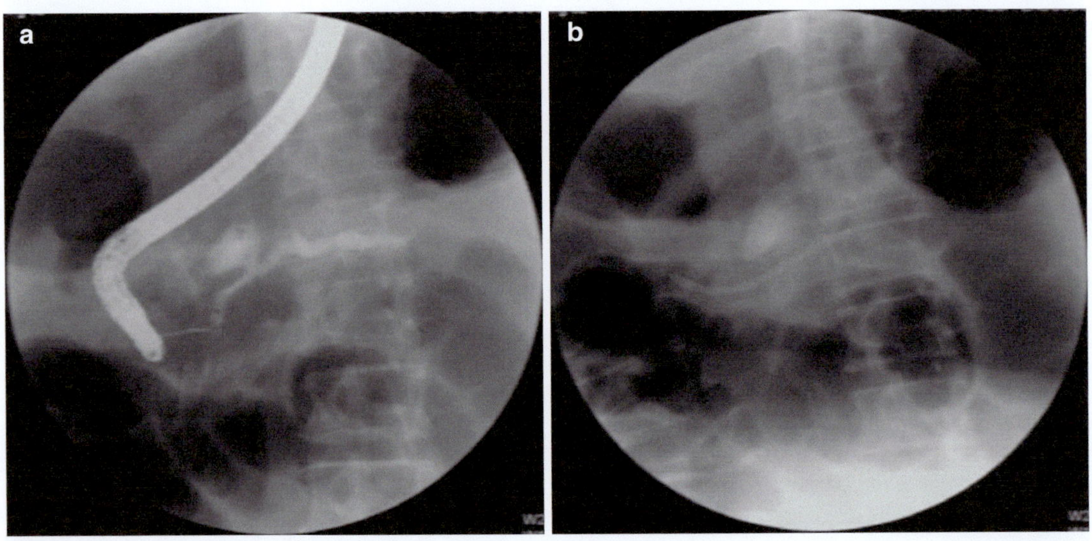

Fig. 13.11 (**a**) After the injection of contrast medium into accessory pancreatic duct, ERCP demonstrated the pancreatic duct well: stricture in the head, irregular distortion and dilatation in the body and tail, and a pseudocyst measuring 5.6 * 4.7 cm that communicates with the accessory pancreatic duct in the pancreatic neck. (**b**) ERCP demonstrated that the stricture in the pancreatic head had been dilated after bougienage and the stent had been placed across the connection between the pseudocyst and accessory pancreatic duct

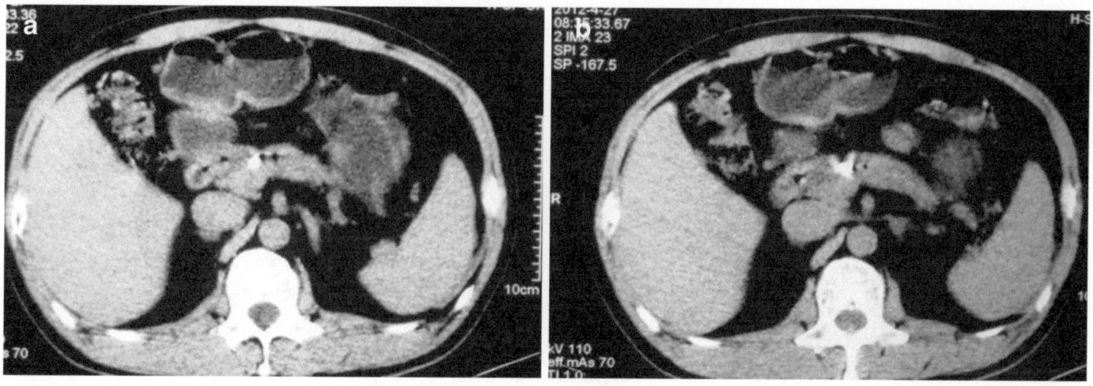

Fig. 13.12 CT revealed a decrease in the volume of the pseudocyst, atrophy in the pancreatic body and tail, and the post-ERCP pancreatic duct after stent placement

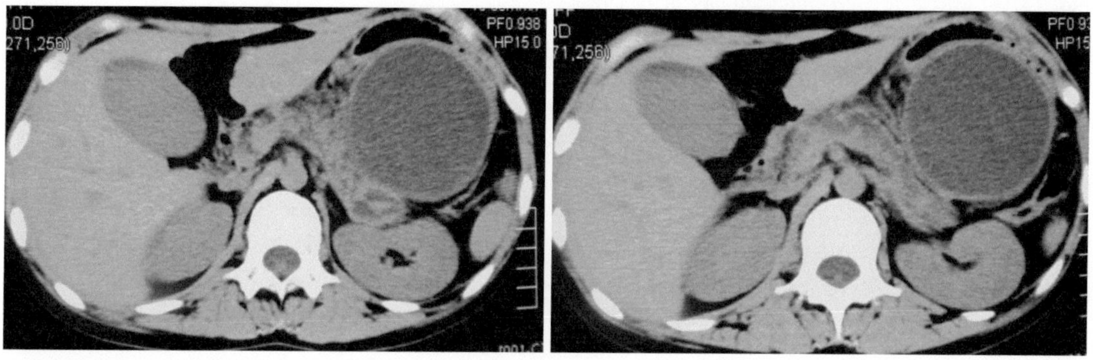

Fig. 13.13 CT revealed pancreatic duct dilatation, multiple low-density shadows in the pancreatic head and tail suggestive of pancreatic pseudocysts up to 7 cm in diameter

4 Typical Case 4: Adolescent Chronic Pancreatitis with Radiolucent Stones

Brief history: a 16-year-old girl complained of recurrent upper abdominal pain for 4 months. In February 2012, she presented with severe and persistent upper abdominal pain under no obvious precipitating causes and was treated according to the diagnosis of acute pancreatitis in the local hospital. In April 2012, the patient was admitted to Xijing Hospital because of a recurrence of pain concurrently with abdominal distention. CT suggested a pancreatic pseudocyst (Fig. 13.13), so ERCP + EPT + naso-pancreatic drainage was performed to drain some brown fluid and decrease the volume of the pseudocyst. Then, another ERCP was carried out to insert the pancreatic duct stent but it failed. Therefore, the patient was admitted to our department for further management.

Physical examination: no significant signs.

Laboratory parameters: total bilirubin 27.9 μmol/L, direct bilirubin 12.1 μmol/L, normal ranges of blood lipid and HbA1c, negative results of CEA, CA19-9 and IgG4.

CT: pancreatic duct dilatation, multiple low-density shadows in the pancreatic head and tail suggestive of pancreatic pseudocysts up to 7 cm in diameter, cholestasis (Fig. 13.13).

MRCP: mild atrophy of pancreas, main pancreatic duct dilatation, and multiple filling defects in the pancreas (Fig. 13.14).

Diagnosis: adolescent chronic pancreatitis with radiolucent stones.

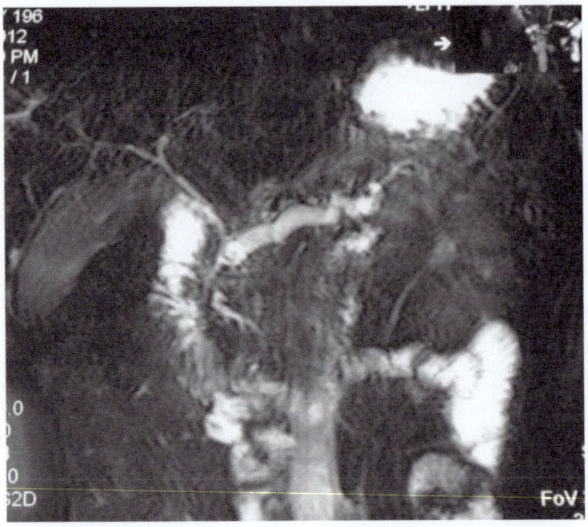

Fig. 13.14 MRCP revealed mild atrophy of pancreas, main pancreatic duct dilatation, and multiple filling defects in the pancreas

Treatment process: ERCP + minor papilla papillotomy + naso-pancreatic drainage was performed on 20 June (Fig. 13.15), followed by ESWL on 21 June and 25 June respectively. Then, the patient underwent ERCP + bougienage of the accessory pancreatic duct + accessory pancreatic duct clearance + stent placement on 27 June (Figs. 13.16 and 13.17) and recovered well afterwards.

5 Typical Case 5: Spontaneous Expulsion of Stones After ESWL

Brief history: a 26-year-old woman complained of recurrent upper abdominal pain for 5 years. In 2007, she presented with paroxysmal epigastric

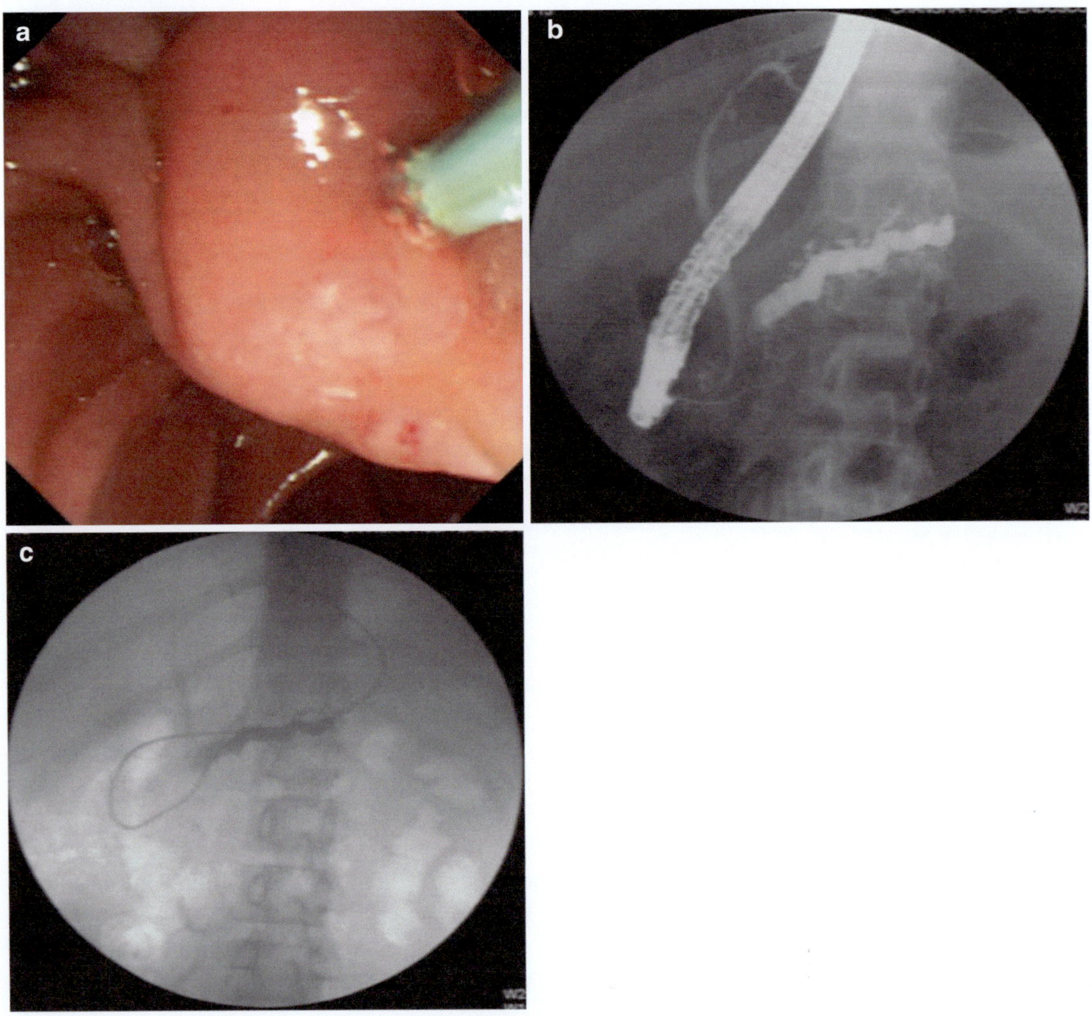

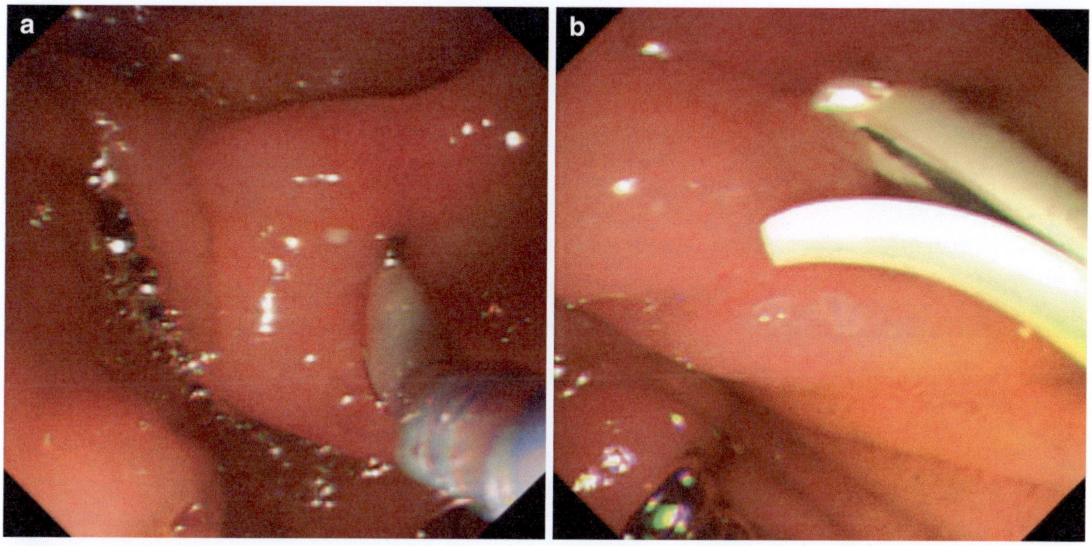

Fig. 13.16 (**a**) Endoscopy showed the stricture near the minor papilla being dilated by bougienage. (**b**) Endoscopy showed stent placement in the accessory pancreatic duct (8.5 Fr, 7 cm)

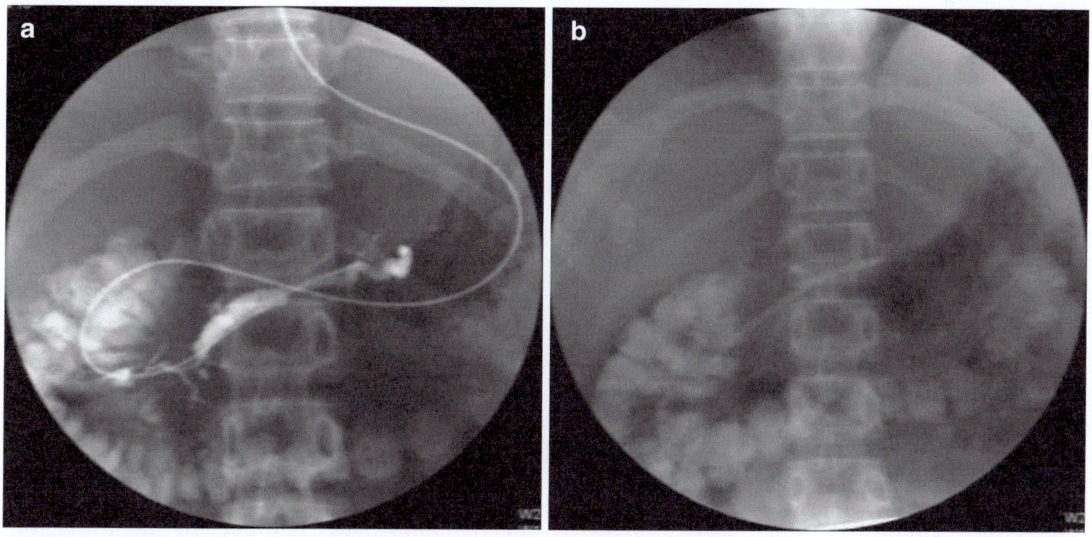

Fig. 13.17 (**a**) X-ray demonstrated the stricture in the pancreatic head, and irregular dilatation in the pancreatic body and tail. (**b**) X-ray demonstrated that the stent had successfully passed the stricture of the accessory pancreatic duct

Fig. 13.15 (**a**) Endoscopy showed the minor papilla on the descending duodenum. (**b**) ERCP demonstrated the accessory pancreatic duct well, distortion and deformation in the pancreatic head, irregular dilatation in the pancreatic body and tail, and filling defects in the pancreatic duct. (**c**) X-ray demonstrated successfully placement of a naso-pancreatic duct via the guidewire

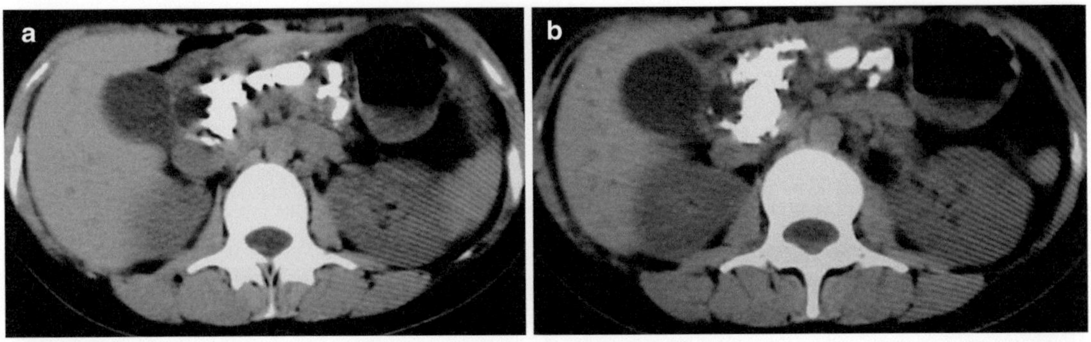

Fig. 13.18 CT before the surgery revealed a large number of patchy high-density shadows in the pancreas, and gallbladder distended

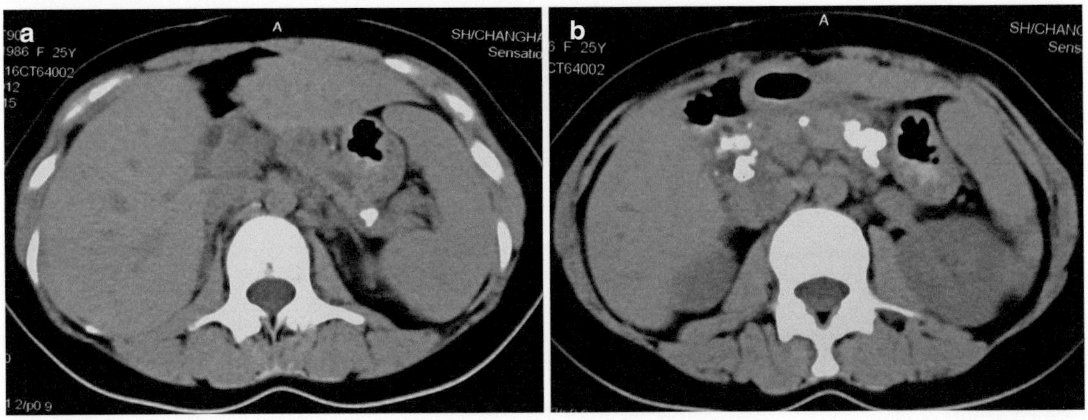

Fig. 13.19 CT in our hospital revealed fewer patchy high-density shadows in the pancreas and no visualization of the gallbladder

colic radiating to the back concurrently with chills, fever and vomiting under no obvious precipitating causes. Cholecystectomy + pancreatolithotomy + pancreatojejunostomy was performed according to the diagnosis of cholecystitis and chronic pancreatitis with pancreatic stones in the local hospital (Fig. 13.18). After the surgery, similar symptoms occurred annually with subsequent hospitalization each time. In October 2011, CT revealed chronic pancreatitis, diffuse and multiple high-density shadows in the pancreas, and main pancreatic duct dilatation in the body and tail. Therefore, the patient was admitted to our department for further management on 28 January, 2012.

Physical examination: soft abdomen without tenderness or rebound tenderness, an 8-cm surgical scar in the upper abdominal.

Laboratory parameters: total bilirubin 21.6 μmol/L, direct bilirubin 9.2 μmol/L, serum amylase 220 U/L, anti-cardiolipin antibody 20.4 RU/mL, normal ranges of blood lipid and HbA1c, a weakly positive result of anti-mitochondrial antibody, negative results of CEA, CA19-9 and IgG4.

CT: fewer patchy high-density shadows in the pancreas and no visualization of the gallbladder (Fig. 13.19).

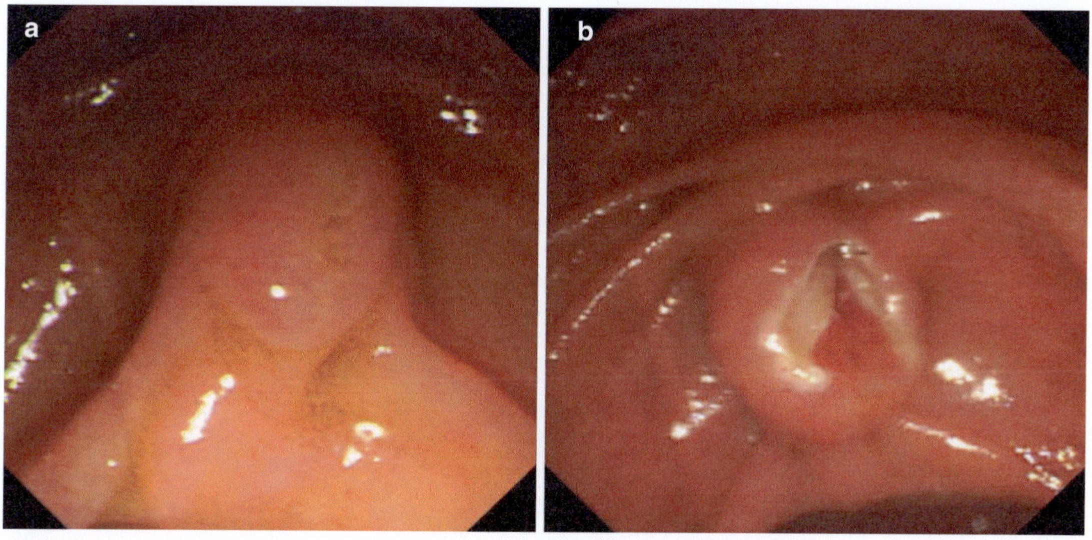

Fig. 13.20 (**a**) Endoscopy showed the major papilla on the descending duodenum. (**b**) Endoscopy showed a 5-cm incision in the major papilla after EPT

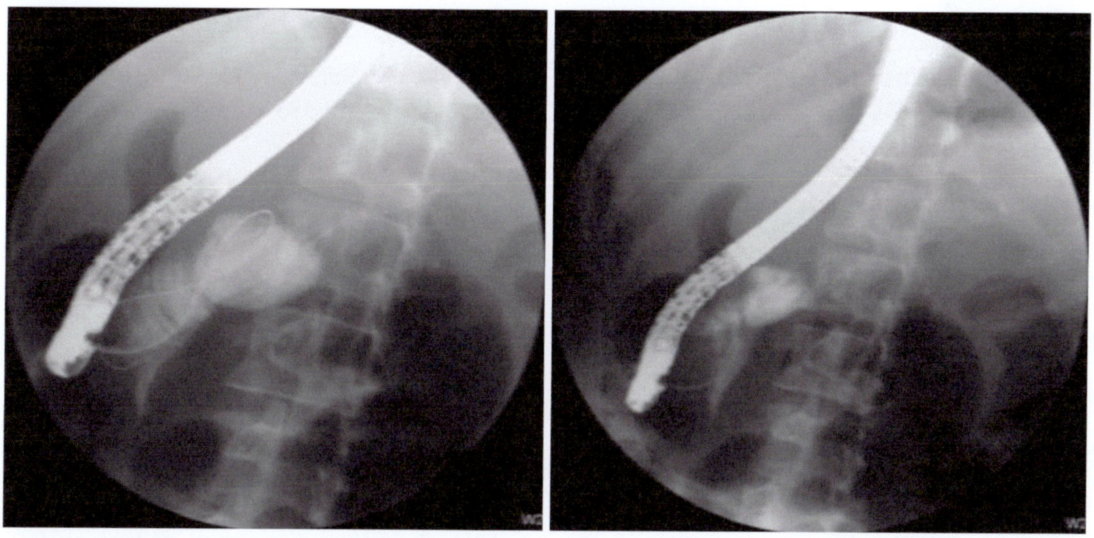

Fig. 13.21 ERCP demonstrated contrast medium into enteric cavity after injection and no visualization of the biliary and pancreatic ducts

Diagnosis: chronic pancreatitis with pancreatic stones, post-cholecystectomy + pancreatolithotomy + pancreatojejunostomy.

Treatment process: ESWL was performed on 30 January, 3 February, 6 February, 7 February and 8 February respectively, followed by ERCP + EPT on 9 February (Figs. 13.20 and 13.21). Stones were collected from the stools 1 week later (Fig. 13.22).

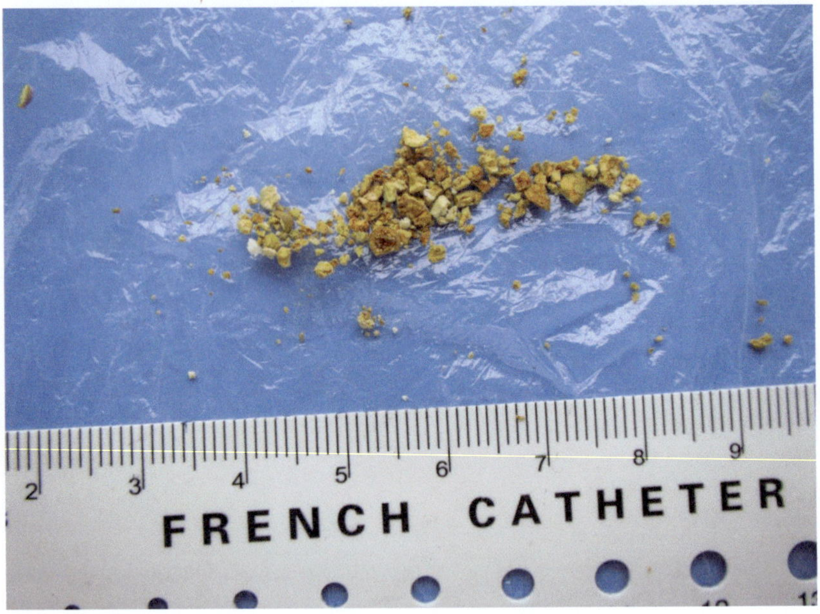

Fig. 13.22 The photograph presented pancreatic stones of various shapes and sizes collected from the stools after ESWL and ERCP

6 Typical Case 6: Autoimmune Pancreatitis

Brief history: a 55-year-old man complained of recurrent upper abdominal pain radiating to the back with jaundice occasionally for 3 years. ERCP + common bile duct dilatation was performed in the local hospital according to the diagnosis of inflammatory stricture of the common bile duct. In July 2010, the pain recurred concurrently with fever and CT in the local hospital revealed the dilatation of both intrahepatic and extrahepatic bile ducts, distal biliary obstruction, and enlargement of the pancreas. Therefore, ERCP + bile duct stent placement was carried out, followed by stent removal 3 weeks later. Shortly afterwards, the patient was admitted to our department for further management.

Physical examination: mild tenderness in the epigastrium without rebound tenderness or guarding, a movable lymph node about 1.0 cm^3 palpable in the right mandible, no significant jaundice.

Laboratory parameters: CA19-9 16.5 IU/mL, IgG4 9.84 g/L, IgE 585 IU/mL, negative results of autoimmune antibodies.

CT: enlargement of the pancreatic body and tail with poorly defined margins, peripancreatic fluid collections, thickening of peripancreatic fatty tissue (Fig. 13.23a), gastric varices (Fig. 13.23b), and abdominal aorta compressed below the opening of renal artery (Fig. 13.23c).

EUS: hypoechoic and heterogeneous area (3.4 * 4.0 cm) in the pancreatic body and tail with poor demarcation, involvement of splenic vein, an enlarged lymph node about 1.0 cm^3 adjacent to proximal pancreatic duct with normal caliber.

FNA: A few pancreatic acini, no tumor cells.

Diagnosis: autoimmune pancreatitis.

Treatment process: after oral prednisone at a starting dose of 30 mg/day for 30 days, the level of IgG4 returned to 4.41 g/L and CT showed normal morphology of pancreas, improvement of gastric varices and the compression of abdominal aorta (Fig. 13.24). Then, prednisone was used by a taper of 5 mg per week. Discomfort had not occurred since drug withdrawal.

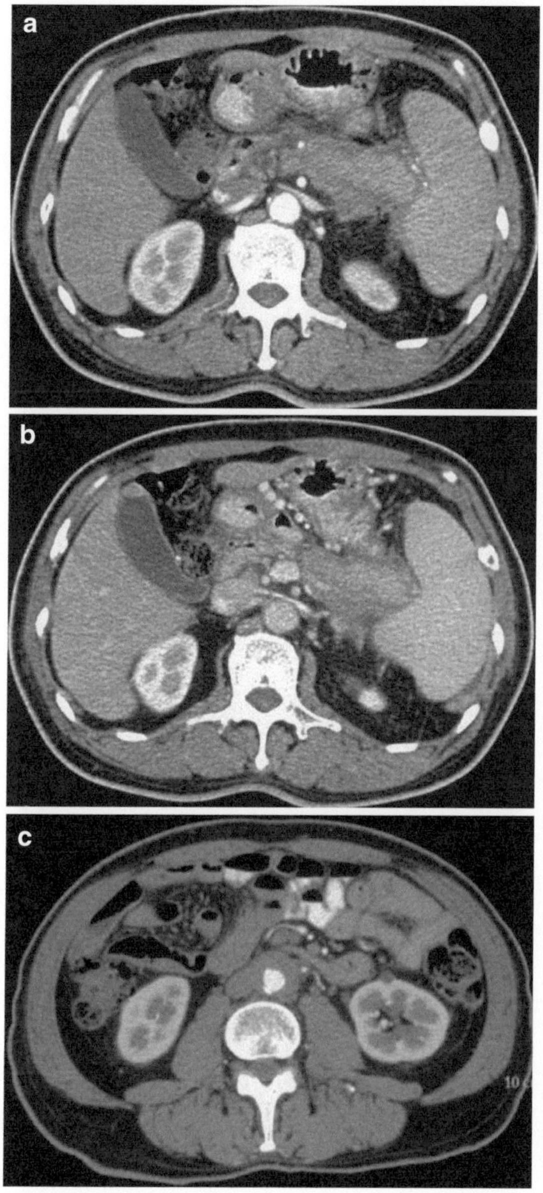

Fig. 13.23 (**a**) CT revealed enlargement of the pancreatic body and tail with poorly defined margins, peripancreatic fluid collections, and thickening of peripancreatic fatty tissue. (**b**) CT revealed gastric varices. (**c**) CT revealed abdominal aorta compressed below the opening of renal artery

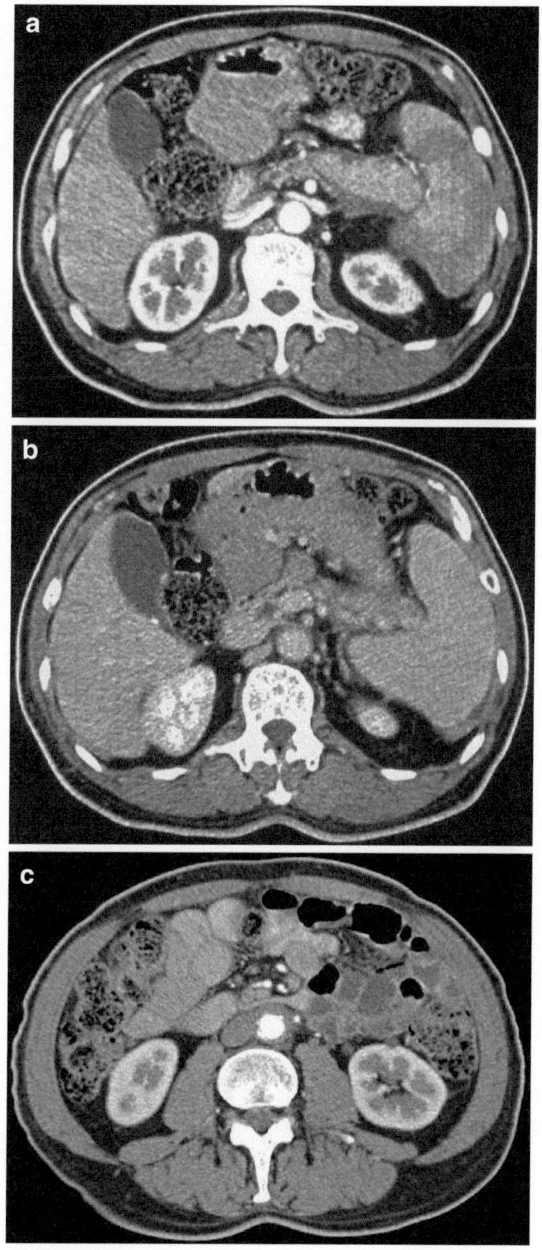

Fig. 13.24 CT showed normal morphology of pancreas, improvement of gastric varices and the compression of abdominal aorta

Index

A

AIP. *See* Autoimmune pancreatitis (AIP)
Alcohol feeding models, 45, 46
Alcoholic(s), 2, 17, 23, 25, 46, 67, 86, 96, 124
Animal models, 18, 30, 31, 34, 41, 42, 45, 47, 48, 51–54, 157, 160, 167, 186
Autoimmune pancreatitis (AIP), 2, 22–25, 50, 87, 107, 110, 116, 146, 150–152, 166, 167, 206

C

Cancer biomarker, 184, 190, 191
Carbohydrate antigen 19-9 (CA19-9), 87, 190, 191, 201, 206
Carboxypeptidase A1 (CPA1) variants, 64–67, 160, 164–166
Cationic trypsinogen mutation, 24, 64, 166
^{13}C-Breath tests, 93–94
CEL-HYB alleles, 64, 67–70
Chronic pancreatitis, 1–4, 7, 13, 22, 23, 29–54, 79–116, 124–126, 141–144, 155, 157, 159–162, 164–166, 171, 172, 183–191, 195–202, 204, 205
Classification(s), 2, 3, 7, 24, 25, 80–83, 88, 95, 106–110, 112, 113, 115, 116, 156, 169
Clinical staging, 9–10
Clinical symptoms, 40, 91, 92, 95, 111, 167
Cohort study, 185
Common alterations, 188–189
Complications, 7, 10, 11, 18, 35, 36, 41, 49, 83, 88, 101, 106, 107, 112, 114–116, 129–133, 135–138, 141, 143, 144, 153, 169–172
Composition, 36–38, 40
Computed tomography (CT), 3, 8, 80–82, 95–107, 112, 130, 137, 147, 148, 165, 169, 195, 197–201, 204, 206, 207
Computer aided diagnosis (CAD), 115–116
Concluding remarks, 54, 163, 164
Conservative management, 123
Contrast enhancement EUS (CE-EUS), 115
CPA1. *See* Carboxypeptidase A1 (CPA1) variants
CT. *See* Computed tomography (CT)
Cytokines, 31, 44, 45, 49–52, 162, 183, 184, 187–189

D

Definition, 7–12, 25, 109, 114, 165, 171
Diabetes mellitus, 10, 11, 21, 22, 41, 51, 83, 87, 88, 111, 126, 138, 143, 152, 170, 171
Diagnosis, 2–4, 7, 22, 79–116, 146, 149, 151, 152, 154–156, 165, 168, 169, 171, 184, 185, 190, 191, 195–197, 200, 201, 204–206
Diagnostic criteria, 3, 79–87, 89, 106, 107, 109, 112, 148–152, 165, 171
Differential diagnosis, 87, 93, 103–105, 107, 111, 115, 184, 185, 190, 191
Drainage, 3, 4, 30, 130, 132–137, 141–143, 167, 171, 201, 202
Duct obstruction models, 42

E

Elastography, 115
Endocrine function tests, 87–90
Endoplasmic reticulum stress (ERS), 64, 65, 167
Endoscopic retrograde cholangiopancreatography (ERCP), 3, 8, 15, 80–82, 95, 99, 105–112, 114, 132, 136, 149, 155, 168, 169, 171, 195–197, 199–203, 205, 206
Endoscopic treatment, 4
Endoscopic ultrasonography (EUS), 3, 80, 82, 83, 95, 106, 107, 110–116, 136, 148, 165, 168, 206
Endoscopic ultrasound-guided fine needle aspiration (EUS-FNA), 148
Endoscopic ultrasound-guided fine needle aspiration/biopsy (EUS-FNA/B), 114, 116
Epidemiology, 7, 8, 13–18, 21, 23, 40, 104, 146, 147, 172, 183, 185, 186, 188, 189
ERCP. *See* Endoscopic retrograde cholangiopancreatography (ERCP)
ERS. *See* Endoplasmic reticulum stress (ERS)
EUS. *See* Endoscopic ultrasonography (EUS)
EUS-TCB, 114–115
Evaluation, 3, 35, 36, 46, 88–90, 92–96, 99, 106, 114–116, 135, 136, 148
Experimental models, 40–54, 67

Z.-S. Li et al. (eds.), *Chronic Pancreatitis*, DOI 10.1007/978-981-10-4515-8

F

Fecal fat analysis, 94

G

Genetic(s), 2, 7, 8, 11, 16, 17, 21, 23–25, 48, 49, 51–54, 63–65, 69, 70, 73, 87, 154, 157, 160, 163–166, 183–187, 191
Genetic models, 41, 48
Genetic risk factors, 40, 72, 154, 157–163, 172
Genome-wide association study (GWAS), 17, 48, 64–66, 69, 73, 158, 161
Glycophophatidyl inositol (GPI), 39, 40
Glycoprotein-2 (GP-2), 37, 39, 40
GWAS. *See* Genome-wide association study (GWAS)

H

Hereditary pancreatitis, 2, 9, 16, 48, 64, 71, 73, 157, 166, 170, 171, 183, 185

I

Idiopathic chronic pancreatitis (ICP), 23, 25, 64–67, 69, 91, 146, 156–159
Immunoglobulins G4 (IgG4), 2, 87, 146–148, 150, 152, 167, 195, 198, 201, 204, 206
Incidence, 1, 13–15, 17, 21, 22, 24, 35, 40, 87, 88, 123, 143, 146, 154, 164, 185, 188
Indirect tests, 54, 93
Inflammatory malignancy, 184–185

L

Laboratory tests, 86, 87, 89, 168
Lactoferrin (LF), 37, 39, 50
Lifestyle modification, 123–124

M

Magnetic resonance cholangiopancreatography (MRCP), 82, 99–103, 106, 107, 129, 136, 165, 168, 196–199, 201, 202
Magnetic resonance imaging (MRI), 3, 22, 34, 42, 82, 83, 99–103, 110, 165, 168, 198, 199
Malignant driver, 185–186
M-ANNHEIM classification, 7, 8, 81, 83, 84
Mechanisms, 2, 8, 18, 21, 23, 29–36, 41, 47, 48, 65, 67, 70, 72, 85, 88, 123, 146, 157–159, 161, 166, 167, 171, 183, 186–188
MicroRNAs (miRNA), 147, 184, 191
MRCP. *See* Magnetic resonance cholangiopancreatography (MRCP)
MRI. *See* Magnetic resonance imaging (MRI)

N

Nuclear factor kappa B (NF-kB), 161, 167, 184, 188–190
Nutrition, 9, 46, 126, 163

O

Osteopontin, 37, 39

P

Paediatric pancreatitis, 164–172
Pain management, 124, 125
Pain mechanism, 29–36
Pancreatectomy, 3, 88, 89, 142–144, 171
Pancreatic adenocarcinoma, 50
Pancreatic cancer, 21, 24, 50, 80, 83, 87, 88, 95, 115, 116, 129, 147–150, 153, 183
Pancreatic endocrine insufficiency, 52, 86, 88, 126, 165
Pancreatic enzyme replacement therapy (PERT), 125, 126, 170
Pancreatic exocrine insufficiency (PEI), 36, 49, 81, 86, 87, 90–95, 115, 125, 126, 165
Pancreatic function tests, 92–95, 107, 109, 111, 169, 170
Pancreatic polypeptide (PP), 89, 171
Pancreatic stone(s), 4, 36, 40, 109, 134, 171, 204, 206
Pancreatic stone protein (PSP), 36–39, 160
Pancreatitis, 2, 3, 8, 9, 15–18, 22–25, 30, 40, 44, 48, 50, 51, 67, 72, 80, 86, 98, 101, 106, 108, 123, 124, 130, 131, 133, 135, 138, 142, 143, 146, 152, 155–157, 159, 161, 164, 166, 167, 172, 186, 189
Pancreatogenic diabetes, 88, 126, 170, 171
Pathophysiology, 30, 41, 45, 48, 54, 90–95, 156, 158, 159, 161, 163, 166
Pathways, 31, 33, 34, 45, 64, 65, 67, 73, 161, 163, 166, 167, 184, 186–188, 190, 191
PEI. *See* Pancreatic exocrine insufficiency (PEI)
Peroxisome proliferator-activated receptor (PPARγ), 184, 189
PERT. *See* Pancreatic enzyme replacement therapy (PERT)
Phenotypic perspectives, 155
Population, 13, 16, 40, 43, 67–69, 88, 147, 153, 154, 158, 160–163, 166, 167, 172, 186, 188
Prevalence, 13, 14, 21, 23, 35, 36, 88, 123, 135, 146, 156, 158, 172, 184
Prognosis, 4, 7, 143, 153, 154, 183, 184, 190, 191
PRSS1, 2, 9, 24, 48, 49, 52, 64–66, 70, 71, 73, 157, 158, 161, 163–166, 183, 185

R

Reactive oxygen species, 188–190
Repeated caerulein models, 44
Risk factors, 7–9, 11, 16–18, 22–25, 66–69, 80, 88, 123, 153, 163–166, 183, 185, 186, 188, 191

S

Secretin test, 80, 92, 106, 111
Serum marker(s), 87, 147
Side effects, 36, 124, 125, 171
Signs, 10, 35, 41, 42, 44, 45, 48–50, 53, 81, 86, 90, 91, 94, 104, 195, 201

Stool tests, 92, 93, 170
Surgery, 3, 4, 30, 107, 125, 131, 133–136, 138, 141, 143, 171, 204
Symptoms, 3, 7, 21, 22, 35, 72, 85, 86, 90, 95, 105, 111, 112, 123–126, 134–136, 138, 143, 146, 165, 167, 170, 171, 196, 198, 204

T

T3cDM. *See* Type 3c diabetes mellitus (T3cDM)
TIGAR-O system, 11–12
Tropical calcific pancreatitis (TCP), 154–164
Trypsin-central pathways, 157, 163
Trypsin-independent pathways, 73, 157, 160, 163, 164
Trypsinogen, 2, 24, 39, 45, 47–49, 52, 64, 66, 70, 71, 73, 157–160, 164, 166, 167, 185
Type 1 AIP, 24, 50, 147–152
Type 2 AIP, 24, 53, 147–149, 151, 152, 166
Type 3c diabetes mellitus (T3cDM), 88–90, 126, 170, 171

MIX
Papier aus verantwortungsvollen Quellen
Paper from responsible sources
FSC® C105338

If you have any concerns about our products,
you can contact us on
ProductSafety@springernature.com

In case Publisher is established outside the EU,
the EU authorized representative is:
Springer Nature Customer Service Center GmbH
Europaplatz 3, 69115 Heidelberg, Germany

Printed by Libri Plureos GmbH
in Hamburg, Germany